Yeah
BABY!

Yeah BABY!

The Modern Mama's Breakthrough Guide
to Mastering Pregnancy, Having a Healthy Baby,
and Bouncing Back Better Than Ever

JILLIAN MICHAELS

WITH EVE ADAMSON

RODALE.

RODALE *wellness*

Live happy. Be healthy. Get inspired.

Sign up today to get exclusive access to our authors, exclusive bonuses,
and the most authoritative, useful, and cutting-edge information on health, wellness, fitness,
and living your life to the fullest.

Visit us online at RodaleWellness.com
Join us at RodaleWellness.com/Join

Rodale books may be purchased for business or promotional use or for special sales.
For information, please write to:
Special Markets Department, Rodale Inc., 733 Third Avenue, New York, NY 10017.

Printed in the United States of America

Rodale Inc. makes every effort to use acid-free ♾, recycled paper ♻.

Photo Credits can be found on page 349.

Book design by Christina Gaugler

Library of Congress Cataloging-in-Publication Data is on file with the publisher.

ISBN-13: 978–1–62336–803–6   paperback

Distributed to the trade by Macmillan

2   4   6   8   10   9   7   5   3   paperback

⚘ RODALE.

Follow us @RodaleBooks on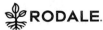

We inspire health, healing, happiness, and love in the world.
Starting with you.

This one is for my beautiful family.
Thank you for being the inspiration behind
not just this book but every day of my life.
Heidi, Lu, Phoenix, and of course
my own beloved mom, JoAnn . . .
I love you to the moon and back again.

CONTENTS

Yeah BABY!

The fact that you have picked up this book is pretty exciting. Obviously, you are either pregnant or desire to be, and that is incredibly fantastic news! So get ready, because I am about to turn everything you think you know about pregnancy upside down. Not to worry. It's all good news! Like this: Research shows us that if you manage your pregnancy properly, not only will you maintain your current level of fitness, but in many cases you can actually improve it! Or how about this one: Recent studies have revealed that pregnancy can be a veritable fountain of youth. Yup! During a healthy pregnancy, your baby can actually give you embryonic stem cells to help you turn back the clock and emerge from this incredible period better than ever! One more teaser: Proper fitness, nutrition, and lifestyle habits can increase your child's athleticism, IQ, likelihood for a healthy adult body weight, and even long-term earning potential.

Bottom line, pregnancy is a magical time, literally and figuratively, where the miracle of life can have tremendous potency and transformative power for you and your little one, if you have the awareness to take the proper actions. There is a lot to know, and a lot to get excited about, and this book is about all that good stuff, including some of the very newest information out there that can help make your pregnancy smoother and help you take advantage of what scientists and doctors know now that they didn't know when your mom had you.

Now, I'd love to continue giving you my best warm and fuzzy, but I am a big subscriber to the "truth will set you free club," and if you are at all familiar with me, I am pretty sure you know that already. So let's be honest: Pregnancy isn't all rose garlands wreathing the heads of cherub-like babies. Your life is about to change . . . and that's incredibly awesome, joyful, overwhelming, and for some (most), scary. Yes, all these emotions can exist simultaneously. And despite all the wonders of modern science, honestly, there are still some parts of pregnancy that aren't all that fun— like morning sickness, mood swings, and swollen ankles. I'm going to walk you through all of it. I'm also going to alert you to some real dangers out there—dangers to your health and to the health of your baby. It is a polluted and not always ethical world, and the sooner you know that, the sooner you can get motivated to do what you can to work around it. That's another big part of this book, as you will soon see.

Welcome to pregnancy and eventual parenthood.

GETTING READY FOR YOUR NEW LIFE

So how is your life about to change? In so many ways! First and foremost, your life is no longer your own. You will soon discover, if you haven't already, that your priorities are utterly realigned. Your emotions will be hijacked, and your body will become a vessel for a brand-new life. All this in just the first 40 weeks—that's some serious S#!+ to contemplate. And the sooner we get real with each other, the sooner I can help you take control, master your maternity, give your kiddo every possible advantage right from the start, and get you a postbaby body to die for.

There. I said it. You can do your absolute best to make a healthy baby *and* be a hot mama, all at the same time. It's the ultimate promise, but I stand by it because I've done it for others and I can do it for you. So why not kick this off with a bang? Together we can make this happen. With the right information, you can make the right choices to exact the optimal outcome for you and yours.

Now maybe you are really looking forward to what I have to say because this is your first baby and you haven't learned that much about being pregnant yet. You are hungry for knowledge because you want to get it right. Great! But maybe you are thinking, "This is not my first rodeo. I've done this before and I'm just looking for the latest info on maternity fitness and nutrition. Otherwise, I'm good." Fair enough, but you are wise to hang with me this time around, because new information is surfacing every day. Even I have been amazed, researching this book, how much has come out in the last couple of years. But guess what? The *Yeah Baby!* "dream team" of experts and I are on top of it. No matter how much you think you know today, by the end of this book, you are going to be even more pregnancy-savvy. You will have more knowledge about what science can do for you, as well as what you don't want to do before, during, and after pregnancy. This will lay the groundwork for genuine good health, now and for the rest of your life as a parent.

Also, I feel strongly that whether it's your first pregnancy or your fourth pregnancy, every pregnancy is different, every kiddo is different, and even you are different with each go-around. The impact on your life as you currently know it will be massive, no matter how many times you've experienced this before.

So let's show you the respect you deserve (a lot!) and appreciate the significance/gravitas of this moment (huge!): You are going to have a baby. Wow. I can't imagine anything more profound than the decision to create a life and guide another human being through this world. I am in awe of you. I wish I could come through these pages and give you a gigantic hug. Or, if I'm being honest, what I really wish is that I could pop a bottle of Dom for you. But that would be inappropriate. So we'll go with the hug.

WHAT DO I KNOW?

The next thing you might want to know is, what do I know about all this? Why should you listen to me? Well, I came to the realization that I wanted to be a parent in my midthirties. That's late-ish, but certainly more the norm these days. Looking back now, with two little ones, I can honestly tell you that nothing is more rewarding, fulfilling, or important than being a parent. And simultaneously, no job in my life has proven more intense, comprehensive, or all-consuming.

All that said, brace yourself for this shocker: I personally have never been through the pregnancy process.

Insert screeching-to-a-halt sound here.

While some of you know this about me, others are likely having a WTF moment right now. You might be asking yourself, "Why the hell did this woman write this book, and why should I listen to her advice if she's never even done it herself?" Here's why: Because one of the people I love the most in this world became pregnant, carrying in her belly another one of the people I love the most—my son. She did the physical labor, but I was there the whole time, inserting my opinions, helping make the big decisions, and obsessively researching every question and grilling every doctor, every step of the way. From the moment Heidi looked me in the eyes and said, "I think I'm ready to have a baby," I was all in. I made it my mission to know everything about every conceivable aspect of pregnancy. (I am an OCD control freak. Another shocker.)

Specifically, I reviewed hundreds of articles and studies in current journals of obstetrics, nursing, and nutrition. I explored every aspect of what conventional medicine and alternative medicine had to offer. I consulted the leading naturopaths, homeopaths, registered dietitians, pregnancy fitness experts, endocrinologists, ob-gyns, and pediatricians in the field (remember that dream team I referenced a second ago?), pertaining to every component of maternity from food and fitness to labor and delivery, from morning sickness and heartburn to prenatal vitamins and acupuncture. I wanted to be sure I had the most current and sound information to ensure the health and well-being of my family. Knowledge is power, and the right information allowed us to make the best choices for us, to optimize the experience and outcome for my partner and my son, and all the while, to feel more in control throughout the whole experience.

I learned a lot—and there's so much to know! The whole time I was collecting this information, all I kept thinking was, "How is this information not mainstream? Why isn't every woman told about this stuff? Why isn't this information standard for all pregnant women? Shouldn't it be in some handy brochure? How come I have to dig through hundreds of studies and then question experts to get this advice? With all the parenting info out there, shouldn't there be a place where you can go to get the real, unadulterated, raw truth?" Turns out, there isn't.

WHAT DO DOCTORS KNOW?
(AND WHAT DON'T THEY KNOW?)

The reason why there isn't a one-stop shop of complete, total, accurate pregnancy information is that there are many approaches and perspectives and opinions on what is true, and doctors and specialists tend to have very specific knowledge in one area, but it may not be the most updated knowledge, and it may not include any knowledge about other, related areas. For example, in our culture, many doctors are not entirely savvy when it comes to the more holistic approach to pregnancy. They don't know a lot about nutrition or exercise science, either. They'll probably tell you to cut caffeine and alcohol. They might say to eat a protein-rich diet and make sure to get plenty of fruits, veggies, and whole grains. But some of them won't even go that far and will tell you that it doesn't matter that much what you eat, as long as you aren't smoking and doing tequila shots. Most will recommend prenatal vitamins and possibly omega-3s, but they won't tell you which ones or what the differences are between brands and compositions. Our doctors are great at many things, but staying up-to-date on the latest food, exercise, or environmental science isn't typically a top priority. They are too busy handling the day-to-day emergencies. And delivering babies. It's pretty amazing how much some doctors know, but it's also amazing what they don't know, which is one of the reasons why it's so important not just to choose a good one but to do your own research as well.

And while I get that every doctor has only so much time in a day, the fact is that in many instances, I uncovered dangerous advice that was being condoned by certain medical professionals, often via major publications and mainstream Web sites. And guess why? A broad and vast influence affects health information in our culture, and it comes from the unfortunate predominance of Big Food, Big Pharma, and the insurance companies that influence what information you get. I probably don't have to tell you how much this sucks. It's outrageous. Unacceptable. No more. No way. Not in my family. Not in yours.

If you have read any of my other books, listened to my podcast, or seen me on television, you probably already know or suspect that I have been raising the red flag for years now when it comes to chemicals and artificial foods and medications that have taken over our food supply and our environment. It's one thing to try to avoid pollution and pesticides and unnecessary medications as a full-grown adult, but when you're creating life inside you, suddenly environmental toxins, fake food, and pollution take on a whole new level of menace.

But I have yet to know of a single pregnant friend who was warned about any of this properly, if at all—pesticides, artificial additives and preservatives and colorings, pollution, adulterated supplements, not to mention the toxic effects of stress. Instead, doctors tend to give the ole textbook spiel, "Avoid the soft cheese, no lunchmeat or raw fish, and be sure to drink water. The end." Whenever I hear it, I can't help asking myself, "Wait, what century are we in, again?" Far more pertinent information should take precedence over "Watch out for the soft cheese." Do you realize that only 500 or so pregnant women get listeria per year in the United States, out of the four million women who get pregnant? There are far greater things we should be concerning ourselves with.

For example, did you know that according to a study commissioned by the Environmental Working Group, the umbilical cord blood of babies born to women in the study contained more than 200 chemicals that shouldn't be there?[1] Yikes! You don't even get to be born with a clean slate anymore. That's how polluted we are. That's how much our environment has been infiltrated with toxic materials. This really pisses me off, and if you are knitting a baby together, or you plan to, then I bet it pisses you off, too.

That's where the motivation and inspiration to write this book was conceived. (Pun intended!) I wanted to share everything that Heidi and I have learned with all the other mommies and mommies-to-be out there, so they could also be armed with information that matters.

Every parent deserves equal access to the latest, most reliable, and honest information about how to nurture the health of both mom and baby. That's the purpose of this book: to empower you with *all* the knowledge, facts, and cutting-edge research so that you can best protect yourself and your baby, personalize this process for an ideal outcome, and craft your own pregnancy and birth decisions for you and your baby.

YOUR NEW PRIORITIES

Pregnancy is a sacred responsibility. So much of what you do, eat, think, feel, and surround yourself with—even what you smell!—during this time can have a dramatic effect on you and your baby. Your behaviors now will impact everything from your delivery and how quickly your body "bounces back into shape" to your child's temperament and behavior, sleep patterns, how your child performs in school, your child's food preferences, life span—and as I previously mentioned, even long-term earning potential. Seriously! Crazy, right?

Like no other time in life, pregnancy is a rare moment when parents have the chance to directly affect the health and future of their child. Now, every pregnancy is unique and influenced by many different variables. While a few things *are* out of your control, such as genetics, most factors affecting your pregnancy are under your direct control. Making smart decisions—such as how you exercise and what you eat, drink, inhale, and absorb, and even your mood—can stack the deck in your baby's favor, building a strong, healthy foundation for his or her entire life.

I also want you to feel reassured that while I definitely have strong opinions, the advice contained herein is not only bullshit-free, it's also judgment-free. I will tell you what's what, but I won't tell you what to do. I want you to know your choices and understand what's happening to ensure you're in the driver's seat. Unfortunately, you'll likely get plenty of judgment throughout your pregnancy, because everybody seems to have an opinion about what pregnant women should and shouldn't do, and once you are a mother with a baby, it gets even worse. While I can't shield you from this, I reiterate my promise—I will never do that to you. When it comes to "mom wars," I am a pacifist. You're safe with me. I respect your decisions, even when they go against my recommendations in this book. I'm here to help. I've got your back.

There is just one society of mothers, and every mother is a part of it, no matter what path she chooses to take with respect to her pregnancy or parenting. We, the members of this club, are heroines. Mothering, nurturing, loving, and caring for your tiny little human is a heroic effort that deserves to be honored and cherished.

Know that I welcome you, salute you, and honor you, my fellow mom-in-arms. I am thrilled to have you as a member of the club!

Now, let's break down what you can expect in the pages to come.

ABOUT THIS BOOK

Yeah Baby! is an information handbook and friendly source of support that will prepare you, both mentally and physically, for the entire process so you have a strong, fit, and healthy pregnancy, from preconception to postpartum. It will simultaneously arm you with the knowledge and the motivation to create the healthiest, most radiant child your body can possibly produce.

First, we'll tackle prepregnancy. If only every woman knew what to do before getting pregnant, we could eliminate a lot of issues. In this part, I'll talk all about how to get ready: what we did, and what you can do, to maximize your fertility and get you in training for the marathon that is to come.

Then we will address the "rules of thumb," as I like to refer to them. Here, we are going to do a deep dive on the most current and optimal pregnancy nutrition and fitness guidelines, as well as lifestyle recommendations and alternative medicine therapies that will help keep you energized and strong while giving your little one every advantage possible for a great future life. We will go way beyond fish oil and folic acid here, so get excited! I'm even going to insert myself into how you decorate your nursery—what type of paint you use on the walls, what kind of bedding goes in the crib, the furniture you buy. Yep, it all matters. Just call me Martha Stewart— Martha Stewart with a high-stakes mission!

Next, we'll address all three trimesters individually. In these sections, we will cover in detail what is going on with your body on a moment-to-moment basis, what's happening with the little growing bean inside of you, what questions to ask your doctor, and how to address any and all symptoms you may be struggling with, to help alleviate any discomfort as safely and effectively as possible. Plus, perhaps most importantly, I will be giving you a separate detailed and comprehensive meal plan and exercise regimen for each trimester in order to take all the guesswork out of it for you and make you and junior bulletproof.

After that, we'll delve into labor and delivery—from doulas and water births to vitamin K drops and placenta eating (can you guess how I feel about that one?). Whatever it is, I've got you covered. This time, in my opinion, can be the most frightening. I'm going to take you by the hand here and guide you step-by-step through all your options so you are empowered and unafraid.

Last of all, we'll cover the equal-parts-exhilarating-and-exhausting "fourth trimester" (the 3- to 6-month period after your child is born). In the fourth trimester, we focus on healing and recovering from the pregnancy and birth, adapting to the new physical and psychological demands of being a mommy, and, quite frankly, getting your physique back into top-notch shape.

Finally, to assuage any last doubts you might have about the legitimacy of my advice, let me just assure you: I know people. No, I don't mean I know people who will come and break your thumbs if you question my authority. On the contrary. I *want* you to question me, and anyone else, if what they tell you doesn't feel right to you.

I mean, one nice thing about being well known in the health and wellness world is that I have access to the best people in the business—aka your *Yeah Baby!* dream team. My endocrinologist, Dr. Katja Van Herle, is one of the best in the country. I know one of the most awesome food experts on the planet, Cheryl Forberg, a registered dietitian, *New York Times* bestselling author, and James Beard Award– winning chef who worked with me as the nutritionist on *The Biggest Loser.* She is brilliant and is with us as part of our dream team to help you out.

I also found the best possible pregnancy fitness expert, Andrea Orbeck, to train Heidi before, during, and after pregnancy. Now she will help inform *your* fitness plan. We've got Dr. Suzanne Gilberg-Lenz on board—an ob-gyn in private practice in Beverly Hills—who is devoted to women's empowerment and public education and who has a ton of training in holistic and integrative medicine. She's here to keep all of our heads screwed on straight when it comes to the craziness and misinformation that so often accompany pregnancy and childbirth. Finally, our pediatrician, Dr. Jay Gordon, is one of the foremost in the field.

Lucky for me (and you), all five have agreed to serve as my panel of experts, weighing in on all the issues and giving us their insider advice on what's true, what's not so true, what's new, and what is age-old and still valid. These are people that, frankly, most of us don't have access to. They are pretty exclusive and pretty well known for good reason. They are the best of the best. And now they are at your disposal. They are truly the cream of the proverbial crop when it comes to pregnancy-related health information. I trust all five of them implicitly, and you can, too.

If you are at all familiar with my previous work, you know that every book I write is inspired by my own personal journeys—be it with weight loss, finding a purpose, self-worth and self-esteem, professional success, or anything else relevant to what I want to tell you. If I've endeavored to achieve it and eventually attained it, I've written about it. Therefore, throughout the book I will be sharing my own personal experiences with regard to my fertility and hormonal history as well as the origin story of how my beautiful family was born—literally and figuratively. And while everyone's journey with fertility and pregnancy is different, some themes always apply. Those of longing, hope, and enduring love are universal.

One more important thought to help you mentally and emotionally frame up this journey. No matter what you may be feeling or thinking at any point in this process, it's okay. If you hate being pregnant, it's okay. If you are feeling vain and worried about stretch marks or "baby weight," it's okay. If you are nauseated, tired, and resenting the hell out of the whole thing at any given moment, that's also okay.

I want to normalize any emotion you may feel, especially if someone tries to shame you for it. If such a thing occurs, the shame is their issue, not yours. There were days Heidi hated being pregnant. There were days she loved it. There were days I was overwhelmed and terrified about how our lives were going to change, and there were days I was overcome with excitement. This is normal. If you should be in maternal bliss for 40 weeks, then fantastic—enjoy! If for any reason you are not, I say again: It's okay. You will be okay. Your baby will be okay. The most important thing is for you to feel safe and validated in any of the emotions you may have. Now that we have gotten that out of the way . . .

Let's jump right in and get to it. You and I have a lot to talk about. We have experts to consult. I have stories to tell. Most of all, I want you to come through this trial-by-fire we call pregnancy feeling your ultimate best for the life you are creating, and for yourself, too. Because you're going to be a mama, and mamas need love and care and nurturing, and I'm going to show you how to do that for yourself so you can do the best mothering job possible.

You've got this and I've got you. Together we can handle anything that might happen. Let's build a healthy baby and make you one hot mama!

PART 1
The Yeah Baby!
BASICS

CHAPTER 1

START ME UP:
What to Do Before You Get Preggers

Time to get knocked up!

It's kind of ironic, isn't it? As younger women, we spend a considerable amount of effort trying *not* to get pregnant. Then, when the time comes to completely reverse that mind-set, it can be a little disorienting. *Please don't let me be pregnant* somehow turns into *Please let me be pregnant*! The average woman in the United States spends 3 decades of her life (not necessarily all in a row) trying to avoid pregnancy and about 5 years trying to get pregnant, being pregnant, and going through the postpartum period, to get the two children most women say they want.[1]

However, during those 5 precious years (for you it may be only 1 or it could be a decade), how you live your life can help in big ways to determine how easily you will become a future mom. Although not everyone does it, planning and prepping your body appropriately for fertility and a healthy pregnancy are essential—both for you and for your baby.

If you are already pregnant, you could skip straight to Chapter 2, but I hope you will read this chapter anyway. You might learn some good stuff that will still be relevant to you. If not, let's start the preparation process for the pregnancy to come. And it is a process—an important one. Maybe you didn't expect that. And maybe you are trying to guess what I am getting at: "I am at a healthy weight." "I have no fertility issues that I am aware of." "What is she talking about?"

Not to worry. I'm gonna tell you.

OUR INADVERTENT PATH TO PREGNANCY PLANNING

I don't want to jump ahead too much, but in an attempt to stress the significance of this chapter let me say the following: Thankfully, Heidi is gay. No, it isn't because we like rainbows and pride parades. It's because we were doing IUI (intrauterine insemination), aka the turkey baster method, which forced us to the doctor *before* Heidi was pregnant and not *after,* like most heterosexual couples I know.

And these doctors asked a million questions, sent her to several other doctors, and ran a battery of tests, which I initially thought unnecessary and inconvenient.

"We're gay," I thought, "not infertile, for God's sake! Get the baster and shoot her up. This is such a waste of time!" I was incredibly impatient and annoyed, until those tests revealed some surprising and extremely significant results.

It turns out Heidi had uterine polyps, a definite roadblock to conceiving naturally. Had we been a typical heterosexual couple, we likely would have tried to get pregnant for 2 years before discovering something was wrong. And had Heidi actually managed to get pregnant in spite of those polyps, she had thyroid issues she was unaware of, which could have caused major complications during her pregnancy, or even caused infertility, had they not been addressed beforehand.

As grateful as I finally was to have had this utterly inadvertent intervention, I was also a bit stunned. I remember thinking, "Why doesn't everybody go through this process?" If a perfectly healthy young woman found these unexpected conditions, wouldn't all couples want to know what their health status is before they start trying? Think of the time and heartache it would save those with fertility issues left in the dark month after month, wondering why the at-home pregnancy tests kept coming up negative.

Even more importantly, wouldn't everyone want to find out if they have any issues that could cause problems during and even after the pregnancy and resolve them *ahead of time*? Why don't all doctors recommend this to all their patients before they try to conceive—not just the gay ones sent to the fertility clinic as a "formality"?

I was also left wondering why a young, healthy woman would be hyperthyroid. And why was her uterus covered in polyps? Heidi saw her ob-gyn for regular checkups. Why didn't somebody catch this ages ago? Why hadn't her ob-gyn asked her if she planned on getting pregnant at any point, so all these issues could have been identified and rectified much sooner? This is really when my gears began turning. How could this whole process be backward for the majority of our population?

But there is much to tell, so let's start at the beginning. Don't worry, we aren't going back to the big bang—I mean the beginning of how Heidi and I came to learn about the importance and necessity of a prepregnancy plan and how we implemented it.

THE BEGINNING

This process started for Heidi and me in early 2010. At this time, I was working on a TV show called *Losing It*. On this show, I would move in with overweight families and coach them back to health. Of course, the families had kids, and for one of the episodes, I moved in with a family in Detroit who had two little girls.

One of the little girls was named Lily, and she was 9 years old. I adored her. I would wake up with them, pack their lunches, help them make healthier dinners, and talk about why we were switching out certain foods for other foods, like whole grain bread for white bread . . . and I loved it. Truly. I enjoyed my conversations with that kid more than any other conversations I was having in my life at the time.

Well, this rocked my world. Until this point I truly never thought I was going to have kids. I was very focused on my career and I had some fertility issues (which I will delve into momentarily), and the combo of the two had me relatively oblivious. After Lily, however, the genie was out of the bottle . . . and she wasn't going back in. Cliché as it may sound, I finally realized that family is the true meaning of life. I love my work, don't get me wrong, but having children transcends it all (in my opinion). They are the point. The whole point. I recognized pretty immediately that I was not going to get to the end of my life and think, *"Wow, I wish I'd spent more time at the office!"* The epiphany swept over me completely, and it altered my perspective forever. So now what . . . ?

At this stage, Heidi and I had been together for roughly 18 months. She was only 28 and her clock was ticking, but not very loudly. Prior conversations about kids were fleeting and brief. They went a lot like this: "Yeah, maybe we'll do that down the road," or "Sure, maybe one day." I didn't want to pressure Heidi, and I didn't know where life was going to take us as a couple, but I knew I needed to start getting my ducks in a row. Now before I tell you what came next, I need to share with you what came first.

YOUR HORMONAL HISTORY . . . AND MINE

I was a "fat kid." You might already know this, as I have written about it in previous books and my "before pic" has been splashed on nearly every talk show I have ever done. But just in case you didn't, I was chubby. To give you an idea of how chubby, at my heaviest I was about 170 pounds at just 5 feet tall. Now, I am 5'3" and roughly 115 pounds. So, as I said, I was a fat kid.

If you're wondering why I am bringing up being overweight in a book about maternity, the answer is simple: My weight and what caused me to become overweight had a significant impact on my hormone balance and my fertility potential later in life. I of course didn't know this at the time, and neither did anyone else, really. It was the '80s, and no one was even talking about whole foods or organic foods, let alone xenoestrogens (chemical compounds that mimic estrogens in your system) or thyrotoxic foods (foods toxic to the thyroid gland) or obesogens (chemicals foreign to the body that disrupt hormone function and lipid metabolism, increasing the tendency toward obesity). Everything I ate or drank was completely processed and loaded with chemicals. Plus, I was relatively sedentary until I got into martial arts at about 13 years old. So not only had I been eating horribly, I also wasn't a very active kid. Insult to injury, I know.

My mom got me into martial arts, not necessarily because she thought I was fat, but because she thought I needed something to be passionate about. And she was right—I loved it. I started going several times a week, and the activity helped me gradually gain self-esteem and slim down. It didn't change my eating habits, though, so the stage was set for what came next. When I was around 15 years old, I had an ovarian cyst burst. This is not a fun experience, by the way. In fact, it is incredibly painful, and I honestly thought at the time, not knowing what was happening, that I was going to die. But I didn't die. They told me I had PCOS, or polycystic ovary syndrome, a hormonal disorder of the endocrine system, and probably endometriosis, a condition causing troublesome and painful periods, in which the uterine lining (called the *endometrium*) tissue spreads and grows outside the uterus, causing the Fallopian tubes to scar and not function properly, if at all. Lovely. As if the teen years aren't difficult enough!

At the time, I was told that PCOS causes ovarian cysts, and that's what happened to me—cysts were growing on my ovaries, then bursting, causing me agony. (Our dream team ob-gyn expert, Dr. Suzanne Gilberg-Lenz, tells me that this is an "old-school" point of view and that actually, my pain was likely due to endometriosis. But at the time this was my diagnosis to explain the cyst formation.) I had always had troublesome menstrual periods, as well as acne and weight gain from insulin resistance—in other words, my hormones were definitely not functioning normally. I didn't know all this yet. All I knew was that my ovaries were "cystic."

Dr. V Says . . .

Our brilliant internal medicine doctor and endocrinologist, Katja Van Herle, MD (I call her Dr. V), has this to say about PCOS. As an endocrinologist, this is her area.

PCOS is likely named incorrectly. It isn't really a problem with ovarian cysts, though when the cysts are present, this often becomes problematic. In fact, many PCOS patients do not have ovarian cysts, but they do tend toward abnormal ovulatory cycles; anovulation (meaning a "period" happens but no egg is kicked out); irregular periods; often androgen dominance (which means higher levels of DHEA and testosterone); acne; hair growth in unplanned places (like the face, belly, and areola); and male-pattern hair thinning. Importantly, PCOS often includes insulin resistance (high insulin levels, prediabetes, or diabetes). This is key when it comes to getting pregnant but also while being pregnant, because it increases the risk of gestational diabetes.

Dr. Suzanne Says . . .

Here is what our awesome and vastly knowledgeable *Yeah Baby!* consulting ob-gyn, Dr. Suzanne Gilberg-Lenz, has to say about PCOS.

Approximately 20 percent of women today have PCOS. It has become rampant, and this has had an important impact on fertility. Early intervention is crucial to preserve fertility, so be sure to get checked for this problem before attempting to get pregnant.

Now the 40-year-old me would have thought, "WTF?! What is PCOS really? And what is endometriosis? What causes these? Do they typically occur together?" (Dr. V says no—they are mostly different processes, but when they happen together, they present a real challenge to fertility.) And what most disturbs me now is this question: Why would an otherwise healthy, active teenage girl have this? How did my body get so out of whack? What is the origin of this issue, and what holistic changes can I make to put my body back in sync?

The 16-year-old me, however, was thinking more along the lines of, "Is this birth control pill they want me to take going to make me gain weight?" I was 16; what can I tell you?

To make a long story short, as I grew older, my knowledge of fitness, nutrition, and endocrinology grew. By the time I was in my thirties, I had a strong understanding of the endocrine system and was incredibly well versed on how to manage my weight, immunity, and overall health via clean and active living. I hadn't had a cyst burst since I was in my midtwenties, and my periods were far less painful. I was able to manage my weight without starving myself and training my body into the ground. Fantastic.

At that point, I never even thought for more than about 5 minutes about ever getting pregnant. I was extremely focused on my career and didn't even know if I would want kids. But because of the PCOS and endometriosis, I figured from a very young age it probably wouldn't be an option for me anyway, at least not without substantial medical intervention. I knew my tubes were blocked from the endometriosis, and I would either need surgery or, most likely, in vitro fertilization. Knowing that I already had cystic ovaries and that I was an "estrogen-dominant" female (having particularly high levels of estrogen in my body), I was concerned that fertility drugs could increase my risk of ovarian cancer and pose other significant long-term health risks. So I wasn't about to go there. I was nervous about messing with my hormones, and I knew that while drugs and surgeries have allowed many women to overcome these issues to bear their own kids, I didn't feel like I could put my body through any more hormonal trauma than it had already endured. I had personally accepted the fact that maybe God had other plans for me. For all those reasons, I began to explore adoption.

Heidi supported me in all aspects of Operation Adoption. We certainly hoped to

Before I Go On . . .

Let's have a little sidebar discussion, shall we? Because I want to clear something up. Back in 2010, I got ambushed by a reporter who asked me if I wanted kids. I responded by saying that I was likely going to adopt. She pressed me, asking, "Why won't you carry the child?" I was caught completely off guard. Instead of just being honest and admitting to issues with infertility, I was suddenly overcome with shame. This prompted my nebulous response, "I don't know if I could put my body through the process of what it would require." I was attempting to imply, without directly stating, that I had fertility issues and was concerned about the side effects of fertility drugs. Although I certainly don't subscribe to the stigma of infertility and I certainly don't find it disgraceful, I admit to suffering from it in my younger years.

Well, this turned out to be one of the worst disasters of my career. The *Huffington Post* had a field day with this headline, which was published on someone's blog in 2010: "Jillian Michaels thinks pregnancy ruins your body!" Which of course I don't think, and certainly never said. They came out with a headline quoting me as saying, "I won't ruin my body with pregnancy." What an epic nightmare it was. I still get backlash from that headline nearly 10 years later, and many people have the completely wrong idea about me because of it.

The reason I bring this up now is not necessarily to defend myself, but because I realize how much shame I had over my infertility and what I thought it meant about me as a woman, let alone as a health expert. If I was so good at my job, why couldn't I have a baby? Blah blah blah. We all know that has nothing to do with infertility, and I am older now and much more mature, so I realize this.

My point, however, is that if any of you are struggling with infertility as well, whether you have been diagnosed with it or you just know, let me say this: It's not your fault, and shame on anybody who dares to shame you for it. You are just as much a woman as every other woman you know. The journey into motherhood is different for everyone, and there is no way of telling where your journey with the process will take you. It will be okay. It will work out exactly how it's meant to. I am living proof of that.

be together long term, but at that point in our relationship, we hadn't officially made that kind of commitment. As time passed, though, and I worked tirelessly to adopt a child, Heidi ended up very involved in the process. By 2011 it became obvious that this adopted child was going to be "ours." We were starting a family—together. But the adoption process can take years, and by mid-2011, there we were, still with no hope or sign of a referral for our child. We were feeling frustrated and hopeless.

Then one day, Heidi looked at me and said, "Babe, what if I try to get pregnant?"

The rest is, as they say, history.

Ha-ha-ha . . . *not*!

For some, getting pregnant is quite simple. You start trying, and bam, you're pregnant. Those who aren't successful with this by-chance approach may have to seek fertility help. For us, the by-chance approach wasn't an option—not because Heidi was infertile, but because, as previously stated, we are a same-sex couple. I'm pretty confident I don't have to state the obvious beyond that point, because you all know your birds-and-bees stuff. Suffice it to say that basically, we just needed our ob-gyn to put the "stuff" up in "there" (aka sperm/vagina). I thought this would be quick and easy. It *sounds* quick and easy. We go in with the goods, they put the goods where the sun don't shine, and whammo, she's preggers . . . right?

Wrong.

THE PRECONCEPTION HEALTH CHECK

I had no idea how serious and significant the process of "pregnancy prep" is for anyone choosing to do IUI or IVF. Straight people just insert sperm, sperm fertilizes egg, egg attaches to uterine lining. Success. So why can't everyone do that?

Simply because instant success isn't as commonplace as you might think for many unforeseen reasons. Even the straight-person method is actually highly unsuccessful most of the time—the chances for a normal, healthy woman of child-bearing age having regular sex is just 20 to 40 percent during any given cycle.[2] And heaven forbid

Dr. Suzanne Says . . .

Although some people choose to go to a fertility clinic for the IUI procedure, a good general ob-gyn will do preconception counseling and diagnosis—but only if you come in before you get pregnant! Also, many well-trained ob-gyns are qualified to perform IUI for you, so a fertility clinic isn't strictly necessary if you have a good ob-gyn.

The 15-Month Pregnancy

You probably thought pregnancy lasts 9 months, but in reality, it takes up a good 15 months of your life: the 3-month period prior to conception, which I call the runway, and the 3-month period after conception, which I consider to be the landing and taxiing back to the terminal. Both count as integral parts of the whole process. Yep, that means that essentially, your pregnancy starts *now*. You can think of this 3-month period as your best chance to get your body into good overall health to help you not only to conceive but to facilitate a healthy pregnancy and deliver a healthy baby. This is the time to "cleanse the temple" that is your body and bring yourself up to all-systems-go status before you get baby on board and take off for the ride of your life. And by the way, Dr. Gilberg-Lenz is totally behind me on this one. She told me that because of epigenetics (the way lifestyle can turn certain genes "on" or "off," affecting your disease risk), prepregnancy health can set the stage for your future offspring's adult health! That means your lifestyle choices now have a real impact, even before you get preggers. How's that for motivation?

you are successful in fertilizing the egg when you have health issues you were previously unaware of, because that can cause a host of problems during your maternity that you really don't want to have to deal with. Like what, you ask?

We first visited the top fertility clinic on the West Coast. Fertility clinics specialize in IUI, so off we went. Because their specialty is infertility, after all, they are trained to look for and solve problems with conception.

The grilling began with our very first phone call to the clinic. We were hit with an onslaught of questions.

"Are you on any medications?"

"Do you have any chronic medical conditions?"

"Do you exercise regularly?"

"Have you already had your thyroid checked?"

"Do you know whether you are ovulating regularly?"

"Do you have any issues like polyps, PCOS, or endometriosis?"

"Have you been checked for HPV?"

"What's your basal body temperature?"

"How thick is your cervical mucus?"

"Has anyone measured your uterine lining yet?"

"We are going to send you 1,000 pages of questionnaires to fill out. Please have them ready when you come in for your consultation." (Okay, I may be exaggerating slightly on this one, but it was intensive.)

When we finally arrived for the first appointment, they began outlining all the tests they wanted Heidi to take before they would even *consider* inseminating her. *Mother of God . . . where is the romance?* I thought. It was all so clinical and overwhelming. And yet, as I've already mentioned, tests revealed that Heidi had uterine polyps that needed to be removed and, even more serious, an overactive thyroid that needed to be addressed.

So, as you see, we made these discoveries about Heidi's health rather unintentionally. There is no protocol in place where doctors regularly monitor your fertility and help you keep up your reproductive health. Yes, you have your yearly checkup (hopefully). And Heidi did this dutifully, but they never checked her egg count, uterine lining, cervical mucus, hormone balance, and so on. The annual physical is a pretty routine yearly check for cancer and STDs, but it doesn't usually address optimal reproductive health, *unless you bring it up!* And then the quality and breadth of information you will get, even if you tell your doctor that you are trying to get pregnant, could vary widely, depending on whom you see.

This got me wondering why nobody ever told me, when I was younger, that my hormonal issues might affect my fertility. Nobody gave me any corrective feedback on what to do about it (barring adding more hormones to the mix with birth control pills). I was too young to know about or think about asking if the condition might impact my future fertility, but it seems insane to me now that nobody ever mentioned that to me or my mother. It's also crazy to me that the majority of doctors aren't helping women prep for fertility, starting as soon as they go in for their first appointment in their teens. Good reproductive health is never a bad thing, whether you choose to have a baby or not. And why aren't doctors instructing their patients long before they want to get pregnant that many necessary steps should be taken in preparation for conception? It should be hammered into women's heads early. Society prepares you to pick a major in college, to choose a career, for crying out loud, but no one really teaches you about maintaining optimal reproductive health for the future. Pregnancy is something that ideally involves physical preparation! It isn't just about romance, emotion, and finances. In my entire life, I have never had one doctor (except Dr. Van Herle, fairly recently) ask me if I planned on getting pregnant or offer any information or guidance on boosting fertility and prepping for pregnancy.

This is a major reason why I decided to write this book. There is a lot you can and ideally should do before you ever start trying to get pregnant, let alone embark on

Dr. V Says . . .

A pregnant woman's body is an amazing thing. Even if you are not optimally nourished and have health issues, the body can use the mother's reserves to nourish the baby. Even if you didn't "prep" before pregnancy, it's never too late to start getting good health habits in place.

However, this is a book about optimizing pregnancy, not just surviving it. It's also a book about optimizing your baby's health, and if you really want to do that, it's a good idea to spend at least 3 months getting ready to "start trying."

First, get a full battery of tests, as described in this chapter, so you can catch and address any health issues you might have now, before you get pregnant. You want the doctor's green light that your body is ready for this journey. Start eating better food now, not once you know you are pregnant, because when cravings and fatigue hit, you want good habits in place. Start taking a high-quality, natural prenatal vitamin up to a year before you start trying to get pregnant, because folic acid in particular is extremely important in the very earliest stages of pregnancy, often before you know you are pregnant, and many women don't get enough without a supplement. Start exercising now, so you can stay active throughout your pregnancy, which will have numerous health benefits for you and the baby. Get in the habit of drinking water and staying fully hydrated now, so you get used to the frequent bathroom trips. Start getting enough sleep right now, and rest whenever you can. Do you need to take a daily nap to get enough sleep? Then start doing that now. Also, get stress management techniques in place now, so when you get overwhelmed during pregnancy, you will have tools to deal with that.

In this chapter, Jillian will address all these things, but what I want you to understand is that during pregnancy, everything gets a little bit harder, so you need to be conditioned and ready. Fill up your gas tank before you hit this road and you will have a much happier, healthier trip.

any official fertilization procedure like IVF or IUI, to maximize your chances of a healthy and successful pregnancy. And that is exactly what I will outline for you throughout this chapter.

So where do you start? The very first thing you should do is inform your:

- Gynecologist
- Family doctor or internist
- Dentist
- Any other medical professional you see regularly for health issues you already have

Book appointments with all of them, tell them you want to get pregnant, and ask them for all the necessary examinations and to run all the necessary tests to be sure you are fit for pregnancy and don't have any hidden health or fertility issues that might hinder the process.

Each of these doctors will see your potential pregnancy from a different angle and will think about and test for different kinds of things. While this may seem excessive, I assure you it isn't. It can save you and your little one from so many potential health risks down the road, as well as thousands of dollars in medical costs due to complications. Even if you have already had a child, I urge you to do this. While mommas with kids know they have the ability to get pregnant, our health conditions can change significantly from year to year depending on many factors. You need to stay completely current with any and all medical issues to maintain the health of your body.

Let's head to the doctor's office!

AT THE GYNECOLOGIST

First thing, pop in for a visit to your ob-gyn. Explain your plans and your health history and get some tests. If you happen to have any issues, you can get them cleared up before you start trying to get pregnant. Some of these tests are screens for risk factors or potential health issues in you or your baby. Others are diagnostic tests, which tell you definitively whether or not you have developed a condition that requires more treatment. Also keep in mind that you may have to have a bit more testing if your pregnancy would be considered high risk. The following factors put a pregnancy into the official high-risk category.

- Very young age at pregnancy
- Age older than 35 at the time of delivery
- Overweight or underweight

- A history of problems in a previous pregnancy
- Health conditions before pregnancy, such as high blood pressure, autoimmune disorders, diabetes, cancer, or HIV
- A pregnancy with multiples

Now, again—none of these situations mean that you *will* have a problem. They simply mean that you have a slightly higher chance of developing some issues, and you and your doctor should be prepared, just in case. Remember: Information is power. Don't be afraid of the tests.

Here's what to do.

Share Your Hormonal History, Including the Details of Your Menstrual Cycle

Did you know that your body's fertility was already being influenced when you were in your mother's womb? That's when hormones first start flowing through you and affecting your development, including what your gender will be, but also much more: how well your organs develop (like your heart, lungs, and brain); how much weight you gain and what your birth weight will be; even when you will be born. What a mother does influences the baby hormonally, too—for example, if she drinks a lot of alcohol, that can stimulate glucocorticoids, which can affect the development of the endocrine system.[3] If she is under a lot of stress, the baby will be exposed to more

Fear Not

One quick caveat before we move on: The information in this chapter and throughout this book could sometimes sound a bit scary and overwhelming to you, especially when I talk about things that *could* happen. I seriously debated doing this because I don't want you to feel scared, but on the other hand, you need to have all the information possible. I want you to know why a test is important, why a procedure might really help, and all the things that vigilance and a healthy lifestyle can prevent. I want you to learn everything I learned when Heidi and I went through it. Please know that almost any physical scenario can be managed with your doctor to facilitate conception and optimal health for you and your child. The key is awareness and preparedness, which is what this section will help you achieve. Let's make a pact to go at this with zero judgment and zero fear. In turn, you can gain a sense of empowerment from all this information and use it to formulate an effective game plan for you and your family.

stress hormones like cortisol. Research shows that when babies are exposed to cortisol in the womb, they are more likely to have a cortisol spike (i.e., major stress) for things like blood draws after they are born.[4] In other words, your pregnancy stress can cause your baby to be stressed out, too! If a mother has diabetes, the child will be exposed to more glucose from the mother's blood and is more likely to be larger than normal at birth or, in severe cases, too small.[5]

After we are born, hormones continue their influence throughout our young lives, and when we hit puberty, they really step it up, launching us into adulthood and our own childbearing years. They affect our weight, sex drive, moods, energy levels, hunger, sleep, and even organ function. Some even argue that they shape your personality.

They also affect our health. Maybe, like me, you have struggled with hormone-related health issues like PCOS or endometriosis. Maybe you have survived cancer and wonder what treatment could have done to your fertility, or maybe you have been lax about birth control in the past and never accidentally got pregnant, so you wonder if you even can get pregnant.

To help you figure out what to tell your doctor, make a copy of the hormonal history form on the following page and fill it out. This might take some time as you think back and remember everything relevant, but it will save you trouble at the doctor's office when you need to know these events and dates.

This will also get you thinking about your entire hormonal life, to help you get some perspective on where you've been and where you are now, which ultimately helps us to get you where you want to go. After you fill this out, keep it in your purse so you have it with you when you go to your first appointment.

Get a Breast Exam, Pelvic Exam, Pap Test, and Pelvic Ultrasound

You probably get these exams every year or two (or you should), but even if you aren't due for one yet, get this standard exam with future pregnancy in mind, to make sure you don't have any suspicious lumps or precancerous cells. Dr. V says you want a normal Pap test, a normal breast exam, and a normal general physical exam. Your doctor can investigate any abnormalities in test results now, before you start trying to get pregnant, because issues with your reproductive organs could, obviously, impact your reproductive health. The pelvic ultrasound isn't part of this standard exam, but it should be! I add it here because this will give your doctor an opportunity to look for uterine fibroids, polyps, and ovarian cysts. Check with your insurance company to see if this is covered—your doctor may need to have a reason to order it—but if you can get it, it can be very helpful. If you have any of the aforementioned issues that a pelvic ultrasound uncovers, it's possible surgery may be required before you try to get pregnant. Heidi did this, and it was no big

(continued on page 18)

My Hormonal History

Was your birth normal? Any complications with you or your mother?

_____

_____

Did you have any health issues as a child? List them, with dates if you know them.

_____

_____

Do you have any family history of genetic health issues, such as cystic fibrosis? (If so, ask your doctor whether you should consider genetic counseling.) Have your parents or siblings had any major diseases or health issues?

_____

_____

At what age did your period first start?

_____

_____

Do you remember any difficulties or issues with your periods as an adolescent?

_____

_____

What was the first day of your last period? (Doctors _always_ ask this, so you might as well figure it out before you go.)

_____

_____

What is your period like now? Do you keep track? Is your cycle regular? Are you a heavy or light bleeder? Do you have a lot of pain? Describe what is typical for you.

_____

_____

As an adult, have you had any serious health issues? List them, with dates if you know them.

_____

_____

List or get a copy of your vaccination history and record it here.

_____

_____

What prescription and over-the-counter medications do you take now? List names, amounts, and when and how often you take them.

_____

_____

What supplements do you take? List names, amounts, and when and how often you take them.

_____

_____

Describe your current diet.

_____

_____

Describe your current exercise routine and/or activity level.

_____

_____

Have you traveled out of the United States recently, or do you plan to travel, especially in areas known for contagious diseases, particularly the Zika virus?

_____

_____

deal—4 months or so after the surgery, she was pregnant! You can also discuss tests for bacterial or yeast infections. These kinds of infections could infect the baby, but most are harmless. However, they can get worse if untreated and make you feel uncomfortable during pregnancy. Not ideal, obviously.

Ask for Standard Sexually Transmitted Disease Testing

No shame, no judgment, but it's always better to know. Many women have STDs without knowing it. Many women also discover that they have one *after* they are pregnant, but it's much easier (and safer) to treat these conditions before you get pregnant. Just find out and deal with it now.

Consider Surgical Intervention

If there is any suspicion that you may have uterine-tissue buildup, scar tissue from endometriosis, or an STD like chlamydia or gonorrhea (which can block your Fallopian tubes), your doctor might suggest you undergo one of two procedures that can help her look at the inside of the uterus and the Fallopian tubes: a special x-ray called hysterosalpingogram (HSG)[6] and/or a laparoscopy, during which your doctor will thread a small camera through a tube into your belly to figure out if you have any abnormal endometrial tissue.[7] These are actually simple procedures that can completely reverse conditions preventing pregnancy. Ask your doctor what is appropriate for your situation.

Bottom line, testing is all part of the whole pregnancy business. Many women struggle with at least one of the uterine or vaginal conditions mentioned here but

Dr. V Says . . .

It is very important to find out where you stand with STDs like gonorrhea, chlamydia, syphilis, hepatitis B and C, herpes, and even HIV. You need to know these things before you get pregnant, because there are many ways to deal with them. Gonorrhea, chlamydia, and syphilis can be treated and eliminated. A vaccine can prevent hepatitis B in the mother from infecting the baby. Herpes includes genital and oral herpes, but genital herpes in particular can be transmitted via contact during birth. With both herpes and HIV, you can take medications a few weeks before the birth to stop transmission to the baby. Whatever it is, you want to know if you have it so you can go into pregnancy with the right knowledge to prevent infecting your baby.

never know it until they get tested. You may think you'd know if you had an issue, but not necessarily! Testing will tell you for sure.

SEE YOUR INTERNIST OR FAMILY DOCTOR

Next, pop in for a visit with your internist or family doctor for a thorough physical. Your general practitioner will help you get a full picture of your overall health. Get any preexisting medical conditions, such as asthma, chronic hypertension, or cardiac conditions, and any autoimmune conditions like lupus or Hashimoto's thyroiditis under control well before attempting conception. These and other conditions can cause pregnancy complications, and you may be completely unaware you have them—just as Heidi was with her thyroid condition. Getting all of this under control with your doctor prior to conception can dramatically decrease any risk of pregnancy complications like birth defects, miscarriage, or preterm delivery.

Here are a few things you will want to have checked.

Check Your Medications and Supplements

Remember that hormonal history form you filled out? Bring it to all your doctor appointments and be sure to ask your regular doctor about all the medications and supplements you are using. Could any of them cause a problem? Are any of them hazardous to your fertility or your future baby's health? Should you wean off anything before attempting conception? Too many people don't tell their doctors what they are taking, and that can cause a lot of issues with reactions to medications, interference with test results, or even serious health problems. If you are on a medication that is hazardous to your fertility or your future baby, your doctor will know and will make an appropriate substitution for you. Here is some general advice, to prepare you.

- **Avoid aspirin and other NSAIDs like ibuprofen (Advil and Motrin) and naproxen (Aleve).** If you take aspirin close to the time you get pregnant and in the beginning of your pregnancy, you may impact fetal growth, experience problems with the placenta, and put yourself at higher risk of miscarriage.[11] However, if you're already taking a prescribed dose of aspirin for a specific medical condition, you may need to continue taking it during pregnancy. Consult with your doctor to see what's best. Acetaminophen (Tylenol) used correctly (not taking too much) is considered safer for pregnancy.

- **Watch cold medicine.** Some cold medicines are safe, but especially during the first trimester, you may want to avoid them all. Ask your doctor about this.

- **Avoid over-the-counter laxatives.** Especially avoid products that contain chemical or herbal stimulants. Most laxatives have not been properly studied for use during pregnancy.[12] Instead, up your water consumption and eat more fiber-rich foods like vegetables, fruit, and cooked whole grains. Dr. Suzanne says magnesium supplements are also safe and very effective.

- **Be careful of "natural" herbs and oils.** The following herbs and natural supplements have been shown to interfere with conception and *should be avoided*[13] when you are trying to become pregnant: arborvitae, beth root, black cohosh, blue cohosh, cascara, Chinese angelica (dong quai), cinchona, cotton-root bark, echinacea, feverfew, ginkgo biloba, ginseng, goldenseal, juniper, kava kava, licorice, meadow saffron, pennyroyal, poke root, rue, sage, St. John's wort, senna, slippery root, tansy, white peony, wormwood, yarrow, yellow dock, and vitamin A in supplement form.

- **Also be careful with essential oils,** often used in aromatherapy, on skin, orally, or in diffusers, before and during pregnancy: The International Federation of Professional Aromatherapists officially recommends only the following oils for use in pregnancy:[14] benzoin, bergamot, black pepper, German chamomile, Roman chamomile, clary, cypress, eucalyptus, frankincense, geranium, ginger, grapefruit, juniper, lavender, lemon, mandarin, sweet marjoram, neroli, petitgrain, rose otto, sandalwood, sweet orange, tea tree, and ylang-ylang. Avoid any other oils right now.

I'll say this again: *Always* run any supplements by your doctor, especially once you get pregnant. People often don't think that supplements are worth mentioning, or they are embarrassed to tell their doctors about the supplements they take, think-

**Pregnant women should
skip flu shots.**

False! With such a hot debate about childhood vaccinations swirling around us in this country right now, it's no wonder expectant moms may be second-guessing whether a seasonal flu shot is a wise idea, too. Fortunately, the flu vaccine is considered safe for women to receive at any point in their pregnancy, and avoiding the flu is a good way to avoid a lot of misery when over-the-counter medications will be limited.

ing the doctors will be critical of them. Don't make the mistake of thinking that herbs are "natural" and therefore not harmful. Be safe and check first!

Update Your Vaccinations

It's ideal to get up-to-date on your vaccinations prior to becoming pregnant. This will not only protect you from contracting an infectious disease during your pregnancy, but it can also help to protect your baby by passing some immunity from you to your little one. Dr. Suzanne says that any live, attenuated vaccinations such as rubella or varicella (chicken pox) should be administered 3 months before trying to conceive. Those made from caspase proteins like the flu virus or whooping cough or hepatitis vaccines can be and are given during pregnancy—but talk to your doctor about what is appropriate for you. Doctors don't all agree about what is appropriate, especially during pregnancy.

Here are the vaccines you will want to discuss with your doctor. You probably won't need them all, but it's good to know whether you do or not, considering your health history, lifestyle, and environment.

- Hepatitis A
- Hepatitis B (if you haven't already checked this at the ob-gyn)
- HPV (human papilloma virus)
- Influenza (the flu)
- MMR (measles, mumps, rubella)
- Pneumococcus/meningococcus
- Rabies

- Tetanus/diphtheria/pertussis (whooping cough)
- Varicella (chicken pox)

If you are pregnant and reading this anyway and you didn't get vaccinated beforehand, don't panic. You can get all of the following vaccines during pregnancy, as long as they are "inactive."[15]

- Hepatitis A and B (Some doctors will advise against this during pregnancy, so check with yours for more information.)
- Influenza injection
- Rabies
- Tetanus/diphtheria/pertussis

After giving birth, all the vaccines are considered safe again.

If you are not comfortable with vaccinations, I suggest talking to your doctor about this or finding a doctor who is on board with your opinions. You can get titer tests to see whether you really need certain vaccinations, but in general, for adults at risk, vaccinations can prevent some pretty serious problems, and the risk-benefit analysis falls on the side of benefit.

Dr. Gordon Says . . .

Jay Gordon, MD, FAAP, is our brilliant and highly knowledgeable pediatrician. This is what he has to say about vaccines during pregnancy.

The TDAP vaccine during pregnancy, especially during the last month or 6 weeks, may create a protective level of antibodies against pertussis (whooping cough) for a newborn. Perhaps the main reasons we have more whooping cough today are that the weakened vaccine creates immunity that wanes over 2 to 4 years, and more people are refusing vaccines now.

As for vaccinations to avoid during pregnancy, I would avoid hepatitis vaccines, both A and B, and also PVC (pneumococcal conjugate vaccine) and meningitis vaccine because they cause some inflammation, and inflammation during pregnancy is not good. I don't know of any "normal" circumstances when these vaccines would be important to a pregnant woman.

Get a Complete Blood Count (CBC)

Are you anemic? Do you know your hemoglobin and iron levels? How is your liver and kidney function? A CBC is a blood test that looks at the numbers of different cells in your blood, including white blood cells, red blood cells, hemoglobin, and platelets. A CBC can tell you if your white blood cell count is too high and you may be fighting an infection; if it is too low, you may be at risk for infection. The number of red blood cells and hemoglobin level can tell your physician whether or not you suffer from anemia, and the number of platelets indicates whether or not you have a blood clotting disorder.[16]

Your hemoglobin level is especially important because it's instrumental in supporting the oxygen level of the placenta, which comes through the hemoglobin in your red blood cells. Your blood volume also increases by 20 to 30 percent over the course of the pregnancy, which increases your body's demand for the iron and vitamins necessary to make hemoglobin. If you start off deficient, you are at a great disadvantage and run a high risk of becoming severely anemic during your pregnancy. This is no good. It will exhaust you and make it harder to fight off infection. Anemia during pregnancy is linked to low birth weight, preterm delivery, and a slight risk of stillbirth. If you're still anemic by the time you deliver, any loss of blood during the birth could leave you woozy and create heart arrhythmia, or even require a blood transfusion. So this is a big one to get ahead of, especially if you are vegan or vegetarian.

While you can boost hemoglobin levels during pregnancy, you're much better off resolving this issue before attempting to conceive, because supplementation during pregnancy is particularly difficult. Iron supplementation is tough because it can cause nausea and constipation, two things many pregnant women really don't need more of in their lives. (As it's always best to get extra nutrients from food rather than supplements, I've listed dietary suggestions for extra iron on page 37.)

Check Your Vitamin D₃ Levels

This is essential for pregnancy! Dr. Suzanne says all prospective moms should have a vitamin D_3 test and should supplement with vitamin D_3 until levels get above 30 ng/ml.

Check Your Thyroid Function

Another very big deal, particularly during pregnancy. The thyroid is a small gland located in the neck that helps to regulate the rate of your body's metabolism. Thyroid disease runs to two ends of a spectrum—hypo (underactive) and hyper (overactive). Some might suggest you wait to see symptoms of either condition before you get checked; I say, err on the side of caution. In my line of work, I have met many women who were completely unaware they had a thyroid condition until they had their levels checked during a routine physical.

Thyroid disease affects one out of eight pregnant women. You supply all your baby's thyroid hormones for the first trimester, so if you're low to start, it could end up having lifelong effects on the baby's IQ and impairing psychomotor development.[17] Thyroid hormones are not only essential in the brain development of your baby, but having too much or too little thyroid hormone can cause pregnancy complications ranging from infertility to preeclampsia (a dangerous rise in blood pressure that is potentially fatal to you and your baby); placental abruption; anemia; postpartum hemorrhage; or other concerns. The key is to know ahead of time if there is a thyroid condition so you and your doctor can closely monitor and/or control your levels before, during, and after your pregnancy.

Check Your Blood Sugar

Many, many people suffer from prediabetes, or even type 2 diabetes, with absolutely no idea they have it. According to the American Diabetes Association, 9.3 percent of the population, or 29.1 million Americans, have diabetes, and of those, 8.1 million are undiagnosed. Plus, 86 million more Americans age 20 and older have prediabetes![18] This is particularly important if type 2 diabetes runs in your family, you live a sedentary lifestyle, or you struggle with weight problems. Diabetes can make it harder for you to become pregnant, so experts recommend that you get your blood sugar under control for at least 3 months before you attempt to get pregnant.

If you get pregnant with prediabetes, you run a higher risk of developing full-blown gestational diabetes, and the overall risks for you and your baby become more

Dr. V Says . . .

If you are healthy, younger than 35, have a regular menstrual cycle, and plan to get pregnant the traditional way, Dr. V says you probably don't need to get your hormone levels checked beyond the thyroid.

A regular menstrual cycle is very useful in helping you to get pregnant and letting you know your due date. However, if you struggle with any infertility issues and/or have irregular cycles, have your estrogen and progesterone levels checked. This information can possibly help your doctor treat the issue.

Dr. V Says . . .

There are three very important reasons why continual monitoring of a woman's thyroid hormone levels is essential before, during, and after pregnancy.

1. Healthy maternal thyroid hormone status (i.e., whether you have normal levels of T4 and T3) is essential for the organ and brain development of the fetus. Low intrauterine thyroid hormone can lead to poor development.

2. If thyroid hormone levels in the mom are too high, early miscarriage and premature contractions and delivery can result.

3. Autoimmune thyroid diseases such as Hashimoto's and Graves' are common, especially with a family history in the mom's lineage. When the female body is growing a developing baby (a foreign body or foreign set of cells, if you will), the mom's immune system can be more prone to autoimmune diseases like thyroid disease. Many women develop high or low thyroid hormone levels while pregnant or during the postpartum period, over the next 9 to 12 months after delivery. Even if you have never had an autoimmune thyroid condition before pregnancy, it can suddenly occur at this time.

For all these reasons, it is very important to check your thyroid hormone levels before getting pregnant and to continue to have them checked during each trimester (or more often, if you are at high risk), as well as in the year postdelivery.

significant (including increased risk of miscarriage, stillbirth, and birth defects such as heart problems or neural tube defects). During the second and third trimesters, your diabetes can make your baby grow too quickly, increasing risks during labor and delivery. Large babies often require Caesarean deliveries or, if delivered vaginally, they are at increased risk for birth trauma called shoulder dystocia. Dr. Suzanne says this is an emergency during which the baby gets stuck because the shoulders are too large; it can cause neurological damage, like cerebral palsy and other serious problems. In addition, a baby's blood sugar can drop very low after birth, since the baby is no longer receiving the high blood sugar directly from the mom. Your doctors, nurses, and lactation consultants will be right on hand to help you manage that situation, so don't worry, but wouldn't you rather get it under control before then?

Check Your Blood Pressure

Most women's blood pressure actually decreases during the first two trimesters, because progesterone and relaxin have made the walls of your blood vessels more flexible to allow for the increased blood volume.[19] But if you enter your pregnancy with high blood pressure, you'll be at greater risk for preeclampsia. Preeclampsia is a high-blood-pressure condition of pregnancy that tends to happen later in your pregnancy. Also known as toxemia and pregnancy-induced hypertension, preeclampsia can cause damage to your organs, including your brain and kidneys, and can increase the risk of preterm labor or a complication called HELLP syndrome, which can cause severe damage to liver function and can interfere with platelet counts and blood coagulation. Preeclampsia with seizures may become eclampsia, an extremely dangerous condition that can be fatal.[20] Depending on the cause of your high blood pressure, your doctor can give you strategies to lower it before you get pregnant, to reduce all these risks.

Consider Genetic Screenings

People can get a little wigged out about genetic testing, but I like to think of it as a high-tech, geeky version of building your family tree. Genetic testing lets you know if your potential baby is at risk for any really serious diseases, and as you do your investigative work, you can learn a lot about your family history, which you can eventually share with your kid! But the biggest motivator here is to find out if any serious genetic or chromosomal issues run on either side of the family tree (yours and your baby's other birth parent's), such as Tay-Sachs disease, cystic fibrosis, muscular dystrophy, sickle cell anemia, thalassemia, hemophilia, or fragile X syndrome. You might already know you have something, and you may also want to discuss with a genetic counselor how likely you are to pass it on, and get your partner tested to see if he is a carrier and what his risks are. Your ethnic background may also put you at greater risk of carrying a disease you don't have, such as:

- Cystic fibrosis, if either of you is Caucasian
- Tay-Sachs disease, if either of you is an Ashkenazi Jew
- Canavan disease, cystic fibrosis, and Tay-Sachs, if either of you is French Canadian
- Sickle cell and thalassemia, if you are of African, Greek, Italian, or Turkish descent
- Thalassemia, if either of you is of Southeast Asian or Filipino descent

For the vast majority, this process just puts the mind at ease, but if one or both of you are carriers for something serious, you will know, and you still have all options available to you.

Dr. V Says . . .

If you have a family history of type 2 diabetes, especially if linked to other elements like high cholesterol and hypertension or insulin-resistant-type PCOS, it is likely that you are carrying the genes that predispose you to insulin resistance and type 2 diabetes. During pregnancy, everyone gains weight, and most people, at least eventually, become at least a little less active, so even if you don't have diabetes now because you are young and have a healthy lifestyle, it is worth paying particular attention to your blood sugar levels before and during pregnancy. The reason for this is that a family history is a risk factor, not only for future type 2 diabetes, but for gestational diabetes.

Get baseline blood sugar testing before you try to get pregnant, so you know where you stand. If your fasting blood sugar is higher than 90, your base hemoglobin A1C is over 6 percent, and/or your fasting insulin is over 10, you don't have much wiggle room to get into diabetes territory once you get pregnant. If this is you, I highly recommend stepping up your healthy lifestyle. A natural diet is important, and regular exercise is extremely important, for managing high blood sugar. Also get your blood sugar tested at every visit. If your doctor balks at this, you can test yourself with supplies from your local pharmacy. Ask your doctor if you can track your blood sugar yourself and send him or her a weekly report, so you can keep an eye on your blood sugar trends as your pregnancy progresses.

Even if you don't have a family history, the occurrence of gestational diabetes is a sign that you probably have the genetic propensity for diabetes. I think of it as an early warning. The good news is that gestational diabetes is treatable—in mild cases through lifestyle alterations and in more severe cases with insulin and/or drugs (like metformin or Glucophage), which you can take during pregnancy if necessary. If you can't make the necessary changes on your own, go to the experts for guidance and ask for help from your partner and friends. It's okay to say, "Hey, I need someone to go on a walk with me" and "Hey, I can't have these foods in the house."

The other good news is that gestational diabetes is an opportunity. Now you know you have this genetic propensity, so with the right lifestyle changes now, you can avoid type 2 diabetes in your future. Had you not known this, you might have been less likely to try to prevent it.

- You can learn about the disease and how to care for someone with that condition, to decide if you want to take it on.

- You can go ahead with the conception and then do prenatal testing to get a definitive diagnosis.

- You can decide to explore alternatives such as adoption or egg or sperm donation (or both).[21]

These can be tough decisions—but your baby (and you) will be much better off if you know ahead of time. I've said it before and I'll say it again: Knowledge is power!

Get a Blood Type Test

If you should ever need blood from a hospital, they will test your blood type and won't just rely on what you tell them. However, it's still good to know your blood type—A, B, AB, or O—and your Rh factor, which tells you whether you have a particular protein on the surface of your red blood cells. If you have it, you are Rh positive; if you don't, you are Rh negative.[22] About 85 percent of us are Rh positive, but

STEER CLEAR OF THE "KITTY LITTER TOXIN"

If you have an outdoor cat, regularly eat raw or rare meat, or garden without gloves, ask your doctor about testing for toxoplasmosis, an infection caused by a parasite that can affect the health of your unborn child. This is why you've probably heard a million times that pregnant women shouldn't change cat litter. Because this test is often not routinely done, and most people with toxoplasmosis don't have symptoms, if you want the test, you will probably have to ask for it. If you do have toxoplasmosis, don't worry. It is easily treated with antibiotics.

The best ways to avoid the parasites that cause the infection toxoplasmosis are as follows:

- Peel fruits and vegetables.

- Cook your meat thoroughly.

- Wear gloves when gardening.

- Wash cutting boards, dishes, counters, utensils, and hands with hot, soapy water after they have come in contact with raw foods.

- Avoid changing cat litter if possible, especially when pregnant. Keep your cat inside. Do not feed your cat raw or undercooked meats.

if an Rh-negative woman has a baby with an Rh-positive man, things can get a little tricky. Don't worry: *Your baby is totally safe.*

The real risk here is to any second or other future baby, because during birth, Baby 1's Rh-positive blood can commingle with her mom's Rh-negative blood. Mom will then form antibodies to Rh-positive blood, and if and when that mom wants to have a second baby with the same dad, her antibodies may attack her second baby's Rh-positive blood. This can cause Baby 2 to develop Rh disease, which can be extremely dangerous. However, science to the rescue—treatments exist to prevent these complications and treat Baby 2's Rh disease. The key is to know all this ahead of time, so you can be prepared.[23] Please test!

VISIT THE DENTIST

You might not have anticipated this one, but believe it or not, your pregnancy can affect the health of your mouth, and the health of your mouth can possibly affect your pregnancy. This might sound weird to you, but what happens in your mouth can get into your bloodstream. Also, hormonal changes in your body during pregnancy can make any preexisting tooth or gum problems worse, and several recent studies have found a strong link between gum disease and pregnancy complications like low birth weight and preterm delivery. Some researchers believe the inflammatory cytokines released by gum infections may be a factor in triggering early-term birth. Women with gum disease—which could be up to 30 percent of us—are at an increased risk of delivering at less than 37 weeks of gestation.[24]

This visit is also a great opportunity to get an overall checkup on your oral health to see if you need any fillings or dental work. If so, get it done now, because you want to avoid doing that during your pregnancy, if at all possible.

CLEARED FOR TAKEOFF? NOW OPTIMIZE YOUR CHANCES

Now that we have gotten all the medical stuff out of the way, we find ourselves firmly planted in my wheelhouse—diet, fitness, and lifestyle strategies to optimize your health and thereby your body's ability to conceive!

Here's your to-do list:

Pull the goalie. As always, let's start with the obvious: If you are on birth control, get off it. Work with your doctor to take you off birth control and ask her when you can expect to begin ovulating again, which has a great deal to do with the type of birth control you were taking. You might begin to ovulate immediately, or it could take several months for your body to adjust and produce its own monthly cycle. (If you were using Depo-Provera, it could be even longer—but not necessarily. Don't assume anything!)

If you are using an IUD for contraception, you will have to have it removed by your doctor, and as soon as it's taken out, your body is ready to conceive. If you have been using some type of barrier method (condoms, diaphragm, or spermicide), the presumption is that you are fertile as long as you don't use them. Many people come

Selling Sickness

Unfortunately, pregnancy is big business. And Big Pharma doesn't want to miss out. The fertility doctors we hired to inseminate Heidi immediately began pimping out drugs to her. "Take Clomid for egg production." "Take home this HCG shot to help trigger ovulation." "Use this progesterone cream after you are pregnant so you don't miscarry."

Here's the deal: As I mentioned, Heidi was not infertile. She was gay and needed a turkey baster. Yet they pushed all these drugs on her that can have significant side effects and should be taken only when completely necessary. Heidi had 15 eggs in her ovaries that we saw on the ultrasound, and the normal range is 15 to 20. She was ovulating normally, which we observed from the at-home ovulation test. And her uterine lining checked out fine. Her progesterone levels were good. She didn't need the progesterone cream.

In many situations people do need these drugs. If you are having fertility issues and are being treated for them, you may need Clomid, HCG, and progesterone. There are good, solid reasons for prescribing these drugs. However, in Heidi's case, none of them were necessary. After we did our homework, Heidi didn't take any of

those drugs, because I was able to get second opinions and determine she didn't need them. Obviously, not all medical professionals try to push unnecessary treatments on their patients and clients, but this approach is so integral to the medical system that it just happens . . . constantly.

The reason the waters are so muddied is because the medical profession does not make money from prevention. It only makes money from procedures and drugs, and that can cloud every expert's judgment, no matter how unbiased they think they are. I'm not telling you to ignore what your doctor says. I am simply telling you that this is an area where you absolutely need to be proactive.

Do your homework. Ask questions. Be mindful. Get a second opinion. And listen to your intuition. If something feels like the wrong thing to do, then maybe it is. You know your body better than anyone, and blind trust in any authority figure can be dangerous. So just keep your eyes open, my friend, and proceed with caution and with your bullshit radar fully functional. Always ask, "Can you explain why I need this?" And be sure you understand and are satisfied with the answer. Do it for yourself and your future children.

off their longer-term contraceptives and use barrier methods until they're truly ready to conceive.

No matter which goalie you'd previously employed, don't panic if you don't get pregnant right away. Just gives you more time to prepare your body!

Quit smoking. NOW. Seriously. If you smoke or your partner smokes, *stop immediately*. I know, easier said than done, but I don't care. Get it done. Dying isn't easy, either. If by some miracle you did manage to get pregnant as a smoker (amazingly, it happens), you do *not* want your little one subjected to the hideous toxins in womb or out. And if you are thinking, "I'll smoke up till I get pregnant and then stop," smoking seriously impacts your fertility as well as your partner's. There is no debate about this. In men, nicotine damages sperm DNA.[25] In women, smoking cigarettes while trying to conceive radically decreases your chances of getting pregnant while also increasing your risk of ectopic pregnancy, miscarriage, decreased follicle count, and potential damage to DNA in the follicle.[26] Dr. Suzanne says that smoking also causes fetal growth restriction and placental dysfunction—yikes! Some estimate that every year you smoke 10 or more cigarettes a day ages your ovaries 4 years. Smokers are more than 50 percent more likely to wait a year or longer to get pregnant than non-smokers.[27] Thankfully, some of these effects can partially reverse themselves once you stop smoking. Did I say STOP NOW yet? Well, I'm saying it again!

The hard part about this one is that you shouldn't use the nicotine gum or the patch while trying to conceive or during pregnancy. Talk with your doctor about a smoking cessation support group. You might want to go through the entire process before you even start trying to conceive so you can take advantage of those tools if you need them. Go online to women.smokefree.gov for some great resources. Find a buddy to lean on. Do anything you can to help yourself succeed. *Never quit quitting.* If you screw up, start again the next day.

Honestly, my friend—you just need to cold turkey this one. Sorry to be so blunt about it, but all that crap is really bad for you. Ask yourself what's more important— your life and your kid or your smokes? Thought so. Now quit and let's move on.

Cut back on caffeine. If you typically have one or two cups of coffee or tea every day, you are okay. But if you are a heavy caffeine imbiber (through coffee, tea, or yuck, soda, or even worse, *diet soda!*), you're going to need to cut back to about 150 milligrams a day, or about one cup of brewed coffee, to improve your fertility.[28] Research has linked *excessive* caffeine consumption (above 500 mg to 1,000 mg, or four to six strong cups daily) to miscarriage or stillbirth. Other research shows no link,[29] but I suggest erring on the side of caution here. That much caffeine is terrible for you, pregnant or otherwise. Why risk it either way? What I can say for sure is that caffeine is a diuretic that washes calcium and other key pregnancy nutrients out of your system before they can be completely absorbed. Caffeine is also a stimulant, so it raises your heart rate and can cause insomnia and contribute to heartburn (which is zero fun). None of this is necessary for you right now, and especially not for your baby.

Another concern is that nonorganic coffee tends to be full of pesticide residue—coffee is one of the most heavily treated crops in the world, and up to 250 pounds of chemical fertilizers douse every acre of conventional coffee.[30] I hope that spoils your appetite for that cheap cup o' joe. It's certainly not something you want to ingest at any time, but especially not while pregnant or while preparing to get pregnant. Start regulating your coffee intake now by cutting it down to no more than one cup a day (roughly 150 mg), and *drink only organic*.

Skip the booze. I know, this one really sucks. I hate to be a stickler, but plenty of current research suggests alcohol can affect your fertility. Your partner should take heed on this as well. I know, I read the research that says alcohol in moderation is

Dr. V Says . . .

If you use any form of hormonal birth control, such as the birth control pill, a patch, or an implant, it's a good idea to stop this at least 3 months before you start trying, and use a barrier method (like a condom) until your cycle is regular again. In some cases, it could take 6 to 9 months or even a year to reset your cycle. If you have an IUD, be sure you are free from any kind of infection and have a clean bill of health after having it taken out, before you start trying. Using a barrier method of contraception is not for health reasons—if you have already had all your tests, you know you are healthy, and your doctor has given you the green light to try getting pregnant, you don't technically need to use a barrier method after stopping your birth control. The only reason to do so is to wait until your cycle is regular again (and this could happen sooner than 3 months, or it could take longer—in which case it is a good idea to see your doctor and get evaluated, just in case there is a problem that can be fixed). This makes it easier to know when you are ovulating, when you have conceived, and when your due date is. But it's certainly not necessary—if you know you are healthy and ready for pregnancy, you can just go for it. If you do choose to wait, this is a good time to focus on getting your healthy lifestyle habits into place while you are waiting for your cycle to get regular again.

okay, and I have heard many women talk about how they were drinking up until the day they knew they were pregnant and had no complications with conception or pregnancy whatsoever. I've heard the stories about the women who had a beer every night or whose European moms drank wine. Sure, it doesn't *always* cause a problem for every person, but some people are more affected by alcohol than others. One Danish study showed drinking between one and five drinks a week can reduce a woman's chances of conceiving, and 10 drinks or more decreases the likelihood of conception even further.[31] A 2009 study done at Harvard University of couples undergoing IVF showed that women who drank more than six drinks per week were 18 percent less likely to conceive, while men were 14 percent less likely.[32] The fact is that alcohol can mess with estrogen and other reproductive hormones, lengthening your monthly cycle and increasing the chances that you won't ovulate at all. No ovu- lation, no egg. No egg, no baby!

Guys are affected in much the same way, with alcohol lowering sperm count and sperm motility. Each ejaculation has fewer sperm, and those sperm that do get in there seem a little drunk—they can't seem to make the long journey to fertilize the egg. No sperm, no baby![33]

The reality is that different things affect different people differently. We all have certain genetic predispositions to certain health issues and conditions that are affected by our lifestyle choices. We have no way of knowing exactly what will impact your individual chances of getting pregnant. With that in mind, if there is a chance it could impede you in any way, is it worth it?

In my opinion, the best thing is to stop drinking alcohol or cut way back to no more than two drinks per week when you decide to try to get pregnant, just as you did with smoking. Some health professionals will recommend stopping about 2 to 3 months before trying to conceive to get the full benefits.

Avoid illegal drugs. Do I have to tell you this? You are an adult, and what you do to your own body is your deal. Obviously they impact your ability to conceive, but more worrisome is if you get pregnant while still partaking and don't know it. Drugs like marijuana, cocaine, Molly, and whatever else the kids are doing these days are all horrible things for a gestating baby, and no, I am not exaggerating. Drugs do all the bad things you might imagine to babies—developmental delays, lowered IQ, mental retardation . . . need I go on? If getting pregnant and having the healthiest kiddo possible is your primary objective, it's time to walk the straight and narrow.

Reduce environmental hazards. Time to do a whole-house overhaul. You won't believe how many pollutants exist in your own home. I'll talk more about this in Chapter 4, where I'll walk you through all the steps for purifying your environment so you can get the chemicals out of your skin care products, cleaning products, lawn care products, and more. For now, just know that when it comes to what you put on your skin, release into your air, or use in your yard, natural is better. Trust me: You're going to want to do this now, before you get pregnant. We didn't, and I nearly had a heart attack when I learned of all the toxins in our home while Heidi was pregnant. From off-gassing of toxic chemicals in our furniture to the biohazards in our hygiene products, I realized we were surrounded by chemicals. Start on this project now to give yourself some more time to deal with it all.

Get to a healthy weight. Sorry to sound like an insensitive jerk, but your body weight has a direct effect on your ability to conceive, the safety of your pregnancy, and the health of your baby. If you are overweight or obese, now is the time to deal, not after you are already pregnant.[34] I know this isn't easy. For some people, it seems like an impossibility. However, if you never had the motivation before, this could be what finally helps you make it happen for yourself.

Current research suggests that being overweight or underweight can each affect your pregnancy—both your health and your baby's.[35] Overweight pregnant women are at greater risk for high blood pressure, gestational diabetes, and sleep apnea, and have a higher rate of Caesarean delivery, while the baby of an obese mother is at greater risk for stillbirth and a variety of congenital abnormalities.[36] That doesn't mean this *will* happen to you or your baby, but getting to a healthy weight first can definitely decrease these risks. Also, underweight women run the risk of a preterm delivery or a low-birth-weight infant,[37] not to mention insufficient body fat to get pregnant in the first place.[38]

If you feel like you can't do this alone (and many people can't, especially if they have a lot to lose), consult with your doctor on what would be a good goal weight prior to pregnancy, then get the name of a great dietitian who can help you form a sensible plan for weight loss—*before you get pregnant*. I can't stress this enough. You *do not diet* during pregnancy. Pregnancy is not a time to eat whatever you want, but it's also not a time to be restrictive. Dieting can cause temporary deficiencies in vitamins and minerals that you and your baby will need.

But you shouldn't be overly restrictive now, either. Diets that cut out entire key food groups (and the nutrients they contain) will not help you right now. If for some ethical, religious, or medical reason you are tethered to a diet that is fairly restrictive, like veganism, for example, or avoiding all grains and other high-carb foods, consult with your doctor on how to supplement accordingly. In the following chapter, I will provide you with some detailed suggestions on what to do and what to ask your doctor about if you are on one of the more common restrictive diets.

Take your prenatal vitamins. This naturally brings me to the subject of prenatal vitamins. While food is the ideal way to get the vitamins and minerals you need, the sad truth is that nowadays, a healthy diet doesn't always cut it. There are many different reasons for this, ranging from a lack of variety in our overprocessed diet to overfarmed soil that has been depleted of its nutrients (thus robbing our food of its innate nutritional power). To prevent deficiency, your doctor will recommend a prenatal vitamin.[39, 40, 41]

If you are already on a good-quality multi and are wondering what the difference is between it and your prenatal, here is the answer: Prenatal vitamins contain more of a specific folic acid and more iron than standard adult multis. A supplement with a minimum of 800 micrograms of folic acid will help prevent neural tube birth

Dr. Gordon Says . . .

Unfortunately, we raise our children in a "toxic soup" because there are so many chemicals in the environment today. One thing you can do about this is to eliminate exposure to pesticides as much as possible. Eat organic food, don't spray your lawn, and if you hate spiders, throw them out the door rather than spraying your home every week for bugs. I also recommend avoiding plastic toys that children will put into their mouths. You might even politely mention to friends who ask about gifts that you would prefer only natural materials. Flame-retardant clothing is toxic, so be informed and buy organic clothing for your baby (and yourself). Also avoid "no-crease" or "wrinkle-free" fabric. It is important to keep chemically laced fabrics off your baby's skin.

defects,[42] serious abnormalities of the baby's brain and spinal cord. Iron supports the baby's growth and development as well as prevents anemia.

While this may seem like a simple directive, choosing the right, high-quality multi isn't as obvious as one might think. I remember the multivitamin our doctor's office prescribed for Heidi. I couldn't believe some of the ingredients in it—a host of known toxins like hydrogenated oils (trans fats), artificial colors (red #40), and dangerous preservatives and chemicals like propylene glycol. I was completely aghast. "How are you giving this to pregnant women?" I barked. The nurse looked back at me blankly with absolutely no idea why I was upset.

I find it so frustrating that doctors have traditionally been required to take only 24 hours of nutrition training in medical school. They are amazing at what they do, but they are not registered dietitians or nutritionists. Knowledge of these types of chemicals and their consequences is typically not part of their expertise. Our *Yeah Baby!* dream team doctors are very hip to this kind of thing, but many are not; this is yet another reason why you definitely have to be proactive in your pregnancy.

Your job is to find a prenatal at a health food store with no artificial ingredients that has 800 to 1,000 mcg (1 mg) of folic acid. I found a brand for Heidi called New Chapter Organics Perfect Prenatal that met all of the necessary nutrient criteria with none of the garbage and by-products. Other brands are also good, but if you want a quick answer, that's a great option.

One caveat: If you have a family history of neural tube defects, talk to your doctor about subbing a higher dose of folic acid. Some doctors suggest increasing the recommended amount in these kinds of cases. If you know you have the MTHFR gene and don't metabolize folate properly (you can find out with a simple genetic test), you may need a prescription for a special kind of prenatal vitamin with methylated third- or fourth-generation folic acid. If you think this describes you, ask your doctor about it.[43] In addition to a prenatal vitamin, I also recommend considering just two additional supplements.

- Vitamin D_3: This is an essential nutrient for pregnancy. You can boost vitamin D_3 by getting about 10 to 15 minutes of sun exposure every day without sunscreen, although this isn't possible for everyone, in which case supplementation may be necessary. Remember that Dr. Suzanne says levels should be tested in mom's blood and supplemented to bring them up to over 30 ng/ml.

- Omega-3 fatty acids: Also essential in pregnancy! Fish or krill oil supplements that are purified so they are free from mercury are great to add to your supplement routine *now*.

Eat optimally. We are going to get into healthy, clean eating in the next chapter (which you should start doing immediately), but here I just want to outline for you some key nutrients that will aid in conception. Just because you are supplementing doesn't mean you shouldn't concern yourself with getting proper nutrition from your foods. Nothing can replace a nutrient-dense diet. The following are the richest food sources of the key nutrients responsible for hemoglobin production (to prevent anemia) and folic acid (to prevent neural tube defects), so enjoy them often when you are trying to get pregnant:

- **Iron:** Oysters, mussels, red meats, enriched cereals, molasses, green leafy vegetables, tomato paste, and dal are all great sources. One note of caution: Don't turn to liver for your iron needs. Liver is best avoided just before and during pregnancy because it contains unsafe amounts of vitamin A, which can cause birth defects.

- **Vitamin B$_6$:** Muesli, whole grains, fortified cereals, tuna, sunflower seeds, lentils, kidney beans, avocado, peas, nuts, and bananas. Note that you can also supplement with 10 mg of vitamin B$_6$ in the early weeks to prevent or diminish nausea. Many B$_6$ supplements also contain zinc, which can help improve fertility. If your multivitamin already contains this much plus zinc, you are covered.

- **Vitamin B$_{12}$:** Poultry, crustaceans, fish, fortified cereals, eggs, and mollusks like mussels, snails, and octopus.

- **Folate:** Spinach, beans, asparagus, peas, lentils, turnip greens, organ meats, oranges, cantaloupes, pineapples, grapefruit, bananas, raspberries, strawberries, corn, tomatoes, beets, broccoli, Brussels sprouts, bok choy, and sunflower seeds.

- **Vitamin C:** Guava, red peppers (sweet or hot), Brussels sprouts, citrus juice, mangoes, papayas, kiwifruit, black currants, cabbage, broccoli, strawberries, lychees, oranges, and fresh sprouts.

- **DHA and EPA:** Ocean-caught wild (not farm-raised) salmon. (Note: Extra EPA and DHA supplementation in the form of fish oil is a great habit to start, even before conception, especially if you struggle with depression or anxiety. Look for brands that are purified to avoid toxicity.)

Relax. I know, you are laughing at me right now because you don't think there is any way you can possibly relax. I am sure that you, like almost everyone else, run around all day long trying to make ends meet, take care of your loved ones, excel at your job, and so on, and now you've got this other giant project going—*trying to get pregnant!* But just about any doctor you talk to will tell you that this step is one of *the most* important.

Stress and tension, whether related to getting pregnant or life in general, can make getting pregnant literally twice as hard. In a study published in the journal *Human Reproduction*, scientists found that, among women who were trying to get pregnant, those with the highest levels of alpha-amylase (a protein in saliva that researchers use as a biomarker for long-standing stress) had more than double the risk of infertility compared with those with the lowest levels.[44] My best proof for this is the journey many of my own friends and family have undergone with conception. My own mom tried for a year to get pregnant. The minute she and my dad decided to "stop trying," just enjoy married life, and do a little traveling, she immediately got knocked up with me.

Many other adoptive families I know went down the adoption path due to an inability to conceive. Then shortly after their decision to adopt, both parents relaxed and accepted their situation—and immediately got pregnant. Sure, this might be coincidence, but I don't think so. Relaxing makes everything in your body work better—Dr. Suzanne says that stress hormones actually interfere with hormonal functions like ovulation, and the stress hormone cortisol increases inflammation—the impact is real, people! Do a little yoga or meditation, get a massage, take deep

Heidi Says . . .

Considering Heidi was the one who was *actually pregnant*, we thought you might be interested to hear her point of view, so you know what she was thinking and feeling through all of this. Welcome to "Heidi Says . . ." boxes, which will appear in each trimester chapter and in the labor and delivery chapter. These are all in Heidi's voice—she wrote them just for you—starting now.

Getting pregnant is a bit fuzzy, but I do remember peeing on many ovulation sticks, refusing Clomid and a shot to stimulate ovulation, and having many follicle-counting appointments. I also remember being told to gain weight, and the ice cream sundaes that followed, thanks to Jillian's insistence. I continued to exercise throughout my attempts and even traveled, trying not to focus too much on the "getting pregnant" part. I think I didn't want to be disappointed if it didn't work.

I attempted IUI twice with no success. Then I visited an acupuncturist and herbalist who had worked with many women attempting to get pregnant, with great success. After a month of acupuncture, some not-so-delicious herbs, those definitely delicious ice cream sundaes, and 10 pounds of weight gain, it was time for the third try. This was the time when I ovulated early, my doctor wasn't available, and Jillian wasn't there to occupy my attention when I was lying on a tilt (normally she would do this by blowing up the condoms and latex gloves like balloons and floating them over to me). And yet, even without all these things in place, this would be the time that would be successful and bring us our little guy.

breaths, and just schedule a little time each day to calm down and be by yourself or relax with people who don't need anything from you. Research suggests it might help, and it certainly won't hurt!

Exercise. Like I wasn't bound to bring this up eventually. But you already know this. There are truly tremendous benefits to exercising before, during, and after your pregnancy, but you want to get a good plan in place before you get pregnant, because then you will be able to maintain it throughout your pregnancy.

We will cover this in Chapter 3, but let me just say right now that exercise has endless health benefits, and increasing fertility is no exception. A review article in the journal *Human Reproduction Update* found that women with PCOS who exercised 30 minutes or more three to five times per week experienced positive changes in their ovulation (and, therefore, increased fertility)—in fact, all the studies that tracked that data showed a similar effect.[45] Exercise is also ideal for achieving a healthy weight, improving sleep, managing stress, lowering blood pressure, and managing blood sugar—all things that help your body get pregnant faster and more healthfully.

However, some data links too much vigorous exercise with lowered fertility. You may have heard of elite runners or other athletes who skip periods during their intense training season. That's because high-intensity exercise can tinker with the normal balance of our female reproductive hormones, shortening the time between ovulation and your expected period, a factor that can reduce your fertility. Also, high-intensity training can literally stress the body, elevating your stress hormones and giving your body the message that now is not the optimal time to become pregnant.

What these findings tell us is that like everything in life, balance is critical. Here are some good prepregnancy fitness guidelines.

- If you aren't exercising now, start a moderate-intensity exercise program, working up gradually to at least 2 hours of exercise per week, preferably closer to 4 hours per week. You don't want to start new things during pregnancy, so get exercising *now*. However, do not exercise with a moderate intensity more than 6 hours a week.

- If you are an extreme athlete who regularly engages in aggressive high-intensity workouts like CrossFit, now would be the time to dial it back and incorporate a more holistic regimen. Consider incorporating more yoga, Pilates, bodyweight training, incline walking, swimming, hiking, and biking. Exercise that is lower stress is the exercise for this stage of your life. Do not exercise with a high intensity more than 5 hours a week.

- If you are undergoing in vitro, exercise at a moderate intensity and do not exceed 4 hours a week.

Consider alternative medicine. It took Heidi three tries before she became pregnant with our son, and while neither of us wanted her taking fertility drugs unless it was an absolute necessity (which it was not), I was open to alternative, holistic therapies, as was she. To be truthful, I think this is what made all the difference.

A few years before I met Heidi, I had fallen off a horse and messed up my shoulder. A trainer friend of mine sent me to his acupuncturist/herbalist. Dr. So is his name, and he's this eccentric Korean man who barely speaks English. I went to see him out of respect for my friend, but I couldn't see how it would help. I told him, "You can't help me. I have a tear in my rotator cuff and I need surgery. Acupuncture won't do anything."

"Humor me," he said, in his thick Korean accent.

I let him do acupuncture on my shoulder for a couple of months—what harm could it do?—and one day I woke up and the pain was gone. I never had to have surgery. My shoulder isn't exactly like it was before, but after 2 years of arm pain, I was back to doing inverted pushups. I had to admit, much as I am a skeptic about these things, that there was something to it. I didn't really know much about chi-and-energy-this and meridians-that, but I couldn't argue with the fact that my shoulder felt better. I also knew that this man was an herbalist specializing in fertility, so at one point I suggested to Heidi that we go and see him.

The first thing Dr. So said when he examined Heidi was, "Your uterus is very cold, very cold. There isn't enough bloodflow." He put her on a course of herbs, started regular biweekly acupuncture sessions, and instructed her to try IUI again after 1 month of treatment with him. Interestingly enough, the next time she tried IUI, she got pregnant.

Coincidence? Maybe. Placebo? Maybe. However, we continued acupuncture treatments biweekly throughout Heidi's entire pregnancy. And by the way, Dr. So knew the sex of our son at 6 weeks, simply from taking Heidi's pulse, and he accurately guessed the exact weight of our son, warning Heidi months ahead of time that she would probably need a C-section (which she refused to accept all the way up to her 27th hour of labor, but we'll get to that later).

Ultimately, if you have the means, I would definitely consider finding an herbalist and acupuncturist who specializes in pregnancy, if that feels right to you. Or consider other forms of alternative medicine if they are more your style, like chiropractic care, massage therapy, or an Ayurvedic doctor. If you already regularly go to a chiropractor, acupuncturist, massage therapist, herbalist, Ayurvedic doctor, or any other kind of integrative health practitioner, you should also tell them about your pregnancy plans. While you can continue to see these health professionals as you try to get pregnant, there may be important ways they adjust your treatment, not just for safety but even to enhance your fertility. Once you are pregnant, these practitioners might also be able to help you with some of the uncomfortable symptoms and could even help to make pregnancy and childbirth a healthier and easier experience for you and the baby.

And now for the wrap-up. Here is everything you should do before you conceive, in a nutshell (or, more accurately, in a handy box for your easy reference).

BEFORE YOU CONCEIVE

- Visit your gynecologist, family doctor, and dentist for advice, testing, and pre-planning. Tell them everything you are doing now and ask what you should do next as you prepare to conceive.

- Stop smoking and drinking alcohol and cut back on caffeine to about 150 mg per day.

- Start taking an 800-mcg folic acid supplement daily to help prevent birth defects[46] or find a good-quality, natural prenatal supplement that includes at least this much folic acid.

- Take vitamin D_3 supplements if a blood test shows you are deficient, and also take fish or krill oil supplements to shore up your omega-3 fatty acid supplies.

- Get to a healthy body weight. If you need help with this, consider my book *Slim for Life* to help you drop the weight and get in great shape.

- Eat nutrient-dense foods, especially those that support healthy blood and provide you with iron, B vitamins, folate, vitamin C, and DHA and EPA.

- Start an exercise plan if you aren't already exercising. If you are an intense exerciser, moderate your plan to be lower stress.

CHAPTER 2

RULES OF THUMB:
Nutrition for Prepregnancy, Pregnancy, and Beyond

While this book is broken down into sections (prepregnancy, all three trimesters, and postpartum), some information is universal. That is what the Rules of Thumb chapters are all about. They provide guidelines for every stage of your pregnancy—before, during, and after—and even for the rest of your life, because they are based on behaviors that nurture health, strength, and stamina. While there are specifics in each trimester and for the postpartum period (as well as prepregnancy specifics you already read about in the last chapter), a large chunk of the information you need to know, be it about food, fitness, or lifestyle, applies throughout this entire process. So instead of my writing the same info multiple times and your having to read it multiple times (I would not do that to you), I created these master chapters called Rules of Thumb. There is one each for nutrition, fitness, and lifestyle. And the very first is about my favorite subject: food.

I love food. I love talking about food. I love writing about food. Though I have a feeling you won't exactly love some of the things I am about to say about *your* food intake, like "no way in hell do you get to eat for two" (mind blown . . . not!), I think you will love the end result of this chapter, which is all about—you guessed it—optimal nutrition for conception, maternity, and beyond.

Nutrition is huge. It can be the root of horrendous health issues, and conversely, it can be a large part of preventing—if not *the* cure for—said health issues. Power eating (as I like to call what I am about to teach you) can help you reverse aging, fend off disease, and in particular, for our purposes now, facilitate conception, the smoothest maternity, and the growth of an über-healthy baby.

The micronutrients (vitamins and minerals) and macronutrients (proteins, fats, and carbs) are quite literally the building blocks for your tiny little human, so it's critical we use top-quality material. In addition, we want to keep you as healthy and safe as possible, and pave the path for a smooth return to your "prebaby body." And while some of you might not be concerned about that, many of you are—so if you are worried, don't be. This chapter has you covered on all the aforementioned fronts.

Okey dokey (yes, I say that sometimes) . . . let's get rolling.

YOUR BABY IS WHAT YOU EAT

Maybe your significant other and family members are already fighting over who gets to "cut the cord." Such an amazing thing, the umbilical cord, isn't it? The fetus (aka your growing baby) is connected to the placenta (aka your body) by the umbilical cord. The cord itself has no nerves, so there is no pain when it's cut. With one vein that carries oxygen and nutrients to the baby and two veins that return waste products and carbon dioxide to the placenta, the cord's sole function is to nourish and sustain your developing child.

Doctors once thought that the placenta was a barrier to substances in the mother's blood that could be potentially harmful. (Those were the days of wineglasses and ashtrays conveniently balanced on third-trimester bellies!) But we now know that it is the size and chemical structure of a substance, not its potential toxicity, that dictates what passes through the placenta from mother to baby. That means the cord can be an incredibly effective conduit to channel all the best nutrients directly into your baby's body. But it also means, very unfortunately, that alcohol, most drugs, chemicals, toxins, and medications can still pass through the placenta and directly into the fetal bloodstream, influencing cell development and genetic expression in your growing baby.

For this reason, nutrition during pregnancy is one of the most direct means that we have to influence the development, growth, intelligence, fitness, and even the life span of our babies. That's why nutrition is Job 1 for the Yeah Baby! program.

Now, in each trimester you will get weekly meal plans and recipes that are carefully designed to do two things.

1. To give your baby the precise vitamins, minerals, and nutrients necessary to maximize each phase of fetal development, from before conception through birth and breastfeeding; and

2. To respond to the needs of your body as it grows and changes, in order to protect your long-term health and help set you up for a killer postbaby body!

But first we must address those general guidelines I mentioned. We'll begin by tackling the "eating for two" nonsense right off the bat.

HOW MUCH SHOULD YOU EAT?

Let me clarify something for you: You are not eating for two. Not before pregnancy, not during pregnancy, not even when you are nursing.

Up until the first 13 weeks, your baby will range from the size of a poppy seed to about the size of a small prawn. In the second trimester, you're still only eating for a tiny human that doesn't exceed a singular pound in total body weight. Even in your third trimester, at the baby's very biggest, your little one ends up the size of a small pumpkin, coming in at around 7 to 10 pounds. That does not justify eating the whole pizza, or a complete second helping of everything on the table. At no point is your child's size even close to the equivalent of eating for another grown, 100- to 200-pound human being. In fact, it takes only around 80,000 calories—in total—to grow a baby. That may sound like a lot, but it's not. Here's how that breaks down per day.

- First trimester: 300 extra calories per day, if you are very active

- Second trimester: about 350 extra calories per day

- Second half of third trimester (last 6 weeks): about 500 extra calories a day

In general, most people should shoot for roughly 1,900 to 2,500 calories a day total. If you are already a bit above your ideal weight and relatively inactive, stick to the lower end of this range to avoid gaining more weight than your baby needs you to gain. If you're fit and very active, you can hang at the higher end of this range, but those extra calories should definitely be the nutritionally dense kind—not candy bars and potato chips!

WHAT SHOULD YOU WEIGH BEFORE GETTING PREGNANT?

Before pregnancy, depending on where you are with your weight, you may want to focus on losing some weight, or you may want to focus on gaining weight. There is a sweet spot of body weight that is ideal for conceiving a child. If your body mass index (BMI) is between 19 or 20 and 24 or 25,[1,2] or you have a body fat percentage between 22 and 25,[3] you are there. (Look online for any BMI calculator to do the tricky math for you. Here is one specifically designed for fertility: attainfertility.com /article/fertility-weight.) However, these standards might not necessarily apply to your individual situation. Your ob-gyn can probably help you identify your ideal weight based on your unique factors; this is just general information to help you ask the right questions, in case your doctor doesn't bring it up.

As a rule, I prefer helping people identify a healthy body weight with the waist-to-hip ratio versus where they fall on the BMI. This is because BMI does not take into account body composition (your percentage of body fat and muscle). According to the BMI, Arnold Schwarzenegger in his prime would have been considered obese! The BMI system just considers weight and doesn't account for those people with higher-than-average muscle mass. Try this method as an alternative to the BMI, to calculate your waist-to-hip ratio and to identify where you fall on the chart below.

1. Using a tape measure, measure your hip circumference at its widest part.

2. Measure your waist circumference at the belly button. (Make sure you exhale before taking this measurement.)

3. Divide your waist measurement by your hip measurement.

4. Your answer equals your waist-to-hip ratio.

Then find your measurement here.

IF YOUR WAIST-TO-HIP RATIO IS . . .	YOU ARE LIKELY . . .
0.71 or under	A bit underweight
Between 0.72 and 0.79	A normal weight
Between 0.8 and 0.85	Overweight
0.85 or above	Obese

HOW MUCH WEIGHT SHOULD YOU GAIN?

How much weight you should gain during pregnancy depends on where you start. If you already have more resources onboard (if you weigh more), you won't need to gain as much weight. In general, whether you have determined your weight level through a BMI calculator, body fat percentage, or waist-to-hip ratio, here is the approximate amount you should probably gain (unless your doctor has different advice for your individual situation).

- If you are underweight, you should gain somewhere between 28 and 40 pounds, or 45 to 60 pounds if you are having twins.

- If you are normal weight, you should gain somewhere between 25 and 35 pounds, or 37 to 54 pounds if you are having twins.

- If you are overweight, you should gain somewhere between 15 and 25 pounds, or 31 to 50 pounds if you are having twins.

- If you are obese, you should gain somewhere between 15 and 20 pounds, or 25 to 42 pounds if you are having twins.

Over the course of pregnancy, the average mom will gain 3 to 6 pounds in the first trimester, 6 to 15 pounds in the second trimester, and 6 to 15 pounds in the third trimester—although keep in mind that everyone is different, and not everyone gains the same amount or at the same rate. Do not be afraid if your weight gain isn't steady—your metabolism will shift constantly, with gains and plateaus as your baby's needs change. Remember, these little creatures are very efficient at taking exactly what nutrients they need from you. Ultimately, as long as you are eating healthfully and exercising safely during your pregnancy, your body and baby will both gain exactly what they need.

If you're having twins, I definitely recommend that you consult with your doctor about the precise weight guideline for you, and I also recommend you contact a registered dietitian to ensure you know how to meet your body's (and your babies') unique requirements, because yes, that requires eating even a little more . . . but you are still not eating for two, let alone three, full-grown adults.

WHEN YOU GAIN TOO MUCH

When hormones begin to fluctuate, stress levels skyrocket, and appetite begins to do strange things, some people find it very hard to eat, and others find it very hard to stop eating. When you are ravenous all the time, or just stress-eating, it's tempting to justify overeating. "I'm pregnant; I can eat what I want, right?"

Wrong.

If you gain an excessive amount of weight (like 50 pounds or more), you will probably experience more consequences than just a lot more to lose after you give birth. You could experience more health problems and pregnancy complications, such as:

- **Hypertension and/or diabetes:** Both of these health conditions can make your pregnancy harder to manage and create potential risks for you and your baby.

- **Discomfort:** Excess weight gain can exacerbate backaches, exhaustion, varicose veins, calf cramps, heartburn, hemorrhoids, and achy joints. And if too many of those extra pounds follow you to labor, they can also make that already-tough experience a lot tougher.

- **Delivery issues:** The heavier you are, the more likely your baby is to be larger, increasing the odds that a vaginal delivery will require the use of forceps or a vacuum. You might not be able to deliver vaginally, as being overweight increases your chances of delivering by C-section, which then makes for a more difficult recovery after your baby is born. And should you choose to have an epidural, excess weight can make the placement of the epidural more difficult.

- **Increased risk of childhood obesity:** Remember the old saying "a fat baby is a happy baby"? Not so. Remember: When you gain, in most cases, so does the fetus—often in the form of fat cells that raise the risk that your child will struggle with and be more susceptible to weight gain as he ages. One study found that, compared with those whose moms gained 18 to 22 pounds during pregnancy, babies whose moms gained more than 53 pounds were an average 5 ounces heavier at birth and twice as likely to weigh more than 8.8 pounds.[4] Another study found that, compared with the children of women who gained the recommended amount of weight, those who gained an "excessive" amount of weight had children who were more than four times more likely to be overweight at age 3.[5] And many studies have shown that birth weight is directly related to later BMI, into adolescence and adulthood.[6]

- **Recovery struggles:** That slammin' mommy body I promised you is going to be much harder to deliver if you let yourself go to pot over the next 40 weeks. Here's a scary bit of info: Studies show that women who gain too much weight and don't lose it within 6 months after giving birth are at a higher risk of remaining obese. I can't tell you how many women come up to me and say, "I just need your help losing my baby weight." To which I respond, "Oh, congratulations! When did you give birth?"

  Seven out of 10 times, they say something like, "Oh, my son is 5." Or 7. Or 13! Then they add, apologetically, "I just never lost the weight." Now, good on them—because it's never too late! But why make the production much harder on yourself and the little one than it has to be?

Pregnancy Weight-Gain Breakdown

Whenever we would go to our ob-gyn appointments, the first thing they would do was pop Heidi on the scale. This was stressful for her, and I had to constantly remind her, "Babe, remember—this isn't 20 pounds of body fat. This is the weight of the placenta, increased blood volume, your uterus, and all of that necessary stuff to make the kid." Reminding her of these things always helped. If at any point you step on the scale and you are struggling, come back to this page and remember how each one of these pounds represents how hard your body is working for you and your baby. Here's roughly how it breaks down.

- 1 to 2 pounds will be placenta
- 2 pounds will be amniotic fluid
- 2 pounds will be uterine enlargement
- 1 to 2 pounds will be breast enlargement

- 2 to 3 pounds will be fluid retention
- 3 to 4 pounds will be increased blood volume
- 4 to 6 pounds will be body fat for milk production
- 6 to 10 pounds will be your baby!

In my 23 years as a weight-loss and wellness expert, I've helped many pregnant women enjoy a fit pregnancy and lose the "baby weight" after giving birth. In that process, I've had many, many conversations with them about the pregnancy and what compelled them to overindulge. The central issues seem to boil down to a couple of things.

- **Comfort:** Being pregnant is hard, and sometimes food is the only vice left.

- **"Freedom":** This one is really interesting—a perceived sense of "newfound freedom" from the judgment of society. If you are stuffing your face, nobody will judge you if they can see you are pregnant. One of my old clients said to me in her first trimester, "I've been hungry for 25 years! Leave me alone, Jillian. I'm finally allowed to eat!"

Here in America, we're constantly bombarded with images in the media of stickthin supermodels and pro-thin propaganda. While it's important to prioritize your health, nowadays many women feel the pressure to be a size 0 to 2, whereas I have known many healthy women ranging up to a size 10.

Then, ironically, during pregnancy, the exact opposite message is propagated—so many pregnancy Web sites and books send the message that it's your right, nay, your *duty* as a pregnant woman to eat, and eat well. I've seen some of those sassy, chatty guides to pregnancy chastise you into eating, invoking the ignorant and damaging adage of "You're eating for two, after all!" or justifying overeating in some other way, stating or implying that you are pregnant, so you deserve to eat whatever you want to eat. I'm sorry, but this is just very wrong.

As much as you may want to think so, it's not because the fetus is craving French fries and milk shakes.

The key to maintaining a fabulous physique before, during, and after pregnancy is to focus on that sense of self-nurture in a positive way. This is not about deprivation— it's about balance. It's okay to have a piece of pizza, just not the whole pie. It's okay to have a scoop of ice cream, just not the whole container. Finding this balance within your pregnancy is integral in helping you maintain a healthy weight during and after. A focus on quality also matters. You know that organic dark chocolate is a lot better for you than a sugar-laden Milky Way; that grass-fed burger is exponentially healthier for you than the one with conventional nonorganic beef that is loaded with hormones, antibiotics, and fillers.

Let's drill down a little deeper into the most important way you can be successful on the Hot Mom, Healthy Baby plan—by paying close attention to the quality of your food.

HOW TO EAT

Now let's get down to the really interesting part: What do you eat? Throughout this book, I'll give you specific advice for the best foods to eat during each of the trimesters and during the postpartum period, but certain rules of thumb apply before, during, and after pregnancy—and ideally, throughout all stages of your life. You can't go wrong with the advice in the remaining section of this chapter. If you generally avoid the "no" foods and focus most of your meals around the "yes" foods, while keeping your portions moderate, you will be in good nutritional shape, and your pregnancy nutrition can focus on tweaking these general concepts for your needs at the moment.

So first, let's focus on what you should eat *in general* . . . no matter what stage you are in right now.

What Not to Eat: The "Obvious No" List

Let's start with the obvious, which you will find in many cases is in small part legitimate and in large part total propaganda, and then work our way into the not-so-obvious, which is where the real truth lies. I bet you already know some of this "obvious" stuff from pregnant friends, your doctor, and pretty much every freakin' pregnancy and baby book, blog, and Web site ever created. Still, I would feel irresponsible not to mention these and honestly set your mind at ease about what listed here is of serious concern and what isn't. So here is what you should *obviously* lessen consumption of or avoid.

1. Easy on the alcohol

This is an interesting one. Have your friends ever confessed that before they knew they were pregnant they were drinking and partying, and now they are filled with guilt and racked with concern that they may have harmed their baby? Inevitably everyone, including their doctor, will say, "Don't worry. This is common. Just stop drinking now." Then a pregnant lady goes to a party and has a glass of wine and all hell breaks loose. She is an evil, selfish, irresponsible woman who will make a horrible mother. WTF? I bring this up to prove a point: So much of the information out there is nonsense—just BS steeped in judgment and misinformation. So which is it? Are six glasses of wine a week prior to knowing you are pregnant fine, but two glasses a week after you know you are pregnant terrifyingly detrimental?

Here are the facts we know: Drinking heavily (nine-plus drinks per week) has been associated with fetal alcohol syndrome—low birth weight, small brain size, distinctive facial stigmata (a certain face shape common to those with fetal alcohol syndrome), psychological and behavioral problems, and the list goes on.[7] But even if you're not pregnant, heavy drinking can result in a lot of health issues like breast and ovarian cancer, heart disease, stroke, liver disease, high blood pressure, learning and memory problems, mental health issues, and so on. Alcohol can also affect your fertility, which is why recommendations vary from stopping drinking completely to cutting back to no more than two or three drinks a week when trying to conceive.

Ultimately, once you are pregnant, be moderate with your alcohol consumption. Thousands upon thousands of studies have been done on drinking during pregnancy, and not one of them has defined a limit for safe alcohol consumption. At the same time, no studies have definitively proven that drinking lightly (one drink up to three times per week) is harmful. According to research recently published, the period your baby is most vulnerable to physical deformities and future behavioral and cognitive issues related to maternal alcohol consumption is in the second half of the first trimester, when crucial parts of the brain and head are forming.[8] The American Medical Association advises that as soon as a woman plans to get pregnant, she should stop drinking. Of course, what you do is up to you, and only you can decide what is right for you, but the bottom line is that science doesn't recommend it, *just in case*.

Heidi chose to go on the wagon as soon as our insemination plans began. And our doctor did give Heidi permission to have the occasional drink, but quite honestly, the thought and smell of alcohol repulsed her the entire 40 weeks, so abstaining was not a challenge for her. She even got pissed when I had a glass of wine, because the smell sickened her. (Remember that detail when I tell you the story of the winery weekend in Chapter 6.) To avoid sleeping on the couch, I went sober for the most part as well.

2. Easy on the caffeine

Interestingly, caffeine is not the real devil in the mix here. It's the pesticides on your caffeine source that are the cause for concern, but let's address these issues one at a time. Once again, there is no hard evidence that caffeine affects fertility. Still, most medical professionals advise no more than 200 to 400 milligrams of caffeine per day even before pregnancy. That's one or maybe two cups of coffee (one for a strong brew, two if the brew is weak) or strong black tea. While some people don't do well with caffeine, others seem to do just fine with moderate amounts, in general, and there are some health benefits, like a high antioxidant content that could benefit your heart and brain and possibly reduce your risk of some cancers. However, if you drink coffee, make sure it is organic! Conventional coffee is heavily treated with pesticides, herbicides, fungicides, and chemical fertilizers (up to 250 pounds of literal poison applied per acre of coffee plants[9]). Although there is some controversy about how much of this residue actually remains in the final fermented, roasted, brewed product,[10] these chemicals and other compounds have been linked to many health issues,

WHAT ABOUT DECAF?

In case you are wondering about decaf versions of your favorite caffeinated beverages, let me fill you in. The three main methods of decaffeinating coffee are the carbon dioxide method, the solvent method, and the Swiss water method. All will result in some leftover caffeine, although a much smaller quantity than that found in regular coffee—regular has 200 mg per cup, while decaf has about 14 mg. Quite a bit less.

The caffeine is negligible, but that actually isn't my primary concern when it comes to decaf—it's the processes themselves that you must be wary of. The chemicals used to pull the caffeine out of the beverage can still be present in the beverage and may pose health risks to you and your unborn baby. If you absolutely must have a cup of decaf coffee, look for beans processed via the Swiss water method and avoid all else.

Decaf-ing your tea is a little easier. If you can't find teas decaffeinated with the Swiss water method, try this: Steep the tea for 40 seconds and pour it out. Then resteep the same tea bag, and enjoy. This trick gets out about 80 percent of the caffeine but still allows the tea to retain some flavor.

from cancer to miscarriage. This is another example, in my opinion, of better safe than sorry. I would advise steering clear. Also, high-quality, organic, shade-grown coffee tastes better (also in my opinion, but it seems obvious to me!).

Now back to the caffeine component. Although most studies show that caffeine intake in moderation is okay, others show that very high doses of caffeine may be related to miscarriages.[11] Honestly, I must have talked to at least five different experts about this one issue, mostly because I love caffeine so much that I can't imagine how one must feel having to give it up entirely, and here is what I extrapolated from their various messages: Your best bet is to avoid caffeine during the first trimester, to reduce a *very* slight chance of a miscarriage.

Also remember that caffeine is a diuretic, which means it can dehydrate you and flush minerals like calcium from the body, so if you do have a morning cup of coffee or black tea, make sure to compensate by adding milk to your coffee or tea, hydrating regularly, and eating more high-calcium foods like dark leafy greens and dairy products.

If you decide to quit drinking coffee, ideally do this before you get pregnant because the symptoms of caffeine withdrawal can be uncomfortable, aka super shitty. You might feel lethargic, grumpy, get headaches, etc., but once you come out of it, you will be just fine. It's worth a try. (It won't hurt to quit while pregnant, but adding discomfort to any pregnancy discomforts might make it harder on your willpower.)

Drinking green tea can be a good way to ease out of your caffeine habit, if you like green tea. It is full of antioxidants and has only about 25 percent of the caffeine of a cup of brewed coffee.[12]

3. No deli meat

Most deli meat is full of salt, nitrates, and fillers, so it's not nearly as nutritious and clean as organic grass-fed or pastured meat and poultry, but that's not where the negatives end. Deli meat can also be contaminated with a type of bacteria called listeria, which can cause miscarriage. These days we hear about salmonella and E.coli relatively often, but listeria has avoided the spotlight. The happy reason is that listeria is extremely rare, with only 2,500 cases reported a year in the United States. That said, pregnant women are way more susceptible to listeriosis, a serious bacterial infection that strikes pregnant women 20 times more often than those who aren't pregnant—17 percent of all cases are pregnant women.[13] So to do some quick and simple math, that means out of the nearly four million pregnancies per year in the United States alone, roughly 500 women will get diagnosed with listeria.[14] Pretty slim odds. But, because listeria has the ability to cross the placenta and may infect the baby, leading to infection or blood poisoning, which may be life-threatening, once again, it's better to be safe than sorry. If you are considering eating deli meats, reheat the meat until it is steaming, to kill any possible bacteria.

4. No unpasteurized milk or unpasteurized soft cheese

Here's the deal: Unpasteurized milk and imported soft cheeses carry the same risks of listeria that deli meats do. While a nonpregnant person with a healthy immune system can eat these and be fine, once you are pregnant, to eliminate any potential listeria risk, steer clear of soft cheeses such as Brie, Camembert, Roquefort, feta, gorgonzola, and Mexican-style cheeses such as queso blanco and queso fresco, unless they clearly state that they are made from pasteurized milk. All soft nonimported cheeses made with pasteurized milk are safe to eat. Hard cheeses are also fine. And skip the raw milk during pregnancy—all dairy should be pasteurized.

5. No raw eggs

Raw eggs or any foods that contain raw eggs should be avoided by everyone because of the potential exposure to salmonella, but pregnant women (as well as children, the elderly, and anyone who is immune-compromised) must be particularly careful. This one is a bit of a minefield because it's not quite as simple as avoiding eggs Benedict or Rocky-style protein shakes. Raw eggs are hidden in many things, such as homemade Caesar dressings, mayonnaise, homemade ice cream or custards, and hollandaise sauce. Although salmonella, unlike listeria, does not pass through to the fetus, coming down with salmonella poisoning would stress you and your baby, increasing your risk of preterm labor. Make sure any recipe involving eggs is cooked at some point, as it will reduce the exposure to salmonella. Commercially manufactured ice cream, dressings, and eggnog made with pasteurized eggs are generally okay.

6. No raw meat or fish

Sorry, sushi aficionados; it's time to avoid the sashimi for a while, and no more rare burgers, either. While sushi and uncooked meat products like beef carpaccio are fine for healthy nonpregnant people, uncooked seafood and rare or undercooked meat or poultry should be avoided during pregnancy because of the risk of contamination with coliform bacteria (like E. coli), toxoplasmosis (a parasitic infection), listeria, and salmonella. The good news is that all concern can be assuaged as long as you cook your meat to 160°F or higher—especially ground beef. No more medium-rare burgers—if the inside of the burger has been exposed at some point, if you don't cook it through, you run a much higher risk of food poisoning.

Pregnancy Cravings: The RD Says . . .

Cheryl Forberg, RD, our expert nutritionist, weighs in on pregnancy cravings:

Hormonal shifts during pregnancy can cause changes in smell and taste perceptions, which may explain why so many pregnant women get cravings for foods they never enjoyed before, or aversions to foods they used to like. These cravings don't necessarily have anything to do with nutritional needs or deficits. They are simply one more example of how hormones can have strange and unexpected effects. However, if you do begin to crave nonfood items like ice, chalk, or dirt (this is surprisingly common!), this could mean you have a physical need for a particular nutrient, most likely some kind of mineral. I once knew a pregnant woman who craved Crisco shortening and ate it by the spoon from the can. Another patient of mine–a man who obviously wasn't pregnant, but the example is still relevant–craved cups of white flour, probably because he needed some of the micronutrients in the fortified flour. Definitely tell your doctor if this happens to you, so you can be tested for mineral or vitamin deficiencies. And if you are just craving ice cream and pickles? It's not going to hurt you, so go ahead and live it up . . . but keep your portions small. (Nobody needs daily vats of ice cream, even if they include pickles.)

7. No pâte

Refrigerated pâte or meat spreads should be avoided because they may contain the bacteria listeria. Canned pâte or shelf-safe meat spreads are okay, but fresh, well-cooked meat is always a more healthful choice.

Now that we have gotten all that out of the way, let's play confessional for a moment: During Heidi's pregnancy with our son, we traveled all over the world for my work. We watched very pregnant ladies in Japan sidle up to the sushi bar, baby bumps in France enjoying a cheese plate (with Brie) and a glass of wine, and mommies-to-be in Italy sipping a latte at an outdoor café. Once in a while, Heidi and I discovered (after the fact) that a food she'd consumed had raw eggs in it or contained an unpasteurized cheese (like the Mexican corn at one of our favorite restaurants in Los Angeles).

My reason for telling you this is not to negate all that I have just said, but to help you avoid paranoia. The chances of food poisoning, especially listeria, are slim. Should you consume something from the above list by accident (or rarely), you and your tiny peanut will most likely be perfectly fine. Obviously, on the very off chance you begin to feel sick or flulike in any way, call your doctor immediately so she can treat you as soon as possible. Quick action will help to prevent transmission or stress to your baby.

The "Seafood No" List

Seafood is a great thing to eat when pregnant as long as you are discerning with which types of seafood you are consuming. It can be a great source of protein, and the omega-3 fatty acids in many fish can promote your baby's brain development. However, some types of seafood are potentially hazardous to your baby's health. Many different types of fish are often contaminated with mercury, which can be damaging in large amounts. I recommend enjoying the right types of fish two or three times a week to reap all the delicious and nutritious benefits with no risk.

In fact, our nutritionist, Cheryl Forberg, recently sent me a new study just published in *Nutrition Journal* that says eating two fish meals weekly is actually not only safe for pregnant women, but can raise the baby's IQ by 3.3 points by age 9. Wow. The study was a kind of cost-benefit analysis, weighing the risk of mercury contamination against the potential intelligence benefits, and two fish meals a week (totaling 8 to 12 ounces), even of higher-mercury fish like canned tuna (which the study says was the most economical choice), turned out to be the sweet spot—keeping mercury levels below toxicity level while maximizing IQ.[15] So while I have always learned and believed that pregnant women should stick to eating mercury-containing fish like tuna no more than once a month, tops, you might want to take this study into consideration (check the endnote reference to look it up and read the study for yourself).

Or, if you really care more about avoiding the mercury and choosing low-mercury fish, below is a more detailed list of mercury content in popular food fish. Totally your call on this one! But do note that salmon, shrimp, and scallops are all low mercury.*

No (or very little) fish with mercury

As I mentioned, mercury consumed during pregnancy can damage your baby's nervous system and has been linked to developmental delays and brain damage. The biggest offenders are shark, swordfish, king mackerel, tuna, and tilefish. Canned, chunk light tuna generally has a lower amount of mercury than other tuna but still should be eaten only in moderation. The bigger and the older the fish, the more mercury it's likely to contain, because the toxins build up in these predatory fish—and tuna are large! Heidi could pretty much take or leave the majority of the no-no foods, but the spicy tuna on crispy rice at our local sushi spot was a true sacrifice. Poor thing. Just remember, it's only temporary.

HIGHEST MERCURY (TRADITIONAL GUIDANCE SAYS AVOID)

Mackerel (king)	Swordfish
Marlin	Tilefish
Orange roughy	Tuna (bigeye, ahi)
Shark	

HIGH MERCURY (TRADITIONAL GUIDANCE SAYS NO MORE THAN TWO 6-OUNCE SERVINGS PER MONTH)

Bluefish	Sea bass (Chilean)
Grouper	Tuna (canned, white albacore)
Mackerel (Spanish, Gulf)	Tuna (yellowfin)

LOWEST MERCURY (GOOD TO GO FOR TWO 6-OUNCE SERVINGS PER WEEK)

Anchovies	Crawfish/crayfish
Butterfish	Croaker
Catfish	Flounder
Clam	Haddock
Crab (domestic)	Hake

* If at any point you are confused about what's safe and what isn't, the Monterey Bay Aquarium has a great Web site to help you identify the toxicity levels of various fish species so you can consume safely: montereybayaquarium.org/cr/seafoodwatch.aspx.

Herring

Mackerel (North Atlantic, chub)

Mullet

Oysters

Perch (ocean)

Plaice

Salmon (canned, fresh—choose wild-caught for fewer calories, higher nutrient values, and fewer pollutants and contaminants[16])

Sardines

Scallops

Shad (American)

Shrimp

Sole

Squid (calamari)

Tilapia

Trout (freshwater)

Whitefish

Whiting

No smoked seafood

Refrigerated, smoked seafood often labeled as lox, nova style, kippered, or jerky should be avoided because it could be contaminated with listeria.

No fish exposed to industrial pollutants

This is primarily for those who fish in local lakes and streams: Avoid fish from contaminated lakes and rivers that may be exposed to high levels of polychlorinated biphenyls. These fish include bluefish, striped bass, salmon, pike, trout, and walleye. Contact the local health department or the Environmental Protection Agency to determine which fish are safe to eat in your area. Remember, this is regarding fish caught in local waters and not fish bought from your local grocery store.

No raw shellfish

The majority of seafood-borne illness is caused by undercooked shellfish, which include oysters, clams, and mussels. Cooking helps prevent some types of infection, but it does not prevent the algae-related infections. Raw shellfish (such as oysters on the half-shell) pose a concern for everybody and should be avoided altogether during pregnancy.

The "Not-So-Obvious" List

Now that we have tackled the obvious, let's move on to the not-so-obvious. In fact, not only is the following information not obvious, it's often swept under the rug, ignored, and at times even condoned—which really pisses me off. I bet you will have read elsewhere (offending sources not listed to avoid a lawsuit) that the following foods and/or ingredients are okay during pregnancy (or ever).

Why would anyone recommend foods that are bad or even dangerous for pregnant women and the developing little ones in their tummies? There are many reasons for this. First, many major Web sites run on advertising. Who do you think spends heaps of dollars advertising online and in print (magazines, etc.)? Big food companies.

Second, the foremost books in this category are years old. Like *over 30 years old* kinda old. That said, some of them have undergone a few revisions, but nowhere near the degree that would accurately reflect the current research. And many of the more recent books in this category tend to be written by traditional doctors whose amount of schooling on nutrition is minimal. The amount of education and time they spend studying the effects of toxins and chemicals in our foods, hygiene products, environment, cleaning supplies, and so on is literally zero. Doctors are taught to treat disease, but their education on prevention beyond "don't eat [stuff on Obvious No List]," "don't eat too much," and "work out" is in most cases utterly nil.

RULES OF THUMB TO AVOID FOOD POISONING

Food poisoning is miserable and dangerous for everyone, but during pregnancy, it is especially hazardous. These general guidelines will cover you for any kind of food. And remember the old adage: *When in doubt, throw it out!*

- *Don't eat fruits and vegetables without washing them.* Make sure to use an organic produce wash to help you avoid any possible chance of food poisoning or exposure to chemical residue of any kind.

- *Don't store or prepare raw meat around any other foods.* Keep raw meat away from all other foods, especially in the refrigerator, and when preparing, use separate cutting boards and utensils.

- *Don't undercook your food.* Cook foods to 160°F.

- *Don't consume food that has been sitting out at room temperature* for more than 2 hours. This isn't wasteful—it's simple safety.

- *Don't share dips or any food* where another person's germs mix with the food you are consuming. There is a reason why double-dipping is rude, even at home. We've all done it—taken a swig from the milk carton, eaten straight out of the cottage cheese or peanut butter jar, and then returned it to the fridge. Bacteria from your mouth can contaminate the food, so teach everyone in the house to play it safe for the next 40 weeks.

Then we have the Food and Drug Administration (FDA), who will approve certain foods as safe despite extremely clear information based on numerous studies that the "food" or ingredient is anything but. (Thank you so much, Big Food lobbyists!) For example, scientists have known for many years that trans fatty acids (like partially hydrogenated oils) are extremely detrimental to our cardiac and neurological health—yet the FDA didn't even attempt to come out against them until 2013,[17] despite the fact that they have been in our foods and wreaking havoc on human health for more than a century.[18] Finally, after decades of research proving how devastating these cheap additives were to the public health, they've been declared "not recognized as safe" and are currently being phased out of the food supply.

Great—one down. Now how many thousands to go?

So here's the deal. This list may sound fringe to some people, but I have researched this stuff to death, and I am telling you that these rules are essential for maximizing the health of your pregnancy. Are you ready?

Rule 1: You must GO ORGANIC

If there was one guideline regarding food quality that I would like in neon, it would be this: *Go organic*. If you've read any of my other books or listened to my podcast, I bet you are not surprised. But before you say, "I can't afford that!" please know that organics are getting much less costly, as more companies are starting to produce basic, store-branded organic products. If you have the means and the access to go 100 percent organic, you could make no greater change in your health. I know

THE DOCTOR-NUTRITION DISCONNECT

Not only are most doctors undereducated about nutrition (meaning the right balance of macronutrients and micronutrients we all need), but most know virtually nothing about pesticides, environmental sources of hormones and antibiotics, endocrine disruptors, obesogens like fake fats, fake flavors, and fake sugars, or any of that, unless they purposefully take the time and money to further their education in those areas. Most doctors are about treating diseases. A few are "upstreamists" who look for the root of the issues (I count Dr. Van Herle, Dr. Gordon, and Dr. Gilberg-Lenz, the doctors on my dream team for this book, among these), but most doctors in my experience are not that way. This isn't because they don't care, but simply because it isn't how they were trained. You get a disease. They diagnose and treat it. Sadly, there is no money in prevention let alone optimal health; therefore, the system doesn't stress it, and it isn't even on the curriculum in medical school.

you've heard otherwise. I'm sure you've read that organic doesn't really matter—that organics are overrated, that their benefits are not scientifically proven, and so forth. This is straight-up propaganda put out into the world by Big Agriculture companies that make these chemicals (pesticides, fungicides, harsh chemical fertilizers, and so on) then sell us their toxic food. I'm sure you've read a lot of it: "Organic food doesn't have more nutrients," "There's no substantial evidence to suggest organic is healthier"—blah blah blah.

Not true.

Going organic is actually more important than anything else you can do for your baby's health. For your Hot Mom bod, you also have to watch calories, of course. But get this: When you're pregnant, I would actually prefer you eat an organic toaster pastry than a container of nonorganic raspberries. In fact, I'd prefer you concern yourself with organics more than you would sugar, salt, saturated fat, starchy carbs, or any other nutrient. (Bet you didn't see that one coming!)

The reason for this is simple: Your body knows what to do with things like raw sugar, whole grain flours, naturally occurring fats, and the like when consumed in moderation (within your calorie allowance). What your body can't process and what are extremely dangerous for your little one are chemicals—the thousands of industrial chemicals that have been added to our food supply without any degree of oversight or control. Many of these industrial chemicals become ingredients in our foods, rendering them nonfoods: fake flavors, fats, colors, sweeteners, preservatives, and more.

The very definition of "organic labeling" denotes foods produced under the authority of the Organic Foods Production Act. USDA-certified organic foods are grown and processed according to federal guidelines that stipulate standards of soil quality, animal-raising practices, pest and weed control, and use of additives. Organic farmers and manufacturers use natural substances and physical, mechanical, or biologically based farming methods to the fullest extent possible. Synthetic pesticides and chemical fertilizers are not allowed, although certain organically approved pesticides may be used under limited conditions. In general, organic foods are also not processed using irradiation, industrial solvents, or chemical food additives.[19]

I would argue emphatically that organic foods have far more nutrients than nonorganic because plants get their nutrients from the soil, and organic soil isn't overfarmed and thereby depleted of nutrients. Still, when you invest in organics, you are paying for what you *don't* get, not what you do. Organic food is relatively free of dangerous toxic chemicals that have been linked to a host of health-related issues affecting you and your unborn little one. Because the burden of proof is not on the chemical companies to prove that their products are safe, we are functioning as lab rats in their grand experiment.

I believe all moms experience that primal need to protect their child, keep her healthy and safe, and give that little spirit every chance and opportunity to make her way in the world. That's why we have to arm ourselves with knowledge, which is what you are doing right now as you read this book.

Here's some knowledge for you that I hope will get you thinking: Incidence of certain childhood cancers has increased nearly 30 percent since 1975.[20] The group Physicians for Social Responsibility reports that 6 percent of cancers are directly attributed to occupational and environmental exposures to specific known carcinogens,[21] and the actual percentage is likely much, much higher—yet we can't find out, because so few environmental chemicals have actually been thoroughly tested. The journal *Environmental Health Perspectives* reports that well over 80,000 synthetic chemicals had been introduced in the United States during the 50 years prior to 2002, with an additional 2,000 to 3,000 new chemicals being introduced each year. Huge amounts of these chemicals are distributed over our air, water, farms, homes, and towns—but according to the National Academy of Sciences, less than half have been tested for their potential human toxicity. And only a stunning 7 percent had ever been studied for their possible effects on childhood development.[22]

Meanwhile, the rate of children affected by allergies continues to skyrocket. The rate of asthma among African American children alone rose 50 percent between 2001 and 2009.[23] Diagnoses of learning and developmental disabilities, including autism and attention deficit/hyperactivity disorder, have also jumped 300 percent between 1997 and 2008, with one in six American children now affected.[24]

Some theories behind the surges of these childhood conditions vary wildly, from radically revised diagnostic criteria and increased awareness to thoroughly disproven vaccine scares. But why are we ignoring the elephant in the room? That overabundance of environmental toxins, antibiotics, synthetic hormones, and chemicals continues to spill out into our soil, livestock, water, and air. In 2006, the Harvard School of Public Health did a systematic review and proved that five industrial chemicals were developmental neurotoxins: lead, methyl mercury, PCBs, arsenic, and toluene. Since then, epidemiological studies have found six more, with others being studied and discovered every day.[25] The *European Journal of Public Health* recently released an analysis that found the European Union spent more than $70 billion in 2008 alone on treating developmental disabilities, asthma, and cancer in children—all caused by their environmental exposure to lead and methyl mercury.[26]

Add to this our culture's massive overexposure to antibiotics that totally wipe out our gut flora, allow unhealthy bacteria (like MRSA) to thrive, trigger systemic inflammation, and have a huge impact on our children's neurological development and function.[27] Then consider that 80 percent of the antibiotics produced in this country are actually pumped into farm animals that we eat (amoxicillin burger, yum!).[28] And finally, the stunner: Despite growing scientific and governmental acceptance of the dangerous reality of antibiotic resistance, the agricultural use of these antibiotics is predicted to increase by *67 percent* globally over the next 20 years.[29]

Not only are these chemicals harming our kids' brains, they're making them fat. One in six American children is obese, and one in three will develop type 2 diabetes. Although overeating heavily processed foods is a large part of the problem, scientists are starting to discover that many chemicals commonly used to grow nonorganic foods are hormone disruptors and tamper with our bodies' natural weight-loss chemistry—what some now call obesogens. Here's the deal. I'm not trying to scare you—but the truth is that this stuff *is* scary. It's become a scary world we live in. But we can protect ourselves. We can shield our families from a great deal of the danger simply by becoming informed. By utilizing the information, guidelines, and recommendations in this book, you are protecting yourself and your child to the best of your ability and setting him or her up for success at conception.

Some organizations are already working on this, and that's the good news. The World Health Organization is in the middle of a massive global study to zero in on the particular biomarkers that can help us determine the effects of this toxic onslaught on our bodies. They're particularly concerned about how these chemicals make their way into mothers—through the air we breathe, through what we absorb in our skin, but mostly, in what we ingest—because many of those chemicals make their way to the fetus directly via the bloodstream and the placenta. And think about the difference in the dose of one of those chemicals. You're a full-size human. Your baby is . . . a poppy seed. And that poppy seed is also trying to grow a brain and a heart and two kidneys—all while trying to protect its tiny duplicating DNA from any chemical onslaught.[30]

Terrifying, right?

Our only defense is to stay as far away from as many industrial chemicals, pesticides, and pollutants as we can. Remember that umbilical cord: *a direct conduit into your developing baby's body.*

In a perfect world, you would adhere to an all-organic, whole-food, minimally processed diet that is calorie controlled (based on calorie guidelines we established previously) and nutrient dense.

In a realistic world, many of you won't have the finances or access to an all-organic diet. You will eat out from time to time, with no guarantee of the food quality. You will need some form of convenience, so a certain percentage of your food will be processed. And while you may have diverse tastes for many different types of foods, it remains extremely difficult to get all the nutrients you need without some form of supplementation.

Given all these factors, the plan, guidelines, and recipes herein will be tailored to create a reasonable marriage of the perfect world and the realistic world. You (and your baby) will have an accessible plan that's affordable and manageable, and that still makes every effort to minimize your exposure to harmful ingredients and maximize your intake of vitamins and minerals. Here are your top priorities.

Do not eat nonorganic dairy or meat. Your first priority when it comes to organics will be meat and dairy. While there are many, many problems with nonorganic meat and dairy, let's start with one that's apropos to pregnancy: lactating cows.

Growth hormones are given to dairy cows to stimulate extra milk production, but the increased milk supply tends to lead to mastitis, or infections of the milk ducts. These cows then get repeated courses of antibiotics, which find their way into our milk cartons and glasses. Those antibiotics make their way down into our guts, where they wipe out all the good bacteria in our microbiomes and allow less beneficial bacteria to proliferate. (Hello, antibiotic-resistant strains like MRSA!)[31]

In case you aren't up on your cutting-edge nutritional science, the microbiome is the gut bacteria you carry around with you and that works with your body to do good things like properly digest your food and improve your immune function—if the bacteria you have are the good kind. There are also "bad" bacteria that tend to contribute to issues like digestive problems, allergies, autoimmune diseases, mood problems like depression, diabetes, cancer, obesity, and autism. Antibiotics in meat and dairy as well as agricultural and other environmental chemicals in food and the environment have a known impact on gut bacteria, killing off more of the good bacteria that benefit human health and encouraging more of the bad guys. This alone is a major reason to go as organic as humanly possible, especially during pregnancy and while breastfeeding, with meat and dairy as well as with vegetables and fruit. Now consider that when cattle are fed pesticide-laden corn, those pesticides collect within their meat—and then we eat them, and the pesticides begin to collect in ours.[32]

So meat and dairy are a great place to start—go organic and begin to nurture your microbiome back to good health before your baby comes through that birth canal—because when the mom doesn't have good bacteria, she can no longer give them to her baby, who literally depends on mom for his burgeoning immune system via the bacteria in her birth canal and breast milk. By the way, some believe this lack of good gut bacteria is directly linked to our country's recent upsurge in autoimmune conditions such as asthma and allergies, celiac disease, thyroid conditions, lupus, and even rheumatoid arthritis.[33] So please, I beg of you, stick to organics. Here are some resources for healthier cuts of meat and organic dairy:

Reduce nonorganic fruits and vegetables. I definitely don't want you to reduce the amount of fruits and vegetables you are eating, but I do want you to cut back on the nonorganic ones. These are heavily sprayed with extremely toxic pesticides, fungicides, herbicides, and chemical fertilizers. One recent major study found that the babies of moms who lived within 1 mile of farms that used pesticides had a 60 percent greater chance of autism.[34] A 2014 Harvard School of Public Health study found that six industrial chemicals (including pesticides) may be triggering recent surges in developmental conditions such as autism, ADHD, and dyslexia.[35, 36] The authors of the study urged regulators to immediately subject all industrial chemicals to neurodevelopmental testing and not call them "presumed safe" until otherwise proven—an absolute ass-backwards practice that has caused tens of thousands of untested chemicals to be released into our environment and our food supply over the last several decades.

Makes you want to hide yourself in a bubble, right? Well, the good thing is, not all of your fruits and veggies absolutely must be organic. You can reduce your and your baby's exposure up to 90 percent by simply avoiding the produce most likely to be heavily contaminated with pesticides. Every year, the Environmental Working Group (EWG) puts out a new list of produce known to be most contaminated for that year, which they call the Dirty Dozen.[37] Eating the nonorganic versions of the fruits and vegetables on the list below exposes you to roughly 20 different toxic chemicals in one shot. Yikes. Here is the most recent list (but keep an eye on their Web site to stay updated: www.ewg.org/foodnews/dirty_dozen_list.php). Note that they have added two bonus areas of caution, so the list really is a little longer than 12:

1. Strawberries
2. Apples
3. Nectarines
4. Peaches
5. Celery
6. Grapes
7. Cherries
8. Spinach
9. Tomatoes
10. Bell peppers
11. Cherry tomatoes
12. Cucumbers
13. Bonus: Be careful of hot peppers
14. Bonus: Also be careful of kale and collard greens

On the flip side, the EWG also publishes a yearly list they call the Clean Fifteen,[38] of the produce items likely to have significantly less chemical exposure and absorption. For these, the nonorganic versions are much safer. Save your money on these guys:

1. Avocados
2. Sweet corn*
3. Pineapples
4. Cabbage

*The EWG also wants you to know that a small amount of the sweet corn, papaya, and summer squash sold in the United States is produced from genetically engineered seed, so if you want to avoid that, go organic for those items as well.

5. Sweet peas, frozen

6. Onions

7. Asparagus

8. Mangoes

9. Papaya*

10. Kiwifruit

11. Eggplant

12. Honeydew melon

13. Grapefruit

14. Cantaloupe

15. Cauliflower

Rule 2: No Artificial Colors, Sweeteners, Flavor Enhancers, or Preservatives

Basically, if they have to add some kind of chemical stew to your food to make it look better, taste better, or last longer on the shelf, you should let it stay on the shelf. Let's break it down.

Artificial colors: You can identify this on any item of food by reading the ingredients. Should you see any color with a number after it (blue #1, blue #2, citrus red #2, red #40), put it right back on the shelf. Originally synthesized from coal tar and now petroleum, food dyes have a long history of controversy—and with good reason. A 2012 UCLA review found that all of the nine currently US-approved dyes raise health concerns of varying degrees. There are many natural alternatives, such as beetroot, turmeric, berries, and other natural dyes that are becoming more commonly used. By the way, organic foods won't have synthetic food dyes, so that makes it easy. Just say no!

Artificial sweeteners: I'm talking about sucralose (the yellow packet), saccharin (the pink packet), aspartame (the blue packet), and any food products containing artificial sweeteners, like yogurt, gum, diet soda, and "sugar-free" desserts. Artificial sweeteners have been linked with a lot of potential health issues, including obesity,[39] and also negatively impact the microbes in your gut by making you glucose intolerant,[40] but the dangers are marked for those who are pregnant. For example, a recent study showed a distinct association between mothers who drank diet soda during pregnancy and babies who were already overweight at age 1.[41] *Age 1, people.* Now, you can find pregnancy Web sites out there telling you that some artificial sweeteners, including aspartame, are safe for use in pregnancy. *Do not believe this.* Many studies have shown no risk, but many other studies have shown links not only to weight gain, hunger, and food effects (ironically, diet soda is likely to make you gain weight), but to issues as serious as brain tumors and leukemia.[42]

Aspartame is still very controversial because there are so many different opinions and even varying research conclusions, but there is significant evidence that aspartame messes with major systems in your body, including amino acid metabolism, neuronal function, endocrine balance, enzyme reactions, ATP stores (which provide you with energy), and mitochondrial action. People have reported aspartame-induced symptoms from blurred vision and ringing in the ears to confusion, memory loss, numbness, and convulsions; from severe depression to heart palpitations, diarrhea to hives, hair loss to hypoglycemia to joint pain.[43]

In other words, you do not want to mess with this stuff. I don't care if every single toxic symptom hasn't been proven yet. Please don't expose yourself, let alone your growing child, to this artificial concoction. Instead, if you have to add sweetener to something, please use organic cane sugar, organic maple syrup, or pasteurized honey in moderation. A lot of people wonder about more natural zero-calorie sweeteners like stevia or xylitol. I have been able to find no research to test the effects of these plant-based sweeteners on fertility or pregnancy, so while they are probably okay, avoid them as well if you don't want to take any chances.

Monosodium glutamate (MSG): MSG is a flavor enhancer commonly found in soups, snacks, salad dressings, seasonings, chips, and most Chinese food. This additive is an excitotoxin, which means it causes hyperactivity through its impact on brain cells. MSG literally overstimulates brain cells, causing them to die. This additive has also been shown to cause many different health issues in certain sensitive people.[44] There is also some pretty good evidence that the glutamates in MSG can break down the placental barrier and overstimulate the baby's neurons.[45] Yikes, and no thank you! It can also make you retain more water, because MSG is a type of salt—hello, swollen feet. Unfortunately, MSG is harder to recognize on labels, as it is disguised by a multitude of names. The best way to avoid MSG is to avoid fast foods, processed foods (even healthy types or those labeled as containing No MSG), and foods that contain a long ingredient list with a lot of additives and preservatives. None of that stuff is doing you or your baby any favors anyway.

Nitrates and nitrites: These additives are used in cured meats like lunchmeats, hot dogs, ham, pepperoni, bacon, and so on. As the meat is cooked, carcinogenic compounds called nitrosamines are released that are highly associated with various cancers. Studies have shown that consumption of cured meats during pregnancy left children at higher risk of developing brain tumors.[46] Nitrates were originally used to preserve meat and prevent botulism, but now, thanks to modern-day refrigeration and more natural preservation techniques for curing meat, they are used mostly for appearance, to appeal to the customers. Nitrate-free meats are still safe and are becoming more widely available. While once you could find them only at health food stores, most regular grocery stores and major brands now carry nitrate-free options.

No trans fatty acids, hydrogenated oils, or fractionated oils: Trans fatty acids and fractionated oils are fats that are processed and altered in various ways. Hydrogenated and partially hydrogenated oils (a major source of trans fatty acids) have a longer shelf life. This is why some of those packaged foods can sit for years without changing. Creepy. You know they are bad because the FDA finally admitted they're bad and not safe for human health, leading to things like heart disease,[47] cancer,[48] and even aggression.[49]

But in pregnancy they are even more dangerous, because they affect your unborn baby and can lead to problems such as hyperactivity, oxidative damage, and molecular changes.[50] The best way to avoid trans fats and fractionated oils is to avoid all the things you're already avoiding to keep MSG out of your diet: fast food, packaged and processed food, and food with long ingredient lists full of additives and preservatives. Even if they don't all contain trans fats (and soon nothing will, because they're being phased out), they are the foods most likely to contain them and are good to avoid in any case. Fractionated oils haven't been proven to have the same health risks as hydrogenated oils and trans fatty acids, but they are still processed and altered from their natural state, so personally I think it is a good idea to avoid them in general. They are in some processed foods.

BHT or BHA: These are food preservatives that the FDA says are safe, but at the same time, the National Institutes of Health says they're "reasonably anticipated to be a human carcinogen."[51] You can find BHA in many fatty processed foods, like fried potato chips, sugary cereals, and in food packaging and petroleum products. Um, no thanks.

Artificial flavors: WTF? Have you ever read the ingredients on a label and it literally just says "artificial ingredients"? What the hell does that mean? For the most part, we don't even really know. The FDA's definition of an artificial flavor is "any substance that does not meet the definition of a natural flavor." But even the term *natural flavor* is still a bit vague. We know it must be derived from something edible, be it a plant, animal, vegetable, or mineral, but that then begs the question . . . *what are the fake flavors made out of?* It must be something fundamentally inedible. Awesome. So just say no. It's not worth the risk when you have so little information.

BPA (bisphenol A): This is another ingredient that the government used to say was safe, but now they have changed their tune. BPA is an endocrine disruptor, and animal studies suggest BPA can do all kinds of disruptive things to the human body,[52] such as cause cancer, heart problems, behavior problems and other brain problems, obesity, diabetes, and ADHD. One study linked BPA content in children's urine with obesity.[53] BPA is also likely to disrupt hormone levels, so it has no business in your life right now. The other really scary thing about BPA is that it has often been used to manufacture plastic, even in items like baby bottles . . . and it *leaches into the baby's milk*. That's criminal, in my opinion. BPA needs to go away, and fortunately, most companies are now phasing it out because of all the bad PR. Just to be safe, however, *never* heat food in plastic containers, never store food in plastic, and avoid canned food with lined cans that could contain BPA. Here's another helpful hint: If the recycling number on the bottom of a plastic container is 3 or 7, it contains BPA. Throw it out! Better yet, stop using plastic for any food use, now and always. Stick to glass, porcelain, or stainless steel for cooking, storing, and serving.

Rule 3: Be Careful of Herbs and Herbal Teas

If you've picked up any "natural pregnancy" book, you may have noticed that there is likely to be a chapter about herbs—the ones that are good for you and the ones that are not. I'm willing to bet that you probably aren't even familiar with half of the herbs listed below unless you are a devout homeopath or a character in a Harry Potter book, but you know me . . . Captain Neurotic here. I want you to have all the info in case.

Here are the herbs to avoid when you are pregnant, and all the way through until you are done breastfeeding: aloe vera, angelica, arnica, ashwaganda, barberry, beth root, black cohosh, blessed thistle, bloodroot, blue cohosh, broom, calamus, calendula, cascara, coltsfoot, comfrey, cotton root, cowslip, damiana, dong quai, fennel, feverfew, ginseng, goldenseal, gotu kola, ipecac, juniper, lavender, licorice root, lily of the valley, lobelia, male fern, mandrake, maya apple, mistletoe, mugwort, nutmeg, passionflower, pennyroyal, periwinkle, poke root, rhubarb, rue, sage, sarsaparilla, senna, St. John's wort, tansy, thuja, uva ursi, wild cherry, wormwood, and yarrow.

NOBODY'S PERFECT

I know this is a lot to digest (or rather, not to digest), but it's critical that you have this information. However, I also want to be sure you understand another very important thing about these "no" lists: They are not meant to give you a panic attack. As I mentioned earlier, it's impossible to be perfect in life, and that includes during pregnancy. Don't freak out if you go out to dinner and the chicken isn't organic, or you had a bite of a cupcake with sprinkles on it colored with red #40. We simply can't completely limit your exposure to toxins, but we can reduce it significantly, and that will make a big difference. The goal is to make sure you are functioning with all the information. From this place of power, the choices you make and the actions you take will yield powerful and positive results—for you and your baby. So give yourself a break and just do the best you can.

Okay, enough with the no-no-nos; let's lighten the mood and start talking about

Wait! You Said to Use Those Herbs Before, Jillian

If you read my books or listen to my podcast, it's absolutely probable that you have supplemented with some of the herbs I mention in this chapter, for reasons ranging from immunity (goldenseal) and bruising and swelling (arnica) to mood boosting (St. John's wort) or calming (kava kava). And while these herbs all have their benefits for the nonpregnant, they are considered unsafe during pregnancy for a multitude of reasons. I could list all the details of all the risks during pregnancy for each one of these herbs, as I have done for so many other foods and practices in this book (as you already know if you've read this far). But honestly, this list would be so long and so full of annoying endnotes that it would waste tons of time for both of us. Dr. Suzanne says that there is almost no data on the safety of herbs and supplements for pregnant women because of obvious restrictions on testing them, so I say better safe than sorry. If you are really in disbelief about any one of the plants listed in this chapter as unsafe for pregnancy, by all means Google it—or just trust me and steer clear. Just wait for those herbal benefits until after you are done being pregnant and are finished breastfeeding. Okay?

That said, throughout the rest of this book, when an herbal remedy *is* safe and can actually help alleviate some kind of uncomfortable pregnancy symptom, I'll be sure to let you know. Also, Dr. Suzanne suggests doing your own research if you want to learn more. She suggests these two resources.

- Motherisk research links at motherrisk.com/women /mothernature.jsp

- Gerald Briggs, pharmacist clinical specialist, who answers many questions on this topic on the Baby-Center Web site: babycenter .com/expert-gerald-briggs

the good stuff. In this next section, we will go over all the stuff you can and should do to optimize your nutrition during pregnancy. Like the don'ts, we will be covering the more commonplace, prevalent info first and then moving on to the lesser-known secrets, tips, and nutrition strategies to really give you an edge!

THE "OBVIOUS DO" LIST

I've compiled information about pregnancy nutrition from the National Academy of Sciences and from other widely available reputable sources for your easy reference. Here's what you need, how much you need, and the best food sources:

Protein (at least 50 grams a day)

Adequate protein during pregnancy provides your body with the resources to build a baby: Muscles and organs are largely formed from protein, so this is no time to skimp. Protein also helps you because it helps to stabilize blood sugar, making you less prone to gestational diabetes. It will also help keep your muscles strong as you temporarily cart that baby around in your belly, and later, when you will be carrying the baby in your arms. Here are the best protein sources.

PROTEIN SOURCE	SERVING SIZE	GRAMS OF PROTEIN PER SERVING
MEAT		
Chicken breast, boneless, skinless	3 oz	28 g
Turkey breast, boneless, skinless	3 oz	27 g
Pork tenderloin	3 oz	21 g
Lean cuts of beef, such as filet mignon, extra-lean ground beef, and flank steak with visible fat trimmed	3 oz	21 g
SEAFOOD		
Fish fillets, most types	3 oz	20 g
EGGS AND DAIRY		
Cottage cheese, low-fat	½ cup	15 g (Note that cottage cheese is relatively high in sodium for a dairy product, so if you have any issues with swelling or high blood pressure, keep your portions small or avoid this one.)
Yogurt, low-fat or fat-free, plain	8 oz	13 g (Note that Greek yogurt has approximately twice the protein, so it is a great choice.)
Milk, low-fat (1% or 2%)	1 cup	8 g (Drink whole milk only if you need to gain weight.)
Medium cheeses (like Cheddar and Swiss)	1 oz	7 g
Hard cheeses (like Parmesan)	1 oz	7 g
Eggs	1 large	6 g

(continued)

PROTEIN SOURCE	SERVING SIZE	GRAMS OF PROTEIN PER SERVING
NUTS AND SEEDS		
Almonds	¼ cup	8 g
Pumpkin seeds	¼ cup	8 g
Pistachios	¼ cup	6.3 g
Sunflower seeds	¼ cup	6 g
Cashews	¼ cup	5 g
Pecans	¼ cup	2.5 g
GRAINS		
Whole grain flour	1 cup	16 g
Oatmeal	1 cup	5 g
Brown rice	1 cup	5 g

Fat: Focus on Omega-3s

Omega-3 fatty acids are essential to prenatal eye and brain development and may even contribute to protecting infants from illness. A study from Emory University[54] found that when women had adequate intake of omega-3 fatty acids during pregnancy, their babies experienced fewer colds and shorter illnesses during the first few months of their lives. In addition to protection against disease, adequate intake of omega-3 has been associated with a number of other benefits, according to a study published in *Reviews in Obstetrics and Gynecology*. Mothers themselves were at lower risk for postpartum depression, and their children had a lower chance of developing type 1 diabetes. I really can't stress the benefits of this enough. And because omega-3 fatty acids can be obtained only from dietary sources, it is essential to include foods rich in these compounds as part of your diet.

Nutrient Roundup

The following chart highlights all the important vitamins and minerals that can help make your pregnancy as healthy as possible. It may look like a lot of information, and it is, but because of this, I have done all the work for you. If you simply follow the recipes and meal plans in the following chapters and purchase from the ready-made shopping lists contained herein, the Yeah Baby! plan will make you and Junior bulletproof.

Yeah BABY! *Nutrient Chart*

NUTRIENT	BENEFITS	DAILY REQUIREMENT[55]	GOOD FOOD SOURCES
Vitamin A (During pregnancy, get vitamin A from food, not supplement sources, beyond what is in your prenatal vitamin.)	Helps with baby's growth of organs and bones Helps with the development of baby's central nervous system Helps you heal from childbirth Fights infection Improves eyesight	5,000 IU	Apricots Butternut squash Cantaloupe Carrots Cereal (whole grain) Dark leafy greens (like kale) Egg yolks Mangoes Romaine lettuce Sweet potatoes
Vitamin B$_1$/ thiamin	Promotes baby's brain development Increases muscle tone in the gastrointestinal tract, stomach, and heart Helps convert glucose to energy Stabilizes blood sugar	3 mg	Avocados Bananas Nuts Peas Potatoes Seeds Whole grains
Vitamin B$_2$/ riboflavin	Can help facilitate successful breastfeeding Aids in digestion of carbs, protein, and fat Helps maintain healthy skin, hair, and nails	2 mg	Beans Cottage cheese Leafy greens Peas Whole grains
Vitamin B$_6$/ pyridoxine	Could help with morning sickness Helps baby's developing nervous system and brain Boosts immunity Helps balance hormones	2 mg	Avocados Baked potatoes with skin Bananas Brown rice Chicken, white meat Chickpeas Pork loin
Vitamin B$_{12}$	Important for fetal brain development Helps with proper cell division Could result in calmer babies[56] Important for healthy nerve function	6 mcg	Eggs Organic meat Organic milk and milk products like yogurt and cheese (not butter) Vegetarian foods fortified with B$_{12}$, like cereal or plant milk

(continued)

NUTRIENT	BENEFITS	DAILY REQUIREMENT[55]	GOOD FOOD SOURCES
Folate (Note that even if you eat a lot of good food sources of folate, it is still very important to supplement with folic acid, starting as soon as possible before you get pregnant.)	Helps prevent neural tube defects in the baby, which affect the brain and spinal cord Boosts immunity Helps prevent infection Helps prevent anemia in pregnant women Could help prevent miscarriage and premature birth	600 mcg	Almonds Asparagus Beets Broccoli Cauliflower Citrus fruits Dark leafy greens Legumes (lentils, pinto beans, chickpeas, etc.) Papaya Peanuts Raspberries Romaine lettuce Strawberries Sunflower seeds
Vitamin C	Aids collagen production, including a healthy placenta Helps with the absorption of other vitamins and minerals Boosts immunity	80 mg (Don't worry too much, but keep your vitamin C supplementation under 2,000 mg per day, to prevent pregnancy complications.)	Bell peppers Berries Citrus fruits Guava Kiwifruit Leafy greens Papaya Tomatoes
Vitamin D	Helps baby grow strong bones and potential teeth Could help prevent gestational diabetes, preeclampsia, and premature birth	400 IU, or more depending on your blood levels. You can safely take up to 5,000 IU daily.	Egg yolks Organic low-fat milk Pork Salmon Sardines canned in oil Trout Yogurt
Iodine	Supports healthy thyroid function for mom Helps brain and nervous system development for baby Deficiencies in pregnancy can lead to decreased intelligence in babies	220 mcg (Make sure this is in your prenatal vitamin, but don't consume more than 1,100 mcg per day.)	Baked potato with skin Cod Mozzarella cheese Navy beans Organic low-fat yogurt Shrimp Turkey Wakame and nori (sea vegetables)

NUTRIENT	BENEFITS	DAILY REQUIREMENT[55]	GOOD FOOD SOURCES
Zinc	Helps produce and repair DNA for healthier cell growth Enhances immunity Deficiencies are linked to pregnancy difficulties	20 mg	Alaskan king crab Canned baked beans with pork Chickpeas Cremini mushrooms Fortified cereal Ground beef (85% lean) Lamb shoulder Milk Pot roast Poultry, dark meat Pumpkin seeds, raw Tofu, firm
Calcium	Essential for developing babies' bones and potential teeth Aids heart, muscle, and nerve function Helps protect against high blood pressure	1,200 mg	Broccoli Calcium-fortified plant milks and citrus juice Cheese Cottage cheese Dark leafy greens Edamame Figs, dried Ice cream Milk Oranges Yogurt
Iron	Helps prevent anemia during pregnancy Helps increase blood volume, which is important for supporting pregnancy	27 mg	Fish Poultry Red meat Plant sources: Blackstrap molasses Fortified cereal Legumes, especially lentils, kidney beans, chickpeas, and lima beans Prune juice Pumpkin seeds, roasted Spinach, boiled Tofu, firm

SPECIAL DIETS

If you are on a special restrictive diet and you'd like to continue adhering to it during your pregnancy, I'm not going to tell you that you can't. However, there are a few things to be mindful of, now that you are getting ready to (or already) have a baby on board. Most special, restrictive diets are not *ideal* for the health of your baby. Can you still follow them and keep both you and your bundle of joy healthy? Yes. It will simply require more diligence on your part to make sure you are getting the key nutrients that some of these diets inadvertently restrict. If you aren't sure about the specifics, I strongly suggest you make an appointment with a nutritionist who is familiar with your special diet to get recommendations more specifically tailored to your exact needs. In addition, here are some general tips on how to proceed based upon your diet of choice.

Vegan

I'm going to be straight with you here—this diet is probably the only one I would strongly suggest you modify during pregnancy. I'm sure saying this is going to make me very unpopular with you if you are a die-hard vegan, but don't get too mad. I am here to help.

If you are vegan, I'm guessing you are aware of the importance of getting enough protein and foods rich in iron, B_{12}, and calcium, as this diet is often associated with deficiencies in these key nutrients. This concern remains during pregnancy, but with greater stakes. All the nutrient requirements in this chapter apply fully to you. You just have a more limited list of sources. That said, you may also be more aware than meat eaters of some less-common sources. Here are some great vegan sources for all the above nutrients.

FOR PROTEIN:

- Almond butter
- Almonds
- Black beans
- Black-eyed peas
- Broccoli
- Bulgur wheat
- Cashews
- Chickpeas
- Green peas
- Hemp, pea, or brown rice protein shakes
- Kidney beans
- Lentils
- Lima beans
- Pinto beans
- Quinoa
- Seitan
- Spinach
- Sunflower seeds
- Tempeh
- Textured vegetable protein (TVP)

- Blackstrap molasses
- Cooked spinach
- Lentils
- Pumpkin seeds

- Quinoa
- Spirulina
- Tomato paste
- White beans

FOR B_{12}:

As you already know from the previous section, vitamin B_{12} is *essential* for healthy nerves and the baby's brain development, and this is the one thing that it is very difficult to get if you don't eat any animal products. This is why it is very important to supplement with vitamin B_{12}—it should be in your prenatal vitamins, but you can also find it in fortified foods. Many whole grain cereals, plant milks like almond milk and soy milk, and some meat substitute products like veggie burgers contain added vitamin B_{12}. Do not rely on nutritional yeast for vitamin B_{12} unless it says on the package that it is supplemented with it. Vitamin B_{12} does not naturally occur in nutritional yeast, contrary to what you might have heard.[57]

ABSORB IRON BETTER

Here are some of my best tips for making sure you are absorbing plant sources of iron more efficiently.

- Eat iron-rich foods along with foods that contain vitamin C, which helps the body absorb the iron. For example, put tangerine slices on a spinach salad.

- Avoid tea and coffee altogether. They contain polyphenols, which can bind with iron and flush it out of the body before you can absorb it.

- Avoid eating calcium-rich foods at the same time as iron-rich foods. Wait at least half an hour after having, for example, a glass of soy milk, before eating your iron-rich meal. Calcium can hinder the absorption of iron.

- Cook in cast-iron pots. The acid in foods pulls out some of the iron from the pot, adding it to your food. Acidic foods, such as tomato sauce, are especially good at pulling iron from your cookware. Cooking foods containing other acids, such as vinegar, red wine, and lemon or lime juice, can have a similar effect.

FOR CALCIUM:

If you don't eat dairy products, you will need to get your calcium from supplements and especially dark-green, leafy vegetables (the chart in this chapter shows you good sources of calcium). Because you are also at risk for vitamin D deficiency as a vegan and vitamin D helps with the absorption of calcium, be sure to get at least 15 minutes of off-peak sun on your bare skin each day if possible and eat vitamin-D-rich foods, like those listed in the nutrient chart in this chapter. Magnesium and potassium also help with calcium absorption. Here is a list of foods with a nice combination of calcium, magnesium, and potassium.

- Almond butter
- Amaranth
- Artichoke
- Blackberries
- Black currants
- Blackstrap molasses
- Broccoli
- Collard greens
- Dates
- Figs
- Fortified nondairy milk (like almond, rice, or hemp milk)
- Great Northern beans
- Kale
- Navy beans
- Oranges
- Raw fennel
- Roasted sesame seeds
- Tahini
- Tempeh
- Turnip greens

Paleo

First the good news: If you are consuming high-quality animal proteins (organic), then you very likely will have no problem whatsoever with your iron, B vitamins, omega-3 essential fatty acids, and protein intake. Yeah! Additionally, part of the paleo diet is an emphasis on natural, grass-fed, or free-range organic meat, which are significantly superior meat choices. Our dietitian, Cheryl, likes to tell people if the cow isn't eating paleo, they're not eating paleo, either. Also consider that if the protein you consume is not organic, you are putting yourself and your baby at risk for extreme overexposure to the dozens of chemicals, hormones, and antibiotics in processed, packaged, or nonorganic meat. So caveat number one is that on this diet, organic animal products fed as closely as possible to their natural diets will be critical.

Another concern is that people who adhere to paleo often avoid dairy products, and this can affect your calcium intake. If you are so inclined, I highly recommend making a few exceptions here. Consider adding organic Greek yogurt and/or pasteurized goat cheese to your diet during this time. If you are adamantly against this, be sure to get plenty of calcium from fortified nondairy alternatives like coconut, hemp, or almond milk; nuts; and seeds; and eat lots of dark leafy greens, like kale, collard greens, chard, and mustard greens. These should be an important part of a paleo diet in any case.

Not all paleo diets are low carb, but most turn out to be that way in practice because people tend not to eat as many vegetables and fruits as would ideally be recommended. In this case, possible side effects of diets that lean toward low carb are as follows:

- Constipation
- Fatigue
- Headaches
- Light-headedness
- Mild dehydration
- Nausea

As you may know, many pregnant women already struggle with the aforementioned conditions in spades, and having them exacerbated by low carb consumption certainly won't help. My suggestion is pretty straightforward. If you are feeling any of the above, do three things.

1. Drink lots of water.
2. Eat at regular intervals (every 3 to 4 hours).
3. Be sure to consume fruit at every meal for energy, fiber, and hydration.

Gluten-Free

If you are gluten-free, I am pretty sure you are aware of what gluten actually is: Gluten is a general name for the proteins found in wheat (durum, emmer, spelt, farina, farro, etc.) as well as other wheat relatives such as rye, barley, and triticale (and in oats via cross-contamination). If you have celiac disease, you must avoid these gluten-containing grains for the rest of your life. In fact, eating gluten could even cause pregnancy complications for you, so definitely avoid it now and always. However, that should not be a problem in pregnancy, because plenty of other grains and other foods are nutrient-dense sources of fiber and carbohydrates.

However, if you are eating a lot of gluten-free junk food (cookies, brownies, refined bread products), you might be low in calcium, iron, fiber, zinc, B vitamins, vitamin D, and magnesium, so it's very important to replace these nutrients through a healthy, balanced diet and appropriate gluten-free multivitamin/mineral supplementation. (Be sure your prenatal vitamin of choice is gluten-free.) Please refer back to the suggested-food charts earlier in this section for foods rich in key nutrients like iron and vitamin D. Choose the options free from gluten. You are safe with all fresh fruits and vegetables, as well as grains that don't contain the offending gluten. Those include rice, corn, millet, and quinoa.

Here are some suggestions for nutrient-dense, high-fiber, gluten-free carbohydrate sources to help fuel you and your little one (and keep you regular). Note that many people with celiac disease have issues with other foods, so obviously tailor this list to your individual needs:

- Corn
- Fruit, all types
- Legumes and beans, all types
- Lentils
- Millet
- Nuts
- Potatoes
- Quinoa
- Rice
- Salads (no croutons)
- Seeds
- Sweet potatoes
- Vegetables, all types

Lactose Intolerant

Lactose is a sugar found in most dairy products. Surprisingly, a large percentage of people have varying degrees of lactose intolerance, which means they are unable to digest it. When they do consume lactose, they get uncomfortable gastrointestinal issues.

If you have this condition and you are avoiding dairy, don't panic. There is really only one main concern, and that is your calcium intake. As we've already established in several of the nondairy diets in this section (namely vegan and paleo), there are plenty of nondairy calcium sources to choose from, as well as lactose-free dairy products, which are widely available (like Lactaid brand). Some other calcium-rich alternatives to dairy include:

- Fortified coconut, hemp, and almond milk
- Dark-green, leafy vegetables like kale and spinach
- Nuts and seeds like almonds and sesame seeds (Don't overeat the nuts and seeds, as they are very high in calories.)

Also, if someone is *mildly* lactose intolerant, consuming a small portion of lactose with another food (e.g., a bowl of cereal with a small amount of milk) may "dilute" its effects and make it more tolerable.

So there you have it. Good nutrition? Check. I know this is a lot to remember, but honestly you don't have to. This chapter will always exist as your go-to reference for whenever you need it.

Plus, each trimester will have even more tailored nutritional information along with superhandy and easy-to-follow meal plans and recipes!

CHAPTER 3

RULES OF THUMB:
Exercise for Prepregnancy, Pregnancy, and Beyond

My goal with this chapter is to completely shatter many of your preconceived notions about pregnancy fitness. I must admit that over the years, many women have expressed concern to me about pregnancy taking a permanent toll on their athleticism (or even their beauty!). Of course, many women don't have these worries, but if you do, let me set the record straight. Actually, quite the opposite is true!

But first, let me assure you (because I know this is also rattling around in your brain) that exercise during pregnancy *will not hurt your baby*. In fact, there is strong evidence that it will make your kiddo fitter and smarter! (I'll tell you more about that later in this chapter.) Furthermore, it will do exactly the opposite of weakening you. Pregnancy will strengthen you! There is even some interesting evidence that the baby's stem cells increase your regenerative abilities. A study showed that women who had heart disease while pregnant experienced much faster and more thorough recovery rates than any other group of heart-failure patients, and research suggests this is because of the regenerative nature of the stem cells in the mother's system due to pregnancy.[1] Yes, pregnancy can regenerate you! As your body builds your baby, your baby revitalizes your body. What a great trade-off!

I want you to know at the very deepest level that as a pregnant woman, you are strong. You are not fragile. You are not broken. You don't have a "disease." You don't even have a "condition." While we must be smart with how you train, in most cases you can maintain your prepregnancy intensity level throughout your entire maternity. If you are healthy, there is no reason why you can't continue to exercise all the way through, and pregnancy will certainly not devastate your level of fitness. In fact, if you are consistent with your exercise regimen, the physiological changes women sustain during pregnancy, like increased blood volume (to hold more oxygen for your muscles) and stronger muscles and bones from carrying around more weight, can even increase athletic performance immediately after pregnancy![2] Even those who have to take it easier because of an injury or a pregnancy-related reason find that they are regenerated afterward and can hit the track, field, or gym with even greater success after giving birth.

For example, British athlete Paula Radcliffe won the 2007 ING New York City marathon 9 months after giving birth to her daughter. Colleen De Reuck, a four-time Olympian, had a string of personal bests and big wins in 1996 following the birth of her first daughter. Yes, I know you are probably not an Olympian, but you get the point: Exercise is awesome for you and the peanut in so many different ways, and the peanut itself may be making you fitter. Hooray!

Now for the reality check. The fact that all this is possible and true and has happened to others doesn't take into account how you may be feeling right now. I appreciate this because I gave the above-referenced pep talk to Heidi in her first trimester, and she practically didn't speak to me for 3 days. (I'll tell you more about this in Chapter 5.)

This surprised me, because Heidi had always been fit. She was an athlete as a kid and a part-time yoga teacher as an adult. She loves to work out. (Weird, right? Those people who love to work out, and also those who order vanilla ice cream—weirdos, all of them! But I digress.)

So you'd think jumping into her prenatal fitness regimen would be a snap for her, right? Well, not entirely. Some days she would go for it, but there were definitely days when she felt exhausted and nauseated and she'd get outraged when I'd ask her to go to the gym with me. The conversation would go something like this.

Me (smiling and nonconfrontational, I swear): "Hey babe, let's go to the gym!"

Heidi: "What the hell's the matter with you? Can't you see that just standing up makes me want to vomit?!"

Alrighty then.

There were also times when she was raring to go and felt frustrated when I would underestimate her abilities in the gym.

Me: "Maybe you should go lighter with the weights. Do you want the 10-pound dumbbells instead of the 15-pound ones?"

Heidi: "I'm not *injured*!"

Basically, each trimester affected her fitness and her mind-set differently, and it was interesting to see this happen, not just as a partner trying to be supportive but also from my point of view as a trainer. Because of this, I brought in Andrea Orbeck early in the process, to step in as Heidi's trainer (and she's here with us now, to help me train you, too!). Not only is she a world-renowned prenatal fitness expert, but she likely saved my marriage.

For the majority of Heidi's pregnancy, she stayed active. She did yoga, lifted weights (not crazy heavy), hiked, jogged, and pretty much kicked ass all around. Ultimately, because of this consistency with exercise during her pregnancy, her body snapped right back into shape. And I mean right away. Within 8 weeks there was zero evidence that she had just been pregnant—except for the baby and the massive boobs.

So I think it's safe to say, times have changed. A lot. In the not-too-distant past, people used to look at pregnancy as a "condition." Pregnant women were considered extremely fragile. They weren't supposed to exert themselves too much, and they were practically kept cloistered throughout their maternity.

Very fortunately, progress has marched on—as has modern medicine—and we know much more about how hardy and strong (and proud) pregnant women can be. Science has proven that exercise during pregnancy is one of the healthiest things you can do for all involved. As long as you follow some commonsense guidelines and abide by certain safety parameters, you can exercise from the first day of your pregnancy right up to (and after) the birth—with plenty of amazing benefits for both you and your baby.

HOW EXERCISE HELPS MOM

In case you need further convincing, research has proven the benefits of regular, moderate exercise before, during, and after pregnancy. By regular, moderate exercise, I mean 30 to 60 minutes of moderate-intensity exercise four or five times a week during your pregnancy, ideally starting 3 months before and extending beyond pregnancy as a new part of your lifestyle. (You will need the strength and energy—trust me!) But you want more specifics? Sure.

Studies have shown us that women who exercise during pregnancy gain less weight and put on less body fat, greatly reducing their risk of (or treating their) gestational diabetes.[3,4] Regular, moderate exercise can significantly reduce typical pregnancy discomforts like constipation, indigestion, headaches, backaches, bloating, varicose veins, insomnia, fatigue, and mild to moderate nausea.[5] Exercise also eases tension, stress, and anxiety and lowers the risk of a premature birth caused by pre-

Andy Says . . .

Pregnancy is a great time to start working out with your partner, if you don't work out together already. Studies show that as pregnant women gain weight, their partners tend to gain weight, too, so keeping fit together can help you both come out of the experience fitter and healthier.

eclampsia (high blood pressure during pregnancy). Women who exercise have significantly shorter push stages (this is the second stage of labor), and their actual delivery and recovery from delivery are easier. Regular exercisers are 75 percent less likely to need a forceps delivery, 55 percent less likely to have an episiotomy, and up to four times less likely to have a Caesarean section.[6] Their chances of struggling with postpartum depression are also decreased (that alone is reason enough to do it, in my opinion!), and exercise generally improves your mood throughout the entire process (and always).

And—I am sure you are going to love this one—working out during pregnancy helps women get their "bodies back" 40 percent faster than those who don't.[7] If you weren't exercising before pregnancy, you might even end up with a better body than you had before you got pregnant.

Clearly, the perks you will experience are awesome, but the benefits don't stop there. Your little one will be better off as well.

HOW EXERCISE HELPS BABY

Exercise during pregnancy has been shown to help your body grow a healthier placenta, due to improved blood circulation.[8] The placenta is the vehicle for delivering oxygen and nutrients to your baby, and it also expels waste products, so a healthier placenta equals a healthier baby. Fit pregnancies also keep the baby at a healthy weight,[9] which is critical to their long-term health. Babies born with excess fat are significantly more likely to become overweight children, and overweight newborns of moms with gestational diabetes are more prone to develop type 2 diabetes later in life.[10] Babies of mothers who exercise throughout pregnancy have about half the risk of fetal stress during labor, with better heart-rate patterns and higher APGAR scores (an assessment of a newborn immediately after birth to determine the baby's health) than the babies of moms who stopped exercising after the first trimester.[11] Indeed, one study found that those moms who continued to exercise until their third trimesters had labors that were an average of 2 hours shorter—now that's some serious incentive![12]

Babies with fit mamas have lower resting heart rates and greater heart-rate variability, a marker of cardiac and nervous system health.[13] Contractions during labor aren't as stressful for your little one, because they are already accustomed to mom working hard physically during the pregnancy.[14] And exercising moms have fewer incidents of tangled umbilical cords and meconium in the amniotic fluid.[15] (This is when the baby prematurely expels stool prior to birth, and it is a sign of fetal distress. The baby can then inhale the meconium, causing respiratory issues.)

The benefits don't stop after your baby is born, either. It's possible that the children of athletic moms may have greater athletic potential. One study found that 20-year-olds who were exposed to exercise in utero performed better at sports than same-age peers whose mothers did not exercise during pregnancy. And babies born to moms who exercised during pregnancy have more mature brain development after birth, perhaps giving them a head start in the smarts department.[16]

Bottom line, babies who have athletic mommies during maternity are leaner, have more efficient hearts, are better athletes, and are potentially even smarter. You'd basically be giving birth to a tiny super human. Okay, I am exaggerating *slightly*, but the point is that the benefits are tremendous. Who wouldn't want to give their kiddo every possible advantage? And exercise does that—for both of you.

Are you convinced yet? Great! Let's start by looking at how to exercise safely.

SAFETY FIRST

Obviously, consult your doctor, share your workout plan with him or her, and make sure all aspects of your pregnancy fitness regimen are safe and appropriate for your individual pregnancy before you jump into something new. Certain medical issues, such as hypertension, heart or lung problems, diabetes, thyroid issues, a history of preterm labor, or a multiple-gestation pregnancy (two or more fetuses in the uterus) may require modifications and/or careful monitoring by your medical team.

During your second and third trimesters, you may develop other conditions, such as placenta previa (when the placenta is lying unusually low in the uterus, either next to or covering the cervix), ruptured membranes (your water has broken), or cervical insufficiency (premature dilation). You may experience vaginal bleeding, just like 40 percent of women during pregnancy. In the majority of these cases, you will continue to carry a healthy baby to term—but it's *critical* that you stop exercising immediately and contact your doctor ASAP so you can do what is best for your pregnancy. In addition, be sure to stop working out and contact your medical team immediately if you experience any prolonged dizziness or faintness, chest pains, persistent headache, calf pain or swelling, fluid leaking from the vagina, muscle weakness, or contractions of any kind. Always be safe rather than sorry—*always, always, always.*

Now that I have once again laid out all the possible doomsday scenarios for you, let me say these conditions are relatively rare and can all be managed should they occur. In almost all cases, exercise makes things *better.* So let's get down to business here and discuss the general guidelines for your pregnancy fitness.

FITNESS RULES OF THUMB

The great news is that the guesswork is out of the equation. *Yeah Baby!* comes with a complete exercise regimen (broken down trimester by trimester), handcrafted by me and trainer extraordinaire Andrea Orbeck, so that you can be as safe and also as fit as possible. That said, should you want to take matters into your own hands from time to time, I am going to tell you everything you need to know so that you get the best results, safely, even when exercising on your own.

But first, in the balance of this chapter, we're going to cover all the rules of thumb for fitness. These rules will apply to all trimesters equally, including before and after your pregnancy, so you'll know you have everything you need to feel totally safe and prepared. We will cover trimester specifics later in the book, in each individual trimester chapter, but for now, let's lay down the basics.

Did You Just Say No to Me?

What? Wait a minute. You say you don't feel like exercising? You don't want to exercise? It's the very last thing you want to do right now? You are exhausted, swollen, nauseated, and achy? If I were your trainer and you weren't pregnant, I might tell you to get up off your ass and get into the gym. But that's not who I am with you, not right now. While part of my job here is to push you to do what is best for you and your baby, I also get it. I completely understand that there will be days when you just flat-out don't feel like you can exercise. No judgment—I'm here for support and information only! I am not going to force you into your running shoes and push you out the door. I promise. But . . . my information says we need to get you moving, so forgive my persistence.

My best advice on these occasions is to try to put it in perspective. First, think of how much better you will feel *after* the workout is over. Think about all the benefits that will pay off, both for you and for baby, in a big way, in the long run. And if all you can manage is 15 minutes instead of 30, or a light cardio session instead of your regular boot camp class, or just a nice walk around the neighborhood or down a nearby trail, know that is totally okay. And if you are really feeling bad? Maybe today you rest, and tomorrow you get back out there. Be kind and loving to yourself. We all have off days where we don't feel like working out, especially during pregnancy. You are your own best expert at knowing what your body can handle right now.

Get Geared Up

"Wear the proper gear!" Really, Jillian? I feel like a bit of a tool giving you this piece of advice, because it's obvious, right? Or is it? I've noticed several trends in the last few years that can be problematic, especially for exercise during pregnancy, so I feel I have to say this. For example:

- **Wear good shoes.** While this trend seems to be dying out, realize that this is not the time to be experimenting with "barefoot" running shoes. No, ma'am. During your pregnancy, you must make sure your body is properly supported with the right shoes that give you arch support and keep your ankles steady as you gain weight you aren't used to carrying, in spots you aren't used to carrying it. Stability is key. If you don't have good shoes, visit a store with experienced staff that can help fit you with the best, most supportive shoe for you.

- **Wear a sports bra.** You are soon to be the recipient of D-cup breasts (or bigger), and those bad boys are going to need some good support. The flimsy, pullover-type sports bras will not cut it before long, so invest in a good-quality, sturdy sports bra rated for medium or high activity.

- **Wear clothes that breathe.** Breathable fabrics that wick moisture (like a nylon-cotton blend) will keep you drier and cooler. Overheating is no fun for you and not safe for baby, either, so dress the part. Also look for workout clothes that are not too tight or binding, so you feel loose and easy and comfortable when you are working out.

Cool It

This one is going to make me sound like an overprotective parent—this is *so* not me, I swear, but in this case, I have to be sure you know that during pregnancy, you never want to allow yourself to get overheated and/or dehydrated. During pregnancy, your body temperature shouldn't elevate above 102°F (39.2°C) for more than 10 minutes. This is particularly important during your first trimester because the developing fetus may suffer defects of the neural tube from an overheated mom. Throughout your entire pregnancy, the fetus can suffer from dehydration if you overheat, so staying cool is important for the duration. Here are some tips to help yourself stay cool.

- Drink plenty of fluids before, during, and after exercise. Keep a water bottle with you and drink from it often. Mixing coconut water in with your regular water is one great way to replenish your electrolytes after or during your workout—better than sugary sports drinks.

Andy Says . . .

If you are feeling dizzy, exercises that require balance can always be done using a bench or chair for stability. The dizziness will eventually pass, so don't worry that you will be permanently off-balance (although you may experience dizziness again after pregnancy, during night feeding).

- Avoid exercising in the heat or humidity. No jogs or hikes outside in the blazing midday sun, please, and stay out of heated fitness classes like spin studios with no ventilation or hot yoga. Don't use saunas and spa baths before or after your exercise session—or at any time in pregnancy, for that matter.

- Immediately stop exercising and take steps to cool yourself down if you have any trouble breathing; feel nauseated, dizzy, or weak; or start to vomit. If you spot any signs of dehydration (your skin gets clammy, you develop a headache, or you suddenly feel unusually tired), stop your workout. Sip ice-cold water and immediately take ice packs or cold washcloths and place them on the back of your neck and your forehead.

Caveats aside, it's very unlikely you'll overheat when exercising, unless the exercise is very strenuous or you exercise in very hot or humid conditions. Our body sweats for a reason—it's our natural, built-in cooling system. So don't worry about this, but do take the necessary precautions to cover all your bases. And during the superhot weather of summer, I highly recommend working out in an environment with a controlled temperature, like an air-conditioned gym.

Easy Does It

The further you get into your pregnancy, the more your center of gravity will shift, and your balance is not going to be at an all-time high. For this reason, be cognizant of where you put your feet, and keep off steep, narrow, or rocky hiking or biking trails for now. Better yet, consider shifting your workouts, at least temporarily, to a gym that has a nice stable floor and padded surfaces. The wrong kind of fall could really lay you up and put the kibosh on exercising, right when you need it.

Taking it easy also means monitoring your exercise intensity. I think we have all seen those pics of women running across the finish line of a marathon, belly bump first, or lifting giant weights on a barbell. But, honestly . . . why? This is just not the time to prove a point. It's like we've culturally spun a full 180 from "take a load off and eat for two" to "I am woman, hear me roar . . . and get pregnant and run a marathon while I'm at it." Whatever happened to balance, people?

While I appreciate that there are women who have performed extreme feats of fitness with a bun in the oven, I simply can't advocate it—nor would any medical professional. Impressive as it may be, why take the risk? You have your whole life to run a marathon, squat 150 pounds, participate in the Spartan race, and let them hear you roar in whatever way you like to roar. Now is the time to take a broader view. Like most things, the safest and most effective plan of action is somewhere in the middle.

How Hard Should You Exercise?

It is important, no matter how much of a badass you are, that you don't work out at an extremely high intensity. The reasoning behind limiting overexertion is that when we work out, our hearts have to work harder to deliver more oxygen (via bloodflow) to our muscles, thereby making our heart rates increase. Due to this fact, there is *some* evidence that women who exercise very intensely during pregnancy could affect their body's ability to pump blood to their baby (during the period of exercise only).

So how do you determine what's safe and what's too much? Back in the day, the general rule regarding a heart-rate limit for pregnant women was 140 bpm (beats per minute). This meant that when exercising while pregnant, a woman would have avoided allowing her heart to beat more than 140 times in a minute.

For those of you who are relatively familiar with fitness guidelines and heart rates, I bet you caught on that a heart rate of 140 bpm is well below the maximum heart rate for a woman between 20 and 40, which would range from a bpm of 160 to 180. While the concern over an extremely elevated heart rate is still legitimate, the guideline of 140 bpm has been thrown out. If a woman is fit entering pregnancy, her cardiovascular system is well adapted to circulating oxygen more easily throughout her body, and she can safely tolerate an intensity level above 140 bpm.

Therefore, today this unilateral heart-rate limit is no longer relevant, because it has been determined that each woman will bear a *different* heart-rate limit based on her current level of fitness. So essentially, one heart rate does not fit all, but every woman does have her own limit.

The current recommendation of the American College of Sports Medicine is that pregnant women exercise only to their prepregnancy exercise intensity level. So if you are a beginner, the recommendation of 140 bpm is a good guideline. If you're an elite athlete, you could go up to 170 bpm.

If you are still confused as to where you fall on the exercise heart-rate continuum, here is a simple guideline that the American College of Obstetricians and Gynecologists recommends, called the talk test. It's as straightforward as it sounds: If you can manage to carry on a conversation while exercising, you are within a safe level of exercise intensity.

The talk test also goes in tandem with another fairly general indicator of intensity called the RPE scale (rate of perceived exertion). This scale determines how intensely you are training based upon how you feel physically when exercising. It is subjective, but it is still a pretty good indicator.

Now pay attention, because in the trimester-chapter fitness sections, I sometimes tell you what RPE you should be working at. Since RPE means "rate of perceived exertion," as you exercise, think about how you would describe your level of intensity. How does it feel to you? Now check out the chart below to see what number corresponds with your perceived intensity numbers (the blank rows are when you feel like you are right between the descriptions above and below). It's generally recommended that when pregnant, you should not exceed an RPE of 14 on a scale of 1 to 20. That rating is based on how you feel on that day, as a pregnant person—not how you might have felt doing that same exercise last year, for example. Here is the scale.

Borg's Rating of Perceived Exertion (RPE) Scale

RATING	DESCRIPTION
6	No exertion at all
7	Extremely light
8	
9	Very light
10	
11	Fairly light
12	
13	Somewhat hard
14	
15	Hard (heavy)
16	
17	Very hard
18	
19	Extremely hard
20	Maximal exertion

How Long and How Often Should You Exercise?

This one is simple: Shoot to work out three to five times a week for 30 to 45 minutes each time. Don't do more than 60 minutes of sustained exercise on any given day, including your warmup and cooldown. The key here is to be consistent enough to get results but not overdo it to the point of exhaustion, which is just plain bad for you, pregnant or not. Now is not the time to push yourself too hard. Remember that rest and recovery are critical components of any fitness regimen, pregnant or otherwise.

What Should You Avoid?

Most sports are fine for you if you are already doing them, but there are a few things to avoid right now:

- **Impact:** From a fall, getting hit with a ball, or impact with another human. Sports like surfing, ice-skating, wakeboarding, gymnastics, horseback riding, and any other activity where there is a high risk of falling should be avoided, especially considering your balance is not going to be what it normally is for a while. Steer clear of contact sports like soccer, basketball, or hockey. This is not the time to be slide tackling a forward or bodychecking a point guard.

- **Elevation:** Sports that occur either above or below sea level should also be considered exempt during pregnancy. Scuba diving can put your baby at risk of decompression sickness resulting from changes in atmospheric pressure surrounding your body. Sports that occur at extreme elevations, like downhill skiing or mountain climbing, are not a good idea now, either. The lack of oxygen at these altitudes may cause altitude sickness for you and your little one. If you are currently living in the mountains of Denver and your body is already adapted to the elevation, then by all means exercise to your RPE tolerance as recommended above—but this is certainly not the time to go climbing Kilimanjaro.

- **Inadequate fuel/hydration:** Make sure you are properly hydrated and your blood sugar is stabilized before exercising. Blood sugar levels can fall rapidly during prenatal training sessions. Have a little snack about an hour before you exercise that has some complex carbohydrates and protein in it. (See the snack sections in the meal plans and recipes in each trimester chapter for good options.) Also, don't forget to hydrate—before, during, and after! Try to drink about 6 to 8 ounces of water for every 15 minutes of exercise, and *never* work out when you are dehydrated. The best way of identifying your hydration level is the color of your urine. If your pee looks like watered-down lemonade, you are good to go; if it looks more like apple juice, hold off until you have had a chance to rehydrate yourself.

What Are the Best Ways to Warm Up and Cool Down?

Warming up before an exercise session, whether you're pregnant or not, is critical to help prevent injury. Warming up gives your heart and respiratory system a chance to accelerate safely, and it lubricates the joints and warms the muscles in preparation for your workout.

During pregnancy, this warmup is equally critical, not only for all the reasons mentioned above, but because your body has released hormones, including an aptly named compound called relaxin, to loosen the ligaments in preparation for bearing and birthing a child. This can make you more susceptible to muscle tears, strains, and sprains. No shortcuts, please!

A simple 5- to 10-minute cardiovascular warmup will be more than sufficient. You'll quite literally prepare your muscles, ligaments, tendons, heart, and lungs for an exercise session to help you be as safe and effective with your workout as possible. Any light cardio works—a light jog, incline walk, stationary bike, row machine, stairclimber, or elliptical trainer will work just fine. You can also utilize the dynamic stretches I have created for you in your exercise index for each trimester.

Similarly, you will need about 5 to 10 minutes to cool down after your workout. The goal here is to slowly and safely decelerate your heart and respiratory system as well as help prevent stiff joints and sore muscles. First, spend about 5 minutes slowing the pace of your workout. A simple walk will do perfectly. This helps to prevent blood from pooling in the lower extremities of your body, causing light-headedness or dizziness (and a possible fall). Then, do 5 minutes of routine stretching, to help with muscle soreness, recovery, and injury prevention during future workouts. The rule of thumb here is to ease into each stretch and go only to the point where you feel the stretch, and no further. Do not bounce in the stretch (ballistic stretching) or attempt to push beyond a gentle stretch. Due to relaxin's effect on your joints right now, it would be too easy to overstretch and pull something. Our fitness trainer, Andy, advises staying well within the outer limits of your range of motion and avoiding crossing your legs frequently, so you don't overstretch your hips or knees. (See your trimester exercise indexes for safe and effective stretches.)

As far as general guidelines go, that's really it. While there is plenty more to know, it pertains to each trimester individually, so I have spread that information throughout the trimester chapters, with specific fitness do's and don'ts based upon where you and your baby are in your awesome pregnancy journey together. You'll also find an appropriate workout schedule and exercise index to make sure you're fully prepped and supported for the best results possible.

Finally: Please don't be afraid to exercise, but at the same time, please don't push yourself to the limit. Be consistent but not zealous. Be strong but not superhuman. A balanced, thoughtful approach is often the best way forward in all aspects of life, and pregnancy fitness is no exception.

CHAPTER 4

RULES OF THUMB:
Environment

So you think you're eating great and working out and you are good and ready for pregnancy? Sure, fitness and nutrition are the obvious subjects for discussion relating to any matter of health, happiness, and well-being—especially during pregnancy. However, another topic also holds great importance for the health of your little one and yourself, and it actually gets very little attention: your environment.

Look around you. Think about where you spend most of your time. What is the environment like in your home, your yard, your workplace? Unfortunately, most of us are surrounded by chemical exposures pretty much wherever we go. Think about what you cook on and in; what you clean with (your home, your car, your clothing); your beauty and hygiene products (from makeup and moisturizer to shampoo and body wash); even your furniture and home decor items (cribs, beds, sofas, carpets, paint). Anything you put on, breathe in, or live around can have a significant impact on your toxin load, and therefore the toxin load your baby will have, even before birth.

This is pretty serious. We like to think our babies come out as clean slates, at least in terms of detrimental exposure to the world. Not so. According to a study spearheaded by the Environmental Working Group, researchers at two separate laboratories found an *average* of 200 industrial chemicals and pollutants in umbilical cord blood of babies born in the United States.[1] This was in 2004—imagine what it might be now! These babies had pesticides; plastic residue; perfluorochemicals used in fast-food packaging and clothing; nonstick cookware chemicals; pollutants from burning coal, gas, and garbage; and more in their blood, including known carcinogens, endocrine disruptors, and neurotoxins, all before even being born. I'm talking about mercury, polyaromatic hydrocarbons, polybrominated dibenzodioxins and furans, perfluorinated chemicals, polychlorinated dibenzodioxins and furans, organochlorine pesticides, polybrominated diphenyl ethers . . . need I go on? It makes me furious to think about newborn babies being exposed to all that crap before they ever take their first breath of actual air or cry for the first time. No, I am not having it, and I hope you are with me on this one! Instead of being victims to our environments, let's be proactive. Let's focus on getting those numbers way, way down for *your* unborn baby—and for you, too, not just while pregnant and nursing but for the rest of your life.

But what kind of action can we take? What are we going to do about our toxic world? The information in this chapter will tell you exactly what to avoid (and what to use instead) to safely, affordably, and effectively protect you, your baby, and ultimately the world all our kids will grow up in. We can't get rid of all the chemicals, but we can definitely make a significant impact in reducing them within the environment you and your baby are living and breathing in most of the time.

OKAY, DON'T FREAK OUT

After Heidi got pregnant, I remember talking with a friend who is a green-living expert. After she congratulated me, she immediately began informing me of all the ways our home could be killing us and harming the baby. I distinctly remember being stunned by all the hidden dangers that were lurking in our home, unbeknownst to us. I started to feel like Howard Hughes! I became so neurotic that I was afraid to friggin' breathe in a room that had just been painted—God forbid it wasn't VOC-free paint! (I'll talk more about that shortly.)

Like me, you might be thinking, "What the hell is she talking about—how can my home hurt me?"

Don't panic.

Like everything, the key to managing your lifestyle is to make as many good choices as possible to help mitigate the toxic things we can't control. You can't avoid it all, but I promise you, when everyone in this country starts to make the kinds of changes I suggest in this chapter, the positive benefits will extend far beyond our bodies and our families. It could save the health of future generations. It could save our very planet (and let's face it, without a functional planet, we are all in pretty big trouble).

So while you read this chapter, don't panic and try not to feel overwhelmed. I'm sharing this info to help you learn how you can minimize any unnecessary exposure to toxins and detoxify your life as simply and accessibly as possible. You can review all the suggestions, weigh what works best for your family, and go from there.

And the great thing about this chapter is that this information will be equally relevant long *after* your child is born—for the rest of both of your lives, to be exact. Once you change these things, they stay changed, and you all stay protected. While greening your routine can be daunting at first, once done, you'll rarely have to revisit these issues again. Steps you take now could result in lifelong changes for the good. For example, if you buy iron pots and pans and you take care of them, you could be cooking in them for the rest of your life (unlike those cheap, toxic nonstick pans that last a year before you have to throw them out and buy more).

First, let's evaluate your home, identify potential hazards, and remove them. No time like the present! If you aren't pregnant yet, this is the ideal time, but if you are, it's never too late to start detoxifying your environment. And remember—don't panic! If your home holds any of these potential hazards, we'll find them and remove them quickly and safely.

Let's begin by overhauling your home—inside and out.

YOUR INDOOR AIR QUALITY

The first thing I would like you to consider is the air you are breathing. According to a study by the California Environmental Protection Agency, every man, woman, and child exchanges between 10,000 and 70,000 liters of air every 24 hours. With this kind of ingestion, you can see that air quality is as important as water and food quality.

Unfortunately, indoor air is far more polluted than outdoor air. According to the EPA, indoor air has two to five times more contaminants and in some cases even as much as 100 times more contaminants than the air right outside your front door,[2] even if you live in a big city.

Here is a list of some of the crap that's in the air of your home.

- **Airborne bacteria and viruses:** These can come from people or pets, wet surfaces, and humidifiers and air conditioners that haven't been cleaned. You can get rid of a lot of this by keeping a clean house and never letting water sit inside humidifiers.

- **Asbestos:** Older buildings can have insulation and soundproofing materials containing asbestos, which can cause serious lung damage. If you live with asbestos, it is very important to get it removed, while you are out of the house.

- **Carbon monoxide:** Carbon monoxide is a dangerous gas that has no color, odor, or taste. Exposure can cause headaches; nausea; dizziness; damage to the brain, heart, or central nervous system; and even death. Minute amounts of carbon monoxide are naturally found in our bodies and in the air we breathe. Large amounts, however, can be released from cars, furnaces, or other fuel-burning appliances. You can also be exposed from cigarette smoke (first- and secondhand), from a fire, or by coming into contact with methylene chloride found in paint removers or other solvents. Many states require carbon monoxide monitors with alarms in private residences, and some also require them in public places.[3] Whether or not they are required in your state, I strongly recommend having one of these, along with a smoke detector, to catch any car exhaust or furnace leaks that might be poisoning your indoor air. The cost is low, and the potential to avoid tragedy is huge, so don't delay.

- **Household furniture and product off-gassing:** This is a big one, possibly the primary cause of indoor air pollution in your home. New carpets, pressed-wood products like particle board and plywood, mattresses, fabrics, glues and adhesives in furniture, and fumes from paint and household cleaners, dry-cleaned clothes, air fresheners, and even home printers and copy machines can all cause major indoor air pollution in the form of volatile organic compounds (VOCs) like formaldehyde.

- **Mold:** Mold can grow anywhere there's moisture, especially if you have had any type of water damage. If you see or suspect mold, call a professional to test for it, and should they find it, have it removed ASAP—this is a job for professionals, not for you and your sponge and dishrag. The most dangerous, albeit very rare, type of mold is called *mycotoxin*, aka toxic mold, the by-products made by mold spores. This can cause many serious

POISON PLAYGROUNDS?

Pressure-treated wood is used to make decks, sandboxes, picnic tables, and play-ground equipment because it lasts much longer than untreated wood in the weather and resists infestation by insects. However, wood used to make these structures was typically treated with arsenic until 2003, when these poison products were phased out. The Environmental Protection Agency says these treated wood products, which are still in many public areas and private homes, are dangerous for children, but you can do some things to minimize exposure. First of all, on your own property, ideally you should replace any older treated wood structures like decks or playground equipment with new, treated wood that is not toxic. If you can't do that, at least replace the parts that children will touch often, such as handrails or surfaces they may sit on or walk on with bare feet. Seal the wood yearly to protect children from direct exposure, and don't pressure wash treated wood or use deck-cleaning solutions, as these can mix with the arsenic and turn it into a more dangerous form (use soap and water instead). And don't store any children's toys or tools that you touch with your hands under the deck, because rain can leach out the arsenic onto items below. If you are eating at a wooden picnic table and you aren't sure if it is treated, cover it with a tablecloth. Other outdoor concerns are pesticides and other lawn and garden chemicals, which can be dangerous for children and pets, as well as for us full-grown adults—more and more natural products are offered every day, both for DIY use and from natural-lawn-care companies. I urge you to check those out if you treat your yard.

health complications, including convulsions and even death. Death by mold? No, thank you! More often, mold that isn't the deadly kind can cause allergic reactions, asthma, sinus infections, rashes, upper respiratory infections, and even anemia. And what about your pregnancy? While no conclusive scientific evidence has linked mold to miscarriage, it obviously would still not be advisable to expose a pregnant woman (or any human, pregnant or otherwise) to mold. It's certainly no good for kids. One Polish study found kids who were exposed to mold in their homes for a long period (more than 2 years) had three times the risk of significantly lower IQ test results than kids without mold in their homes.[4] So get the mold out.

- **Radon:** Radon is a cancer-causing, radioactive gas that unfortunately is undetectable—you can't see, taste, or smell it. It is actually the second-highest cause of lung cancer after cigarette smoking! Radon is created naturally from the decay and breakdown of uranium in the ground. Radon can be found in soil, well water, and building materials like granite and cement and is believed to be the second-leading cause of lung cancer among people who've never smoked.[5] Just to have peace of mind and be 100 percent safe, do a radon test. There are companies you can hire to do this (it generally costs about $300), or you can test for it yourself by purchasing a DIY test kit at your local hardware store for about $20 to $30. You can also get a test online at radon.com or radon.info. If you find that your home has high concentrations of radon, don't worry. Most radon problems can be fixed by a do-it-yourselfer for less than $500— well worth the money. If you want or require the assistance of a professional, simply check out a list of "certified radon mitigators" in your state at radon.com/radon/radon_map.html.

- **Smoke:** Whether from cigarettes or chimneys, automobile exhaust or even improperly vented heaters, smoke and the toxic by-products it contains can be a major indoor air pollutant. Please don't let anyone smoke in your home (does anyone still *do that?*), and see my more detailed discussion of fireplace smoke later in this chapter.

I feel like going over all the possible dangers of the above for you and your baby would be obvious and redundant (and maybe get everybody more upset than is necessary!). Suffice it to say that the above can cause everything from cancer to brain-development impairment in your baby. Without beating a dead horse further, let's go over how to safeguard yourself and your loved ones with better indoor air quality.

- **Ventilate.** Open the windows whenever possible so any toxic fumes can get aired out.

- **Get a green thumb.** Houseplants actually do make a real difference in your indoor air quality. NASA scientists found that one potted plant every hundred square feet can help remove harmful contaminants from the air in your home.[6] The best varieties are bamboo, English ivy, gerbera daisy, and green spider.

- **Just say no.** Ban smoking of any kind from your home.

- **Air it out.** Air your dry cleaning *outside of the plastic wrap* for 4 hours outside your home before putting it in your closet or wearing it. (I'll talk more about dry cleaning later in this chapter.)

- **Quit the chemicals.** Don't use or store harsh chemicals in your house or attached garage. Not only will this improve your indoor air quality, but it will remove potential serious hazards for small children and pets. (Later in this chapter, I'll share some great natural alternatives with you.)

- **Furnish and clean your home greener.** I'll talk more about keeping a greener house later in this chapter.

- **Clean your air.** There are several ways you can actually clean the air in your home. Installing a true HEPA filter with a VOC filter in your furnace will get a lot of the impurities out, including allergens like dust and mold spores. You can also get HEPA filters for your vacuum cleaner. A good-quality air purifier is also a great addition, especially for the bedrooms in your home, including

A NOTE ABOUT PETS

Some people might say that a truly clean home is pet-free. Not me. If someone in your family has a severe pet allergy, then of course you have to consider that, but in my opinion, the value that a beloved and well-cared-for pet adds to the family is incalculable. For example, kids who grow up with pets learn compassion and responsibility, and according to a recent Swedish study of more than one million children, they are less likely to develop asthma when they reach school age if they were exposed to animals regularly before the age of 1.[7] Personally, I would much rather clean a little more often and get good-quality air filters than get rid of my pets. If you are an animal lover, you probably agree—so while you are worrying about your indoor air, don't worry about your pets. The stress relief they provide when you sit and relax and pet them or take them out for a brisk walk certainly outweighs any worries about what pet dander might be doing to your indoor air quality.

the nursery. We all spend a lot of time sleeping and breathing deeply, and air purifiers do a good job of keeping the air cleaner than it would otherwise be. Air purifiers can't take out everything—for example, they won't remove radon or carbon monoxide—but they definitely make a difference in cleaning out the stuff that could be irritating or cause allergies or even asthma in your home.

HOME DECOR

Your home is your haven, your sanctuary, your . . . chemical stew? While homes contain a lot of pollutants, you can detox your home through many different methods, some requiring very little effort. This is so worth any effort at all, however, especially if you are planning to be pregnant or are already there. As you raise your children, you will constantly encounter sources of toxins, and this is not a reason to freak out or fear life, but it is a reason to seek out cleaner options for your home and lifestyle. In that spirit, I would like you to consider all the ways that your home decor can introduce poisons—or not. Whether you are painting, carpeting, or buying furniture for the nursery, here are the things to think about now, rather than later.

Remove lead.

I'm sure I don't need to tell you how toxic this stuff is, and developing babies can be exposed to lead while in the womb. Lead can cause brain damage, or even death, and once kids are walking around, lead exposure can cause developmental delays, brain damage, decreased muscle and bone growth, and kidney damage.[8] You know all those jokes about kids chewing on paint chips? No joke, people. Clearly, we need to get any lead out of your home ASAP!

The EPA has stated that more than 80 percent of the homes built before 1978 likely contain some lead, because lead was not banned from paint until that year. If you suspect there might be lead in your home, the National Lead Information Center (epa.gov/lead/forms/lead-hotline-national-lead-information-center) offers a list of EPA-certified labs near you where you can send paint chips to be tested. They'll also provide you with a list of lead-abatement specialists who can seal or remove the lead. Or you can contact leadlisting.com.

Important: Do *not* try to remove the lead paint yourself! And be sure you and your family are out of the home while it is being removed.

Reconsider the carpet.

If you have carpeting or are considering putting it in your home and/or nursery, keep these few things in mind. Wall-to-wall carpet can be a haven for dust mites, which can cause allergies and asthma for you and your little one. In addition, carpeting and carpets are often made of synthetic materials that "off-gas" toxic fumes, such as from the stain-resistant treatment or the chemical adhesive that binds the carpet together.

If you already have carpeting and it's been around for a while, it may not be off-gassing too much anymore, and it's better not to replace it now, unless you plan to replace it with natural flooring like tile, wood, or bamboo, with a natural-fiber throw rug you can toss into the washing machine. If you have to have carpeting, I recommend natural-fiber, eco-friendly materials such as abaca, raffia, or seagrass.

To manage those dust mites in your current carpeting, install a high-quality disposable filter in your central air system, if you haven't already. Airborne dust mites will be circulated through a central air system and can wind up in any room of the house, but a good filter will catch them and trap them. HEPA filters and filters made for catching allergens are best. Also consider the air purifiers I mentioned in the previous section, especially for bedrooms, and vacuum that carpet once a week with a quality vacuum containing a HEPA filter.

Air out your paint.

Have you ever walked into a freshly painted home and been darn near knocked out by the smell? The reason for this is that VOCs—vapors like benzene, ammonia, formaldehyde, kerosene, and a host of other known carcinogens and toxins—are off-gassing into the home. The dangerous health effects of VOCs can compound with repeated exposure, and young children are particularly susceptible to risks from VOCs due to increased time indoors, where the concentration is higher than in the outdoor air.[9] According to the EPA, VOCs not only cause irritation to your eyes and respiratory tract, but they can cause loss of coordination, nausea, and headaches and could damage vital organs like your liver, kidneys, and central nervous system. They have also been shown to cause cancer in animals, and levels of VOCs are typically 10 times higher inside than outside.[10] You don't want to mess around with VOCs.

So before you slap that coat of baby blue or pink or yellow or green on your future child's walls, make sure you get "VOC-free," "no-VOC," or "zero-VOC" paint, which is almost completely free of carcinogenic chemicals. The option we used for our kids' rooms was a non-VOC, milk-based paint called Safecoat. Check it out at afmsafecoat.com.

Although VOCs are typically thought of as paint related, paint isn't the only thing that releases them into the environment. They are also in paint strippers and solvents, wood preservatives, aerosol sprayers, cleaners, air fresheners, automotive products, hobby supplies, and your dry-cleaned clothes. I'll talk about some of these other

GREAT RESOURCES FOR NATURAL, GREEN FURNISHINGS

You might be thinking, "How in the heck am I supposed to know what glue a piece of furniture is put together with?" Understandable. Luckily, these concerns are becoming much more mainstream, and many products now include this information if they are green and natural. Also, someone has done this research for us. Check out the following sites for great information and green-living supplies:

- greenguard.org is a certifying organization that ensures furniture is low toxicity. They list many different product suppliers on their Web site.

- greenguide.com is a great resource for green building materials.

- ecochoices.com is an online store with great green products, from organic-cotton beach towels to natural mattresses to maple furniture and eco-friendly jewelry, art, and baby nursery supplies.

- furnature.com is another online natural furniture store that also has mattresses and other bedding accessories, as well as natural fabric, if you like to make things yourself.

- greenhome.com is yet another green-living store that has cleaners, plumbing supplies, and stuff for both home and business, as well as green-living information.

And for the nursery . . . if you are specifically looking for green, nontoxic products for your nursery, check these out. You'll find everything from organic crib mattresses to baby toys and clothing. Some sites have only baby stuff; others have sections on their sites for this category.

- abundantearth.com

- babyworks.com

- ecowise.com

- humanityinfantandherbal.com

- facebook.com/Little-Merry-Fellows-151171319043/

- simplybabyfurniture.com

- shepherdsdream.com

- theorganicmattress.com

categories later in this chapter, but if you have decided to go with hardwood flooring in your home (or somewhere else like a deck or patio), when treating it, staining it, or sealing it, choose a water-based product instead of a solvent-based product. Check out environmentalhomecenter.com for greener, cleaner options.

Choose your furniture carefully.

No, you don't have to throw away all your furniture! But when decorating your nursery and adding new pieces to your home, it doesn't hurt to have the facts so you can make the best choices. Ideally, choose furniture options that are low toxicity, which means they would be free of:

- PVC
- Formaldehyde-based glues
- Toxic flame retardants
- Wood stains that contain the industrial chemical perfluorooctanoic acid (PFOA)

Synthetic materials or natural materials treated with synthetic substances can off-gas chemicals, just like paint can, including VOCs. Instead, look for furniture made with natural materials like hardwood, bamboo, organic cotton, and naturally tanned leather, untreated or treated with natural substances.

CLEAN UP THE KITCHEN

Next, let's head into the kitchen. You have a lot more than food in your kitchen. You also have toxins, like cleaning products, nonstick cookware, and plastic—and I'm not even talking about the processed food! Specifically, I want to zero in on the things you use to cook, serve, and store food that are potentially hazardous to you and your baby.

Upgrade your cookware.

When it comes to cookware, be sure to avoid Teflon and all other "nonstick" pans. The chemicals they use to make pans nonstick are made from PFAs, which is an acronym for poly- and perfluoroalkyl substances. These have been linked to serious health concerns, like infertility, thyroid problems, and even organ damage in animals.[11] The EPA also says they are probably carcinogenic, and nonstick cookware (as well as anything else that is stain resistant or waterproof) probably contains chemicals in this category. For cookware, these synthetic polymers release toxic fumes at high heat that can actually kill birds and cause flulike symptoms in humans.[12] We had a cook plate on our stove that we didn't realize was Teflon. Heidi made pancakes on it one morning without thinking, and our parrot became incredibly ill. Fortunately, our vet was able to save her and we figured out the problem immediately, but can you imagine? That's how toxic that stuff is. Plus, the nonstick coating tends to scratch and flake off in food, and although these particles are supposedly inert, those inert flakes may be made with PFA and may contain it residually. Some research suggests that PFA could mess with your hormone balance, reproductive health, and even fetal development.[13] Do you really want to eat it? I don't think it's worth the risk, just so your omelet slides out of the pan. Instead, opt for stainless steel, cast iron, ceramic, or glass cookware instead, and add a little olive oil. You'll be good to go.

Lose the bleach.

Don't we all just love bright, blinding-white paper towels, paper plates, coffee filters, and napkins (not to mention toilet paper and baby wipes)? How do you think they got so white? Paper is made from trees, right? And are trees white? Nope. Those paper products we are so used to seeing in their snow-white form are bleached. Chlorine is toxic mainly because when it binds with anything made of carbon (like paper), it produces extremely toxic dioxins and other pollutants.

Although the really toxic bleaching that all paper mills used to do has largely been replaced by less-toxic methods (at least in the United States and Canada), many companies still use chlorine compounds[14] that are at best damaging to the environment and at worst a health risk for the end user (you and baby). Instead, choose the unbleached version of any paper product in your home whenever possible. That means paper products that use only nonchlorine bleaching processes, favoring oxygen, peroxide, or ozone bleaching methods instead. The very best choice is PCF paper: processed chlorine-free. These products are chlorine-free and use chlorine-free recycled paper. Put simply, get the brown paper towels and coffee filters instead of the white ones.

Plastic storage containers.

Never, ever store food in plastic containers, and especially never *heat* food in plastic storage containers. Plastics are a whole chemical hazard unto themselves. I wrote about this extensively in *Master Your Metabolism,* and you can go there if you want even more gory details, but here are the basics you should know: Plastics are linked to a host of health-related issues like cancer, endocrine disruption, birth defects, and the like. For these reasons, we want to remove as much plastic as possible from your life. Some are more dangerous than others. I will go over it for you below, but you can also use checnet.org as a resource on safe and unsafe plastics:

- **UNSAFE: Polyvinyl chloride (also labeled as V or PVC), recycle #3:** Found in cooking-oil bottles; cling wrap; clear wrap around meat, cheese, deli meats, and other food items; plumbing pipes; and toys. This one is truly the worst, both for its environmental impact and for how it accumulates in the human body. It contains hormone disruptors and carcinogens, which are released into foods when this type of plastic is heated. You can recognize it by the recycle #3 symbol. Instead, choose non-PVC cling wrap, store food in glass, and buy cooking oil in glass bottles.

- **UNSAFE: Polystyrene (also labeled as PS; extruded type commonly known as Styrofoam,** although, fun fact, Styrofoam-brand cups no longer exist), recycle #6: This is an extruded (forced out of a machine) type of plastic found in disposable coffee cups, take-out containers, foam egg cartons, meat trays, packing peanuts, and foam insulation. There is also a nonextruded type found in CD jewel cases and used to make disposable cutlery and transparent take-out containers. Polystyrenes include benzene, butadiene, and styrene, which are all known or suspected carcinogens, especially when heated, and polystyrene is also an endocrine disruptor. You know those old-school cups of noodles you heat in the microwave? Polystyrene soup, anyone? These and the kind in plastic bowls from Chinese takeout contain toxins that bind with fat and will set up shop in your body tissues. To avoid it, never drink hot drinks out of foam cups, eat food from foam containers, or use conventional plastic cutlery on hot foods. Let restaurants know you care about their take-out containers and look for those that use paper-based containers or those made from corn or sugar instead of polystyrene. If you do end up with takeout in a polystyrene container, put it in glass or ceramic as soon as you get home.

- **USUALLY UNSAFE:** "Other plastics," or the recycling category #7 for plastics that don't fit into the other descriptions. These include dangerous PC (for polycarbonate) and harmless PLA (for polylactide, a plastic made from corn, potatoes, sugar, or other plant-based starch): Found in baby bottles, micro-

DOING GOOD WITH GARBAGE

The use of polystyrene in insulation is actually an environmental boon: Eighty-five percent of an insulation called Rastra is made of recycled polystyrene, creating a very energy-efficient building material out of the waste of one of the world's worst plastics.

wave ovenware, stain-resistant food-storage containers, medical storage containers, eating utensils, plastic liners of almost all food and soft drink cans, Lexan containers, old Nalgene or other hard plastic water-drinking bottles, 5-gallon water jugs, and building materials. PC is the bad stuff—it contains bisphenol A, or BPA. I've talked about this already in this book, but some 700 studies, mostly on animals, have linked BPA with endocrine-disrupting effects like early puberty, abnormal breast tissue and prostate growth, lower sperm counts, and neurological effects like hyperactivity. BPA leaches into the tissues at an extremely efficient rate, even before birth—it's been detected in human urine, blood, amniotic fluid, placenta, umbilical cord blood, and breast milk.

BPA is especially dangerous for babies and young kids; laboratory research has found that animals subjected to BPA, even at low doses, before and directly after they're born have a higher chance of being overweight, insulin resistant, and leptin resistant as adults. To avoid it, use only glass baby bottles, or if you use plastic bottles, do not put them in bottle warmers. Drink from water bottles lined with stainless steel or ceramic and avoid lined aluminum and steel cans, which often contain BPA. Also never wash BPA-containing plastic in the dishwasher, as this will degrade it further. If it gets cloudy, throw it away—it is disintegrating. Common sense note: If you ever smell plastic in any liquid or food, *don't drink or eat it!*

PLAs, on the other hand, are awesome. They are created from plant materials and are 100 percent compostable. Many natural food stores and restaurants and also many enlightened, more mainstream stores and restaurants are switching to these compostable take-out containers.

- **SAFER: Polyethylene terephthalate (PET or PETE), recycle #1:** Found in bottles for cough syrup, ketchup, salad dressing, soft drinks, sports drinks, and water. Also found in plastic pickle, jelly, jam, mustard, mayonnaise, and peanut butter jars. These are pretty inert, with no known health hazards, and are easily recycled into fleece and polyester fabric. This is also a good choice for baby bottles—these are the colored, opaque, or less-shiny ones. Don't reuse water bottles made from this kind of plastic, though—they can attract bacteria when reused.

- **SAFER: High-density polyethylene (HDPE), recycle #2:** Found in toys, shampoo bottles, milk jugs, yogurt containers, margarine tubs, recyclable grocery bags, trash bags, laundry detergent bottles, composite lumber, Tyvek building material, some Tupperware products, sanitary products, original Hula-Hoops, and some shrink wrap. This type also contains no known endocrine disruptors or carcinogens and is easily recycled, but don't microwave food in it, put hot food into it, or leave it out in the sun. Also, this type is made from oil, and it's not an efficient process, so know that it is a wasteful product, environmentally speaking.

- **SAFER: Low-density polyethylene (LDPE), recycle #4:** Found in grocery bags, bowls, lids, toys, six-pack rings, trays, power cables, liners, cling wrap, sandwich bags, food coloring bottles and other squeezable bottles, and bottle caps. Another safer, inert choice, but again, don't warm it up, and know that many recycling centers don't accept this type. When you are done with it, you will just have to throw it away, and it will end up in a landfill.

- **SAFER: Polypropylene (PP), recycle #5:** Found in plastic utensils, cups, thermal underwear (such as Under Armour brand), clear bags, diapers, safe baby bottles, some yogurt containers, and condiment bottles. This one is not known to be hazardous to end users, but don't heat it up, and know that it is not generally accepted at recycling centers.

Okay, that's a lot of plastic talk, but finally, I would just like to say that although plastics are certainly handy and hard to avoid completely, it's almost always better to use something else, if you can, for the sake of both health and the environment. I try to live as plastic-free as I can, and I hope you will, too.

GO AU NATUREL IN THE YARD

While you might think I'm telling you to run around naked in your yard (and if that's your thing, who am I to stop you?), what I mean here is that there is no reason to put any chemicals in your outdoor living space. The yard is not often the first thing you think of when removing toxins from your home, but many different dangerous chemicals can be used on your lawn without your even knowing—94 percent of households report using some kind of pesticide.[15] If you hire a landscaper, a pool guy, or an exterminator, chances are their tool kit includes some pretty ferocious chemicals. Have you ever seen those little signs on people's lawns advising you to keep children and pets off the grass because it was just treated? This is what I'm talking about. Whatever that crap is, if they have to put up a warning sign, then you don't want it on the grass where you might walk or garden or where your dogs play, and where, in the future, you will likely play with your child. Keep it clean and pure, folks. It's nature. It doesn't need chemical intervention.

Specifically, it is very important to avoid:

- Chemical weed killers like Roundup
- Chemical pesticides like Bug Clear, Plant Rescue, and Raid Ant Killer
- Chemical fertilizers like Miracle-Gro

These types of chemicals not only contain a bunch of synthetic materials and chemicals, but many of them (or the companies they support) have been guilty of environmental violations, including mislabeling products to make them seem safer than they really are, as well as other shady safety and business practices.[16, 17, 18, 19] It's big business, folks. They don't have your health as priority one, I can tell you that! All these outdoor chemicals contain substances that can cause extreme endocrine disruption and even death in just about every animal they come into contact with, from frogs to bees, and have been linked to developmental diseases like autism. Don't subject yourself, your baby, or the planet that is your baby's future home to these potent toxins. Instead, check out facebook.com/safelawns.org for tons of useful tips to accomplish all the above as safely as possible.

SKIP THE FIRE

Admittedly, I am a sucker for a fire on winter nights, but have you ever gotten a headache from one? Watery eyes? Nagging cough? This may have been because burning wood can emit carbon monoxide, dioxin, arsenic, formaldehyde, and potentially other toxic VOCs. Children living in wood-burning households have higher rates of lung inflammation, breathing problems, pneumonia, and other respiratory diseases. Although the *idea* of a fire is nice, keep your wood burning to the occasional outdoor campfire, if that. My advice is to avoid being around wood-burning fires entirely when pregnant, if possible. If you do decide to have one, here are some ways to make it safer.

- Use only *untreated wood* that has dried out for at least 5 to 6 months—it will give off less smoke.

- Or use Java-Log fire logs, which are the least toxic of the manufactured fire logs and are widely available.

- Have your chimney cleaned and serviced yearly, so there is no buildup of creosote (a wood-tar combination that can cause a chimney fire) and toxic smoke doesn't end up filling your living room.

- Ideally, if you must have a fire, consider switching from a wood-burning fireplace to one that burns natural gas, or a pellet stove.[20]

NOW ABOUT THOSE CLEANING PRODUCTS . . .

You knew this was coming, right? Because every time you clean the toilet or spray the furniture, you wonder . . . is this *bad for me?* I remember when I was a kid, my mom believed that keeping a spotless home was good for your health. She would religiously use gnarly chemicals like bleach and ammonia to "kill the germs." Well, guess what? A lot of those germs are a lot less harmful than the chemicals we tend to want to use to get rid of them. When we inhale those fumes and get those products on our skin, their chemicals get into our systems and set up shop.

Unfortunately, we have only recently become aware of this, but at least now we know how dangerous those harsh chemicals really are. We know that many of the ingredients in standard household cleaners can cause everything from acute exposure emergencies (many involving children under 6 years old who swallow or spill these cleaners[21]) to long-term hazards like asthma, lung damage, and heart damage to more minor issues like allergies and headaches. Many contain endocrine disruptors that interfere with fertility and could cause birth defects and cancer . . . and don't even get me started on what these do to the environment we would all like to preserve for our children. After all, cleaning chemicals have to go somewhere when you flush them down the toilet or send them down the drain. From our laundry detergent and dish soap to our toilet bowl cleaner and floor polish, it's time to examine and make over our cleaning protocol and supplies.

I'm not going to list all the dangerous chemicals, their effects on health, and products that contain them, because it would literally be hundreds of pages—it would be an entire book on its own. Instead, let's use a solution-based approach. Here is what I do to find less-toxic options. This is my list of the products and brands that are better for you, and some DIY solutions to help you green up your cleanup.

DON'T FORGET: NO KITTY LITTER!

I've already mentioned this in an earlier chapter, but it seems apropos to remind you here: When your cat uses the litter box, it can deposit a parasite in the litter that can lead to toxoplasmosis, a parasitic infection that can make you feel "fluish." It's not going to kill you, but it is definitely dangerous if passed on to your baby. Then it can lead to vision or hearing problems. That means, lucky you, during pregnancy you now have a totally legitimate excuse to have your partner or a friend clean the cat litter for you. It won't hurt *them*. Now, if you didn't know this and you have been cleaning out the litter box, and you feel you could have been infected, just contact your doctor and ask. The simple treatment for toxoplasmosis is antibiotics—some types are safe for use during pregnancy, and your doctor can advise you about this.

Look for the Buzzwords

I always look for words like:

- Ammonia-free
- Biodegradable
- Free of dye or perfume
- Noncarcinogenic
- Non–petroleum based
- Nontoxic

Buy the Proven Brands

These are the brands I have personally investigated and found to be cleaner, greener, and purer than conventional cleaning chemicals.

- Bona, for hardwood floor cleaner
- Ecover, for dishwasher tablets, laundry detergent, and laundry stain remover
- Honest Company, for laundry detergent, floor cleaner, toilet cleaner, and glass cleaner
- Method, for furniture polish and toilet cleaner
- Mrs. Meyer's, for powder surface scrub and liquid hand soap
- Shaklee, for a multipurpose cleaner
- Simple Green, for an all-purpose carpet cleaner
- Skoy, a cloth to replace bleached paper towels and sponges

Try DIY Cleaning Products

There are tons of totally safe products in your own kitchen and bathroom that you might never have considered as excellent cleaners. Here are some of the things I've tried, but this is just the beginning. You could fall into the Internet rabbit hole of safe, natural, make-it-yourself cleaning product "recipes" and stay there for hours, but start here and see what works for you and your household. This list contains the main ingredients that most homemade cleaning products are made from. Once you have these on hand, you can find endless ways to use them to clean, deodorize, shine, unclog, and refurbish just about anything in your home. Pretty soon, you'll wonder why you ever spent a bunch of money on cleaning chemicals.

- Baking soda, usually used for cleansing and deodorizing
- Club soda, which removes rust and crud from anything and everything
- Hydrogen peroxide, often used in combination with white vinegar as a sanitizer
- Lemon juice, a great substitute for bleach

- Olive oil, an excellent natural furniture and floor polish; it also gets the fingerprints off stainless steel appliances
- Salt, a multipurpose mineral that can do everything from remove stains and mildew to deodorize and even deter ants
- White vinegar, diluted, is great for cleaning floors, windows, mirrors, showers, etc., and when combined with baking soda, it can help unclog a sink. (Pour in the baking soda, then pour in the vinegar and watch it fizz. Kids love to watch this.)

DRY CLEANING

If you are in the habit of dropping off your business clothes at the dry cleaner on a regular basis, you may think you can't live without it, but don't do this when pregnant. Just don't. Instead, why not rethink your wardrobe? I appreciate that this may seem impossible to you. Maybe you are thinking, "Sure, Jillian, your business suit is workout clothes, what do you know about the executive wear I need for my job?" Fair enough, but the fact is that the chemicals used to dry-clean clothing are very toxic. There are some other good alternatives, which I'm listing here.

And aren't you going to be wearing maternity clothes pretty soon, anyway? You might as well get used to a more casual look now. Who knows, you may get hooked. I'm not saying you're going to start wearing spandex to the office, but many machine-washable clothes can look quite professional, and they tend to be more comfortable, too.

Here are some possible alternatives for cleaning your clothes:

- Steam your clothes without dry cleaning. A clothing steamer isn't very expensive and does a great job.
- Brush-clean with a microfiber cloth.
- Hand wash in nontoxic soap and air-dry.

If none of these work for you, other less-ideal but also less-toxic options are:

- Find a "wet" cleaner as an alternative. These guys use cleaner, greener soaps to get the job done.
- Locate a "green" dry cleaner. These eco-friendlier companies will use pressurized CO_2 instead of the chemicals used in traditional dry cleaning.

If you absolutely must dry-clean something and wear it, be sure to remove the plastic cover and air the clothes out, outside, for at least 4 hours prior to wearing— pregnant or otherwise.

ON TAP: GETTING THE BEST WATER

You probably drink it all day long, but you also cook with it, bathe in it, and clean with it. Basically, humans can't live without it, and we are in contact with it all the time, so what do we do to make sure the water we use is as pollutant-free as possible?

Unfortunately, all water today contains some level of contamination, no matter where you get it. For example, I pulled this paragraph off the public health Web site for LA County: "All water—regardless of its source—contains some contaminants. A mountain stream, for example, might contain significant amounts of animal waste; a remote underground spring may have high levels of radon (a radioactive material present in certain types of rocks and soil that can seep into ground water)." They also go on to mention that water can contain everything from arsenic to mercury to E. coli and the like. Doesn't exactly make you want to drink up, right? It's true that bottled water isn't the perfect solution, and it doesn't make you immune. In fact, tap water is far more regulated than bottled water, and even if you buy the best bottled water on the planet, that's purified, alkalized, and infused with minerals and electrolytes (like Aqua Hydrate—I invested in this company for that very reason), you still wash your food and your body in tap water.

MORE PROOF THAT ENVIRONMENTAL CHEMICALS ARE HURTING US ALL!

Right before I finished the final edit of this book, I found out about a new article that recently appeared in a journal called *Environmental Health Perspectives.* This "Consensus Statement" came from dozens of united scientists in many different disciplines who all came together to demonstrate the extreme danger to children from many common environmental chemicals to which all people in the United States are regularly exposed. They say that these chemicals, many of which are commonly found in household products, medications, and in agriculture, place children in the United States "at an unacceptably high risk of developing neurodevelopmental disorders."[22] Yikes! The chemicals they list include many of those I mention in this chapter, including phthalates in plastics and common medications and lead and mercury in fertilizers. The main point that impressed me was that so many scientists all came together to get the word out about how detrimental the situation is, how vulnerable children are to these common compounds, and how urgent it is for the next generation that we take action to solve this critical problem. It is a call to action, and we should all listen!

Tap water is not all created equal. Some parts of the United States have excellent-quality tap water, but other parts do not. Municipal water suppliers must provide an annual report to their customers, and this report provides information on local drinking-water quality, including the levels of various contaminants found in the local water. Water quality reports can be obtained by contacting the supplier directly or through the EPA's search tool for your local water supply: epa.gov/ccr/ccr-information -consumers.

But even if your water checks out, I still recommend filters. Sadly, it's impossible to test for all potential contaminants—even though public water suppliers screen for more than 200 potential pollutants. And even if your water is good, your pipes might be leaching chemicals into your tap water. Yikes! So filter your water. There are many options, but the two I recommend as the most effective are:

Reverse osmosis filter on the house

Faucet-mounted carbon filter

Use them both for best results, and your tap water may be higher quality than that bottled water you've been buying (which is often just filtered tap water anyway).

LAPTOPS, CELL PHONES, AND OTHER ELECTRONICS: DANGEROUS FOR BABY?

Some people fear that electromagnetic fields (EMFs) or electromagnetic radiation (EMR) from laptop computers, cell phones, even televisions and clock radios are dangerous for health. This is a controversial subject, and there is no 100 percent solid evidence that these things affect human health, but some studies suggest that there *could* be health concerns.[23] A lot of the concern is probably hype meant to get you to buy products, and plenty of studies have shown no problem with these devices at all.[24] However, some studies suggest that there might be issues with constant exposure to these devices, especially for fetal health.[25] This may be an area where you want to be a little bit careful, just in case.

- You can buy radiation protection pads to put under your laptop if you frequently actually rest it on your body.[26]
- Don't rest your laptop on your pregnant belly, even with a pad.
- Don't keep electronics within a few feet of your body while you sleep.
- Don't set your cell phone on your pregnant belly, and keep it from making direct contact with your body most of the time, if you can. This is what the speaker-phone button and earbuds are for, people!
- Try not to spend more time than is necessary sitting in front of a screen, large or small. Whether or not the EMFs are harmful, there are healthier, happier

things you could be doing, like taking a walk or actually engaging in real human conversation. If you have a screen habit (scientists know screens are addictive!), it's probably better to break it now anyway, so you can set a good example for your future children.[27]

PERSONAL HYGIENE

For this section of the book, I defer to the great wisdom of my makeup artist and personal favorite green-beauty expert, Paige Padget, author of *The Green Beauty Rules*. Many personal-hygiene and beauty products are full of chemicals that soak into your skin and get into your system, but there are also many cleaner, greener choices. How do you know what to use? First of all, Paige says to avoid the Three Ps.

Parabens (prefixes: methyl, ethyl, propyl, butyl, and isopropyl) are used in about 99 percent of beauty products to prevent oxidation and kill bacteria and other living organisms harmful to humans. They are rapidly absorbed into the skin and metabolize and accumulate in the body. Parabens disrupt endocrine function by mimicking estrogen. Improper endocrine function can adversely affect metabolism, the nervous system, and blood sugar levels.

Perfume (fragrance, parfum) is a ubiquitous term often used to mask the use of hundreds of toxic chemicals. Fragrance can help a woman feel sexy, but it's loaded with petrochemicals and, often, chemicals called phthalates. Phthalates are endocrine disruptors. They mimic hormones and interfere with normal hormone production. Phthalates are linked to a birth defect in boys[28] in which the urethra opening develops on the underside of the penis rather than the tip. It occurs in roughly one of every 250 male births. Phthalates have also been linked to reduced sperm counts in men and early puberty in girls. Fragrance is in a wide variety of beauty products from moisturizers to makeup. Expecting mothers can reduce the risk by reading the ingredient label. If it contains the words *fragrance, perfume*, or *parfum*, avoid the product.

Petrochemicals can be identified by looking for the abbreviations PEG, DEA, and SLS, as well as *eth* and ingredients with an *x* or *y*; for example, ethylhexylglycerin. Petrochemicals appear on labels as mineral oil, petrolatum, and paraffin. They may contain known or suspected human carcinogens and harmful breakdown impurities from the manufacturing process that are not listed on labels, such as dioxin, posing health and environmental risks. Petrochemicals and their by-products have been known to cause or have been linked to serious health problems, including cancer, neuro- and respiratory toxicity, birth defects, and endocrine disruption. They can also cause allergic reactions and skin irritation.

Look for natural hygiene and beauty products without any of these P-words, and you are already on the right track. If you want more guidance, look for products that are EWG Verified. This means the Environmental Working Group has given them the thumbs-up because they are free of the chemicals the EWG believes are dangerous to human health and the environment, they disclose all their ingredients, and they follow good manufacturing practices.[29] The EWG also has a page that lists every kind of hygiene and beauty product it has approved. Find it here: ewg.org/skindeep/search .php?ewg_verified=products.

Paige's Picks

Want to do beauty like Paige does? Here are her favorite products and companies. Each of them meets her very high standards for chemical-free beauty. In the Resources section at the back of this book, you can find a much more extensive list of Paige-approved products and companies. This is just to get you started:

SKIN CARE

- Derma e Microdermabrasion Scrub
- Mad Hippie Vitamin C Serum
- Osea Eye Gel Serum

MAKEUP

- Beautycounter Color Define Brow Pencil
- Mineral Fusion Eyeliner
- W3ll People Narcissist Foundation Concealer Stick
- Burt's Bees Lip Crayon

HAIR CARE

- Shea Moisture Organic Raw Shea Butter Moisture Retention Shampoo
- John Masters Dry Hair Nourishment and Defrizzer
- Rahua Voluminous Hair Spray

BODY CARE

- Andalou Naturals Aloe Mint Cooling Shower Gel
- Burt's Bees Mama Bee Belly Butter

- Burt's Bees Mama Bee Leg & Foot Creme
- Burt's Bees Naturally Nourishing Milk & Shea Butter Body Bar
- Hugo Naturals Vanilla and Sweet Orange Massage and Body Oil
- Moom Natural Wax Strips

NAIL CARE

- Acquarella Water Color
- Burt's Bees Lemon Butter Cuticle Cream
- Deborah Lippmann Intensive Nail Treatment
- Scotch Non Toxic Nail Polish Remover

BABY CARE

- Burt's Bees Baby Bee Nourishing Lotion, Fragrance Free
- Burt's Bees Baby Bee Diaper Ointment
- Burt's Bees Baby Bee Shampoo & Wash, Fragrance Free
- Burt's Bees Baby Bee Wipes, Fragrance Free
- Butt Naked Baby Soothing Bath Soak
- California Baby Diaper Rash Cream
- Waxelene: The Petroleum Jelly Alternative

And that's a wrap for this chapter! It's possible these changes might seem daunting to you at first glance, but here's the good news: Once you change these things, they stay changed . . . forever! And you can feel good about the purity and quality of your environment, both during your pregnancy and as you raise your babies. Best of all, they will learn how important it is to live as chemical-free as possible, so they can teach future generations and maybe even save this beautiful planet of ours and all that call it home.

PART 2

The Yeah Baby!
HEALTHY PREGNANCY

CHAPTER 5

YOUR FIRST TRIMESTER:
The Eagle Has Landed!
(or the Grumpy Sleep Alien)

And here you are—pregnant. Right now, as you may be battling morning sickness or exhaustion, you may feel both envy and pity for me, knowing I have never had the experience of personally being pregnant. I will tell you now that this is one of the great regrets of my life, never to have had the privilege of growing an actual human. I wouldn't trade my kids for anything, but if life were a fairy tale and I got one wish, it would be to have grown them inside my belly. If and when the going gets tough at various points over the next 40 weeks, try to keep one amazing fact in mind: You are growing a human being, buddy. *Wow.* I am in awe.

But as you already know, I was at Heidi's side the entire time she was doing this most important job. Day in and day out, I was her cheerleader, confidante, and (intermittently and infrequently) her punching bag. (Okay, she never actually punched me, but admits to wanting to whenever she heard me chew during the first 3 months. I did get a solid shove once, during a particularly virulent bout of hormonal rage. Such is life. That story still makes for great dinner conversation. I suspect I am lucky to have gotten out of the whole experience alive. But I digress.) It is an honor to accompany you on your journey through this book and an honor to share my story with you as well.

It has begun. You did it. You are preggers, and you are probably looking ahead at the next 9 months with a combination of elation and trepidation. Even though you don't have a baby bump yet, there are major changes going on inside you during this trimester. You are growing your baby from a freaking zygote, a single fertilized cell, to an embryo that plants itself in your uterine wall, to a plum-size fetus sprouting arms and legs. Pretty cool, right?

Having said that, there are a bevy of "side effects" you could possibly experience during this time, like nausea (morning sickness, which doesn't necessarily happen in the morning), tender breasts (or even possibly tripling your cup size), food aversions, constant peeing, headaches, mood swings, fatigue, and many other symptoms that I'm sure will make you feel just completely overjoyed. The good news is that you might not have any side effects during your first trimester—and I have yet to meet a woman who suffers with *all* of them. Typically, women get hit with four to six of the traditional symptoms, and by the end of the trimester, they pass. Now, this is just my personal observation, based on having watched nearly all of my dearest friends go through the process, from first trimester to giving birth to beautiful babies. None of them have been hit with *every* symptom.

For us, I was convinced Heidi's body had been invaded by a sleep alien. She was *exhausted*. She would wake up, eat, take a nap, eat, take a nap, eat, konk out on the couch. She could barely keep her eyes open. I would literally be midsentence, and I'd look over to find her passed out, mouth agape, sawing away. Location was irrelevant. She could be sitting on the couch, the passenger seat of my car, the movie theater— anywhere, anyplace, anytime she could and did knock out.

Then came the spidey senses. The woman had the nose of a bloodhound. She would just blurt out things like, "Do you smell ballet slippers?" in the middle of a movie—at the movie theater. When I gave her my utterly confounded, are-you-insane look, she would begin questioning our neighbors in the theater for validation. (That did not go over well.) She even made the manager of a restaurant call the gas company one night because she was positive she smelled a gas leak.

Needless to say, we were not the most popular couple during this time period.

The onslaught of odors that affected her mood ran the gamut. Some could actually make her dry heave and others just "really pissed her off." Beer and dog food were the worst offenders. After she yakked in our kitchen sink while attempting to feed the dogs one night, that job was delegated to me—permanently. (I often wonder to this day if it was a ploy to get out of pet duty.)

I personally thought the cravings thing was hilarious. Some of them lasted her entire pregnancy, like ice chips—but *only* ice chips from Coffee Bean. I once made

Yeah Baby! REMEDY Headaches

If your head is aching, you may need more calcium and magnesium in your diet. For more calcium, try adding organic (or at least hormone-free) pasteurized cheese, yogurt, and dark leafy greens to your diet, as well as fortified coconut or almond milk. For magnesium, eat more pumpkin seeds, sesame seeds, pine nuts, almonds, beans and lentils, bananas, figs, brown rice, avocados, and up to two or three Brazil nuts per day.

Heidi Says . . .

My recollection is that the first trimester was pretty painless and nausea-free, although I don't remember much of it because I'm pretty sure I napped more than I had ever napped in my life. I was incredibly tired, but also overwhelmed with excitement. I didn't initially have any cravings, but then suddenly, the only things I wanted to eat were apples and oranges. Pretty boring, I know! My mind was also so focused on the baby growing inside of me. Was he the size of a pea, or a lentil, or a grape? Would I shake him loose if I ran too fast? No wine or caffeine for me, only organic food, and maybe some Häagen-Dazs peanut butter ice cream now and then. I remember that I did feel slightly like a crazy person.

When we traveled to Japan during this time, I longingly stared at the sushi until I discovered pumpkin ice cream and pumpkin curry. Jillian was afraid to even touch pumpkin curry after I professed my love for it—I wanted it all to myself! My emotions were all over the place, too. I may have shoved Jillian off the sidewalk and into the street at one point after one too many friendly taps on the bum, but I am not officially admitting this!

I also remember looking in the mirror and noticing a change in my stomach. I took many pregnancy photos. It's a strange feeling to have no control over what your body is doing and to just let it put on weight where it needs to. I quickly got over that issue, however, after I saw the bouncing little grape in the ultrasound. After that point, I grew to love my ever-growing bump and quickly changing body.

the mistake of bringing her crushed ice from our icemaker, and she looked at me like I was the world's biggest asshole. Others were fleeting, but momentarily all consuming. One night, she had to have pizza from our local pizza joint, with pineapple and feta cheese. But by the time I brought it home, she was crying because the thought of it suddenly made her want to gag.

Which brings me to the mood swings. I believe I alluded to this earlier when I mentioned she wanted to punch me for chewing my food. Don't be surprised at how the smallest things can elicit the biggest emotions during the first trimester. The Budweiser commercial with the puppy and the horse would bring her to hysterical sobs—which is ironic, considering how much she suddenly loathed the smell of beer.

And then there was the infamous "shove" incident. One night I playfully swatted Heidi on the bum, like I had done at least, oh, about 100,000 times before. Sexist, I know—but as a woman, I'd always managed to get away with it!

Until that day.

Before my hand even recoiled off her butt cheek, she spun around on her heels, eyes possessed, and shoved me with the strength of 1,000 demons escaping the ninth circle of hell. She launched my unassuming ass across the street and then rushed to hover over me. As I sat there stunned, I watched Heidi transform into Linda Blair from *The Exorcist* as she growled, *"Don't do that."*

Needless to say, I never did again.

Luckily, her nausea was minimal, but she had back pain, both upper and lower. She would constantly gaze at me with the puppy dog eyes and prod me to "rub." And there I found myself, rubbing tight shoulders and a sore lower back—for hours on end. Funny enough, no matter how tired she was, the one thing that was sure to wake her up was when I *stopped* rubbing. To this day, I still have thumbs of steel.

Now that you are good and excited about what's to come, let me preface by reiterating that all the symptoms *will* pass—they did for Heidi, and they will for you, too. In the meantime, in the following pages, let's take a closer look at what's happening to you—and to your baby.

Yeah Baby! REMEDY *Morning Sickness*

If you are suffering from morning sickness, vitamin B_6 may help you feel a whole lot better. Great food sources are turkey, chicken, brown rice, bananas, wild-caught salmon, blackstrap molasses, avocado, and pumpkin seeds. Certain types of herbal teas are also helpful. Try ginger, lemon, mint, or chamomile tea when your stomach is feeling the heave-ho.

Ginger in particular is probably the most effective of the herbal teas for nausea. Some Canadian researchers recently decided to analyze the medical research to see what real evidence there was for this reliable rhizome alleviating the wooziness associated with morning sickness in the first trimester of pregnancy. Scouring the combined results of six different studies where 508 women were randomly assigned to use ginger daily to relieve their upset stomachs, the researchers found that using ginger for 4 days straight was associated with a fivefold likelihood of improvement in symptoms.[1] You can make your own ginger tea by boiling 1 tablespoon of chopped raw ginger in 2 cups of water for 5 to 10 minutes. Strain before drinking.[2]

QUICK LIST: WHAT TO ASK YOUR DOCTOR IN THE FIRST TRIMESTER

If you didn't visit the doctor before you were pregnant, definitely see your doctor or nurse midwife by the 8th week of pregnancy and then every 4 to 6 weeks after that. If you are newly pregnant and have only a primary care physician, this is also the time to do some research to find a good ob-gyn and, if you also want to use one, a midwife and/or a doula. Ask for recommendations and talk to people you know, including your primary care physician, about who would be good to enlist for your birth team. Keep in mind that you will want someone whose philosophies are in line with yours—for instance, if you want a more natural birth experience, make sure your doctor will be open to your preferences. Here are a few things to review and some additional suggestions:

- During this trimester, your healthcare provider will screen you for anemia, determine your blood count and blood type, and check you for diseases (such as hepatitis and STDs) as well as immunity to rubella.[3] You will be notified of any abnormal results, but you can also ask if you are worried.

- List your current medicines (both prescription, supplement, and herbal) and ask if they are safe for baby.

- If your doctor does not counsel you about pregnancy diet and exercise, mention your current meal plan and fitness routine and ask for suggestions and advice.

- Go over your current vaccinations. If you are missing any, ask whether it's important to undergo them now or whether you should wait until after your baby's birth.[4]

- If you feel incredibly nauseated or fatigued or are having any other symptoms that worry you or don't seem normal to you, mention them. Don't be nervous— your doctor has already heard it all. Also ask for advice on relieving these symptoms without harming your growing baby.[5]

- Talk about your birth plan to make sure your physician and you are on the same page. For example, if you hope to have a natural childbirth or a water birth, check to see if your physician is supportive of that. If you aren't sure, ask about birth options.

- If you bleed at all during this stage of pregnancy, mention it to your healthcare provider. Some spotting is normal, but it never hurts to get it checked.

- Ask for your due date.

- Find out how much weight is healthy for you to gain throughout your pregnancy.

- If you are on a special diet (such as vegetarian or vegan), mention it and ask your doctor if any special supplements are needed.

- Mention any family history of genetic conditions such as cystic fibrosis and ask about the pros and cons of genetic counseling for someone with your family background.

DEVELOPMENT IN THE FIRST TRIMESTER: WEEKS 1 TO 4

We think of pregnancy as a process that typically lasts 40 weeks, or just over 9 months—from the time of your last period to the moment of childbirth.[6] We talk about these 9 months in terms of trimesters, but here's a little known fact: The trimester system actually stems from the famous abortion case Roe v. Wade! The lawyers argued that dividing pregnancy into trimesters allows doctors to more easily discuss and compare the development of the baby and the health of the mom.[7] However, when it comes to tracking your baby's rapid growth and development, I think it's easier to look at it week by week.

In these sections, I just want to take a second to appreciate all the cool changes that are going on inside your body—what a miracle!

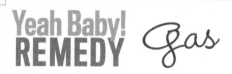

Yeah Baby! REMEDY *Gas*

Nobody will point it out, but you may suddenly be feeling extra gassy these days, and those early pregnancy rips can really clear the room! To avoid the embarrassment, not to mention the discomfort, eat more foods containing good bacteria to feed your gut and digestive enzymes to help your body process your food without so many gastrointestinal . . . hiccups. You can take a probiotic supplement, but even better, eat more yogurt and kefir. For digestive enzymes, add papaya, pineapple, mango, and pasteurized honey to your diet. You could also try alfalfa tea and peppermint tea, both of which are known for reducing intestinal gas.

What's Happening to Me?

Some women don't even realize they are pregnant during this early stage (all the more reason to take great care of yourself as soon as you start trying to get pregnant). If you're really tuned into your body, you may experience symptoms like tender and swollen breasts as early as 1 week after conception. Within 6 to 12 days of conception, as many as 25 percent of women have slight bleeding that is a lighter color than their regular period, which is caused by the implantation of the fertilized egg.[8] It's nothing at all to worry about!

Once your body realizes that an egg is fertilized, you start to produce more estrogen and progesterone. These hormones help prepare your womb to house the fetus and encourage the milk glands to develop in the breasts. But these extra hormones can already make you feel a little nuts—they can cause headaches, mood swings, and food cravings or strong aversions to some foods. To support the baby, your body will need a lot of extra blood, so you will produce human chorionic gonadotropin to increase blood volume—and all this extra bloodflow may make you feel tired and dizzy and constantly needing to pee in these early weeks.

Also, your stomach starts preparing for the food to be diverted to your growing fetus, so your stomach takes longer to empty, allowing nutrients additional time to absorb into the bloodstream and head toward your baby. This digestive slowdown may give you heartburn or constipation (the bane of up to 38 percent of all pregnant women).[9, 10] Morning sickness is common during this trimester and will probably vanish by the 4th month of pregnancy. Until then, some doctors suggest you eat frequent, small meals to keep your blood sugar stable.[11] Other ways you can help alleviate morning sickness are to stay hydrated, avoid artificial sweeteners (I hope you've already quit the stuff anyway), and consider trying seasickness wristbands like Sea Band or Travel Eze that stimulate antinausea acupressure points. Heidi never took these off for the entire first trimester. She swears by them.

Another common symptom is fatigue. If you feel sleepy and wiped out, give in to the urge to nap whenever possible. Lack of sleep during pregnancy can disrupt your immune system, leading to a lower birth weight, University of Pittsburgh research has found.[12] And if you just feel like total crap with severe nausea, vomiting, and fatigue, so much so that you are losing weight, feeling faint, and getting dehydrated, it's possible you have an uncommon condition called *hyperemesis gravidarum*. This is a fancy term for extreme morning sickness, and it can sometimes necessitate a quick visit to the hospital to replenish fluids and nutrients or receive medication to reduce the nausea and vomiting.[13] This is what briefly hospitalized Kate Middleton, the Duchess of Cambridge, during both of her pregnancies, but everything turned out just fine both times. If this does happen to you, you are in royal company.

What's Going On in There?

Thanks to advanced home pregnancy tests and ovulation kits, you may know you are pregnant long before your body gives any indication. These early stages of pregnancy are very tender, and you need to baby yourself. Nature makes sure the conditions are really optimal before she commits, in order to ensure the health of the mommy and the health of the baby. For this reason, miscarriage is very common. As many as half of all pregnancies can end in miscarriage (often, before anyone ever knew there was a pregnancy), and up to 25 percent of recognized pregnancies end in miscarriage, most within the first 3 months.[14] And it's not your fault. It happens. It's heartbreaking. Should you endure this, please know that you are not alone, and I stress again, it's *not your fault*.

If you are wondering what you can do to be proactive and prevent this from happening, you are already doing it. By following all the guidelines to reduce exposure to harmful chemicals and toxins that I outlined in the earlier chapters, as well as working with your doctor to control diabetes and high blood pressure, you are optimizing your body's ability to create a nurturing environment for your baby to develop in your womb.

As for what's happening inside your uterus, the sperm and egg are getting busy, uniting to form a zygote. This can take up to 2 weeks. If you got pregnant using infertility treatments, add 2 weeks to the date of conception to determine the gestational age of your fetus (your fetus has a head start!).[15]

Once fertilization occurs, the zygote travels down the Fallopian tube to the uterus and begins rapidly dividing to form a cluster of cells that will become a blastocyst. Around week 4, the blastocyst divides into two sections—the inner group of cells becomes the embryo, and the outer group of cells nourishes and protects the embryo. The blastocyst nestles into the uterine wall (implantation), and the placenta forms.[16]

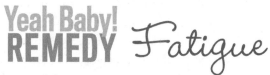

Yeah Baby! REMEDY Fatigue

Feeling dead to the world? B vitamins and iron to the rescue! These are known to provide energy, so load up on B-rich and iron-rich foods like beef, pork, chicken, turkey, lamb, wild-caught salmon, sunflower seeds, pumpkin seeds, bananas, and brown rice. Dehydration can also contribute to fatigue, so up your water intake to about 10 cups per day. You may find you can face the day much more easily when you are fully hydrated.

TRUE or FALSE If you have no morning sickness, you're more likely to be carrying a boy.

More likely to be true (but not a guarantee)! According to a British study that examined the medical records of close to 10,000 women who experienced a form of extreme morning sickness called *hyperemesis gravidarum,* women affected were more likely to be carrying girls than boys.[17] However, experiencing no morning sickness at all doesn't necessarily mean you're carrying a boy—you're just lucky. (And again, Kate Middleton, the Duchess of Cambridge, had this condition during both pregnancies and had a boy first and then a girl, so . . . not always true!)

At the end of this month, your embryo is ready to start the intense work of growing into a fetus!

DEVELOPMENT IN THE FIRST TRIMESTER: WEEKS 5 TO 8

Things are gearing up, and you are starting to notice. Here's what's going on inside.

What's Happening to Me?

When week 6 hits, you may feel the side effects of pregnancy in full force—all those earlier twinklings of tiredness and picky eating now morph into extreme fatigue, tender aching breasts, and full-on morning sickness (complete with your daily visits of nausea and sometimes vomiting).[18] During the 7th week, you develop the aptly named mucus plug—a blob of mucus that plugs up the opening of the cervical canal to seal off the uterus, keeping your fetus safely protected. That handy mucus plug will stay firmly in place until the cervix dilates during labor.[19]

If you haven't already met with your doctor, this second month is when you absolutely must get in there. Your caregiver will assess your overall health and set a schedule for regular checkups (usually every 4 to 6 weeks).[20] Be prepared to discuss your family history and schedule various screening tests.

What's Going On in There?

The 5th week is when the real fun begins: Your baby's brain, spinal cord, and heart begin to develop.[21] The embryo consists of three parts:

- The ectoderm, or top layer, will become skin, nervous systems, eyes, ears, and connective tissues.
- The mesoderm, or inner layers, will turn into the heart and circulatory system, bones, muscles, kidneys, and the reproductive system.
- The endoderm, or inner layer, will morph into the lungs, intestines, and bladder.[22]

Crazy, right?

By the 6th and 7th weeks, the gastrointestinal tract begins to develop and teeny-weeny buds emerge where arms and legs will soon form. But right now, the embryo is still tiny, measuring $\frac{1}{25}$ inch long.[23] (Seriously, imagine that—1 inch separated into 25 pieces. Just *one* of those pieces is your kid!)

Eyes and ears start to form, and the miniscule heart manages to find a regular rhythm circulating blood through a very basic system.[24] In week 8, the arms and legs have grown enough to distinguish tiny hands and feet, but the fingers and toes are still webbed. The lungs begin to form while the brain continues to develop.[25] The upper lip and nose are formed, and the eyes are visible.[26] Unbelievable.

DEVELOPMENT IN THE FIRST TRIMESTER: WEEKS 9 TO 12

You are almost at the end of your first trimester—a major milestone! This is when many women finally start telling people they are pregnant.

TRUE or FALSE If you have heartburn, your baby will be born with a full head of hair.

Maybe a little bit true? Surprisingly, there may be some evidence to support this old wives' tale. Doctors at Johns Hopkins in Baltimore followed a small sample of 64 pregnant women and asked them to rank the severity of their heartburn. Most of the women reported some degree of heartburn, and the amount seemed unrelated to the baby's gender or any common characteristics the mothers shared related to their age or weight. However, when the researchers asked an independent panel to evaluate photographs of each newborn in the study to assess how much hair the babies had at birth, the heartburn-hair connection was significant. Most of the women who reported moderate to severe heartburn gave birth to babies with average or above-average amounts of hair; those lucky women who were heartburn-free were more likely to have baldies.[27] Don't ask me why!

Dr. Suzanne Says . . .

Noninvasive Prenatal Testing, or NIPT, is a great new option for expectant parents because it is a simple blood test that is 99.9 percent accurate in determining Down syndrome risk, as well as certain other genetic conditions, and carries absolutely no risk to the mom or to the pregnancy. It can also tell you the baby's sex at just 10 weeks, long before an ultrasound could tell you.

NIPT is an interesting test. It looks at fetal cells in circulation in the mom's blood, and we can identify which cells are the mom's and which are the fetal cells. The fetal cells are then examined for missing or extra chromosomes. If you were to have a positive result, then this would suggest the need for amniocentesis or chorionic villus sampling (CVS) to confirm. Otherwise, these invasive tests would be unnecessary.

Today, anyone over age 35 should be offered this test, and some offices (like mine) offer it to everyone, at any age. If your doctor doesn't offer it to you, just ask. I am of the belief that all pregnant women should be able to benefit from the information this test reveals.

What's Happening to Me?

As early as 10 weeks, you can do a noninvasive prenatal test (NIPT) that tests your blood to look for signs of genetic abnormality in the fetus. Dr. Suzanne Gilberg-Lenz, our resident ob-gyn, says that the NIPT is actually replacing most of the more invasive preliminary screening tests like chorionic villus sampling (CVS) and amniocentesis. The reason this test is so great is that a clear result can mean you don't have to worry, and you never have to put your pregnancy at even a tiny risk due to testing. The NIPT is especially important if you are older than 35 or have genetic issues in your family, but Dr. Suzanne thinks it should be offered to every pregnant woman because it is completely safe—just a simple blood test.

If, however, there is any indication of an abnormality on the NIPT test, this is a good reason to do CVS or amniocentesis, depending on the nature of the results. These tests are both more invasive but are definitive in diagnosing genetic abnormalities (the NIPT is more of a screening test).

The CVS test involves taking a sample of the chorionic villi from the placenta, which is done through the vagina or through an incision in the abdomen. This can let you know whether your baby has a chromosomal condition, such as Down syndrome or cystic fibrosis. This test is done earlier than other tests that provide this information (like amniocentesis), which is preferable in case the information would affect how the parents choose to manage the pregnancy.

There are some cases where you might want to jump straight to the CVS test without first doing NIPT:

- If you and your partner are both carriers for cystic fibrosis or Tay-Sachs disease or you both carry any other serious or life-threatening genetic disorder that is autosomally recessive (you both need to have the gene), and you want to know whether the baby will be affected.

- If either you or your partner has a known history of a serious life-threatening autosomal dominant genetic disorder (such as hemophilia), and you want to know if the baby will be affected.

In either of these cases, CVS can cut to the chase. (Simple blood or saliva tests can determine whether you or your spouse are carriers of these genetic diseases.) Your doctor would likely schedule the CVS between 10½ to 13 weeks, according to Dr. Suzanne.

What's Going On in There?

This month, your tiny C-shaped embryo will begin to look more like a fetus. In the 9th week, nipples, hair follicles, and organs begin to form, and elbows and

 TRUE or FALSE Avoid hot baths, which can cause birth defects.

Partially true. Here's an example of one myth that's rooted in a bit of truth. Because a core body temperature more than 101°F can present some risks during pregnancy, most experts agree that pregnant women should avoid prolonged soaks in hot water during the first trimester when certain heat-related birth defects are possible. However, for the average healthy pregnancy, a short soak in a warm bath can be an ideal way to relax and unwind. Hot tubs, on the other hand, which are usually set to maintain a steady temperature of 104°F, are far more likely to lead to this sort of rise in body temperature and are best avoided throughout pregnancy.[28, 29] So skip the hot tub. They are full of chemicals to keep them from growing bacteria anyway, so best not to soak in that chemical stew right now, no matter what the temperature.

toes are visible.[31] By the 10th week, the fetus begins to form a face, with eyelids and ears taking shape.[32] The head becomes more round and a neck begins to develop.[33] Once you reach the end of this 10th week, you officially end the "embryonic period" and begin the "fetal period." During the 11th week, the body of the fetus will grow rapidly—limbs are long and thin, although the head still makes up half the size of your baby.[34] The eyelids are fully formed, and red blood cells sprout up in the liver. His or her little penis or vagina will also start to develop![35] By the end of this trimester, all of your baby's major organs will have formed, as well as limbs, hands, and a nose. Your baby will even have soft fingernails by week 12.[36]

FIRST TRIMESTER NUTRITION

Yes, you are eating for two now . . . but, no, I am not talking about calories. Hopefully you recall from our Rules of Thumb nutrition chapter that it takes only about

80,000 calories to make a baby—which breaks down to just a few hundred more calories a day (depending on the trimester). That's not much, folks.

What I am referring to when I say "eating for two" are the foods that comprise the Yeah, Baby! meal plan. These foods not only help you achieve optimal health, manage any pregnancy symptoms, and facilitate an easy rebound to your "pre-baby" body, but they also support your little one in every way to grow and develop as healthy and strong as possible. So eat the good stuff. Here are some do's and don'ts for you to remember at this crucial developmental stage of your pregnancy. Let's start with the don'ts and get that negativity out of your life right away.

First Trimester Nutrition Don'ts

- **Don't: Eat any of the chemicals or crap** we covered in the Rules of Thumb nutrition chapter.

- **Don't: Eat a ton of processed carbs** like white flour, white rice, white sugar, or the like. These types of foods spike and subsequently crash your blood sugar, leaving you feeling completely wiped out. Dr. Suzanne says they can also increase rebound nausea. (Processed foods are usually loaded with preservatives and crap that should be avoided regardless.)

- **Don't: Consume foods that are high in sodium.** High-sodium foods cause water retention, which will make any part of you that's swollen and bloated that much more swollen and bloated.

- **Don't: Get too full—or too hungry.** An empty tummy can increase feelings of nausea, but so can an overly full belly. Make sure to eat balanced, regular portions of food every 3 to 4 hours.

- **Don't: Consume greasy foods** or a large amount of saturated fat from animal protein. These foods can increase symptoms of "morning" sickness (ha! more like "all-day" sickness) as well as expand your waistline. Lean proteins, such as chicken or turkey breast or leaner cuts of grass-fed beef, lamb, or pork, are best at this time.

- **Don't: Eat "dangerous" foods.** Remember, while it's always a good idea to prevent illness and disease, it's particularly important to take special precautions now. As a result, steer clear of soft cheese made from unpasteurized milk, raw eggs (no sneaking bites of raw cookie dough or cake batter!), sushi and other raw fish or shellfish, unpasteurized juice or milk, unpasteurized honey, raw sprouts, and store-bought salads that may contain E. coli, listeria, and other bugs.[37]

First Trimester Nutrition Do's

Now for the good stuff. Here's what to build your meals around. I've already talked about a lot of these in the Rules of Thumb nutrition chapter, but these are the particular foods and nutrients to focus on right now:

- **Do: Eat complex carbohydrates and high-fiber foods** in their most natural state, with their nutrients and fiber still intact. Think whole grain breads, pastas, and cereals, beans and legumes, fruits, and vegetables. In other words, you want foods in or close to their natural forms that have not been stripped of their nutrients. Their high fiber content ensures they break down more slowly, giving you a stabilized release of blood sugar and therefore a stable energy supply. A Harvard study of more than 13,000 female nurses found that eating at least 28 grams of fiber a day may help prevent gestational diabetes, which can cause preeclampsia.[38] Particularly great sources of fiber include all legumes (pinto, black, white, Great Northern, split peas, lentils, and kidney beans) and raspberries (8 grams per cup, more than some beans and bran cereals, surprisingly!).[39] And remember, this added fiber will also help minimize constipation.

- **Do: Eat iron-rich foods.** Foods rich in iron help to fend off fatigue, headaches, and shortness of breath, as well as improve your mood. In addition, women who are anemic run a greater risk of a preterm delivery, so keep the iron coming.

Yeah Baby! REMEDY *Constipation*

If you are feeling a little stopped up lately, it's probably because so many things are changing in your body right now that your digestive tract can't quite keep up. The remedy is more fiber, magnesium, and probiotics. For fiber, try prunes, beans, lentils, peas, sun-dried tomatoes, artichokes, broccoli, chia seeds, hemp seeds, carrots, whole grains, berries, oatmeal, and organic air-popped popcorn. Also drink more water! A magnesium citrate supplement every evening can also help to get the action going, but magnesium-rich foods like seeds and nuts, dark leafy greens, beans and lentils, avocados, bananas, figs, and brown rice will also help. Finally, add more probiotics with yogurt and kefir, and pour a little more extra-virgin olive oil on your salads.

Iron is also essential in the production of hemoglobin in red blood cells, which brings oxygen and nutrients to your baby. Remember that your body is in the process of increasing your blood volume, and iron supports that. Vitamin C is well known for helping increase iron absorption, so many of the Yeah, Baby! recipes include citrus with an iron source. (See a list of iron-rich foods on page 73 in the Rules of Thumb nutrition chapter.)

- **Do: Be sure to get enough vitamin D,** which promotes healthy birth weight and bone formation and strength. A 2012 Spanish study found that low vitamin D during the first and second trimester was linked to lower cognitive and motor skills scores in babies at 14 months of age. Other studies from the same researchers found a lowered risk of attention deficit disorder in children whose mothers had higher levels of D.[40] Vitamin D also helps your body maintain healthy levels of bone-preserving calcium and phosphorus. Canadian researchers found evidence that low vitamin D in the first trimester predicted the risk of gestational diabetes, which ups your risk of preeclampsia and preterm birth, and you *and* your baby's risk of developing type 2 diabetes later in life. Your prenatal vitamin will likely have vitamin D, but ask your doctor about additional supplementation as well. Also, get some vitamin D the natural way: Get outside for 15 minutes of direct sunlight! You can also get extra D from salmon, fortified milk or almond milk, egg yolks, and shiitake mushrooms.[41]

- **Do: Consume potassium-rich foods** to help flush out bloat, keeping electrolytes and fluids in balance as your blood and other fluid volume increases.

Cheryl Says . . .

Our crackerjack registered dietitian, Cheryl Forberg (who would probably never eat Cracker Jack!), has this to say about iron supplementation.

I'm always careful not to recommend iron supplementation until I know the medical doctor recommends it due to an iron deficiency or anemia. Don't self-dose with iron supplements while pregnant, ever. Your prenatal vitamin probably contains just enough, and too much iron can interfere with your body's ability to absorb other minerals, cause gastrointestinal symptoms, and create other issues.[42]

But don't worry about potassium supplements—find a balance through food, because too much potassium causes its own problems.[43, 44] Ginger has 8.3 mg of potassium per teaspoon, doing double duty to help manage morning sickness. Beets, tomato paste and puree, halibut, winter squash, pork loin, cantaloupe, canned clams, leafy green salads, yogurt, avocados, and bananas are all rich in potassium.[45]

- **Do: Choose foods rich in vitamin B$_6$ if you have morning sickness.** Studies have found 30 mg of B$_6$ helpful in preventing and easing the nausea and vomiting of morning sickness.[46] B$_6$ may also prevent preterm birth and miscarriage. Familiar healthy-food staples—chickpeas, sockeye salmon, spinach, banana, avocado, pistachios, pumpkin seeds, turkey, and chicken—are all good sources of B$_6$. Even marinara sauce has some![47]

- **Do: Have plenty of foods high in folate**—but also take your supplemental folic acid (the supplemental form of folate). Although, in general, bodies tend to absorb vitamins from food more readily than from supplements, there is some evidence that folate is an exception.[48] That's why the supplement known as folic acid is so important. Still, it doesn't hurt to have dietary backup. Folic acid helps prevent megaloblastic anemia in pregnancy, which can be caused by folate deficiency sometimes brought on by morning sickness, so it's good to have an increased amount of folate right now, when your baby needs it for nervous system development.[49] Folic acid will also give you some extra energy in this exhausting first trimester. One surprisingly good source of folate is that satisfying favorite, avocado.[50] (See many more folate-rich foods on page 72 in the Rules of Thumb nutrition chapter.)

- **Do: Get enough calcium and magnesium.** Shoot for 1,000 mg of calcium and 350 mg of magnesium to help relax muscles and fend off any headaches or leg cramps, regulate blood sugar, and prevent preeclampsia. These minerals also support your baby's nerve development, as well as his or her ability to grow strong bones and teeth. Magnesium contributes to normal functioning of more than 300 enzymes in the baby's body. You can get calcium from dairy products, kale, bok choy, canned sardines (eat the soft bones), and tahini. Good magnesium sources include quinoa, almonds, cashews, spinach, peanuts, and edamame.[51, 52] (See page 76 for more calcium- and magnesium-rich foods.)

- **Do: Eat enough foods that contain provitamin A (carotenoids from plant-based foods).** Carotenoids from fruits and vegetables are important during the first trimester. Vitamin A facilitates a host of very important processes during your baby's embryonic growth, including protecting the process of cell division itself. Foods like melon, dark leafy greens, sweet potatoes, carrots, tomatoes, apricots, peaches, and red peppers are rich and safe sources of carotenoids, which your body converts to vitamin A.

Note of caution: Do not attempt to get excessive amounts of vitamin A by taking beta-carotene supplements. High doses could cause birth defects for baby and liver toxicity for you. Eating carotenoid-rich food such as fruits and vegetables carries none of this risk, so this is definitely a place to go totally natural with food instead of supplements.

- **Do: Consume foods rich in DHA and EPA or omega-3 fatty acids.** We've discussed this quite a bit, but your baby's brain and eyes are worth it! Lamb is a good source of DHA. Wild salmon, sardines, anchovies, trout, and walnuts are also good and safe sources of EPA. Flaxseed is a good source of ALA (alpha-linolenic acid), which your body can convert to omega-3, but this is not as complete a form as what you will get from fish, plus it's not the most efficient conversion process.[53] If you can eat animal sources of omega-3 fatty acids, you will be getting a more sure and consistent source.

- **Do: Be sure you get your iodine.** Iodine contributes to the production of thyroid hormones, which are critical for development of the fetal and neonatal brain. The fetus is dependent on its mother's stores of iodine and thyroid hormone in early pregnancy. A deficiency can result in mental retardation, physical retardation, and deafness.[54] Thyroid hormones also help promote bone formation and fetal growth and prevent low birth weight and preterm birth.[55] Iodized sea salt, seafood, and dried seaweed are all good sources.

- **Do: Try to eat foods rich in vitamin B$_{12}$,** which is vital for brain development. Organic meats like beef and lamb are the best way to go on this one. If you are a vegan, be sure to eat foods fortified with B$_{12}$, like some nut milks and cereals.

- **Do: Hydrate often.** Drink water until your pee is almost clear, like watered-down lemonade. Proper hydration can help fend off fatigue, headaches, and bloat. Noshing on ice chips and sipping (and smelling!) lemon water have also been shown to help manage nausea.[56]

The Yeah Baby! MEAL PLANS

We covered the majority of our eating guidelines in Chapter 2, Rules of Thumb: Nutrition for Prepregnancy, Pregnancy, and Beyond, and the entire Yeah Baby! menu plan and all the recipes have been created to reflect those rules, while adding foods that are particularly good for providing the specific nutrients you and your baby need right now, in your first trimester. I've tried to keep the menu plan as simple and satisfying as possible, so you can maximize your napping time and minimize any time in the kitchen.

To keep things ultra simple, I have listed which weeks to use each week of recipes. For example, the first week of recipes is for Weeks 1, 5, and 9. This way, you won't ever get tired of those particular recipes, but you will also get more familiar with them; after you've made them a few times, they will feel like second nature to make. You might also notice that some recipes are repeated more than once in the different charts—these are some of my favorites that I think are particularly delicious, nutritious, and easy to make, so I use them a little more often. I know you will find your particular favorites, too.

Which brings me to another point: You do not have to adhere to the menu plan as the be-all, end-all. Although this is an excellent nutrition plan to follow when you need one, of course, I still want you to be able to go out to dinner, try other recipes from other books and mommy Web sites, repeat your favorites from this plan more often than I have listed, and just continue to eat your favorite healthy foods in general. I don't want you to obsess over this list or feel like you have to be "perfect"! Take it easy on yourself. Simply use the nutrition Rules of Thumb as your general guide about how much and what types of foods to eat, as well as which foods and chemicals you should try to avoid. Think of your trimester meal plans as a foundation to build upon, a secret blueprint to giving your baby every edge available to be smarter, stronger, and healthier, for life. Feel free to swap in any week for another week, if you find a particular week or recipe hits all the right craving notes for you.

Please refer to Appendix A starting on page 271 for the recipes. Also, if you need more recipe ideas, check out our nutritionist Cheryl Forberg's cookbook *Flavor First*. All of her scrumptious recipes are *Yeah Baby!* friendly and use only natural ingredients to support mama's health and baby's growth.

Meal Plan 1 Weeks 1, 5, 9

	BREAKFAST	LUNCH	SNACK	DINNER
MONDAY	B4 Power Parfait	Mediterranean Chicken Sandwich	Bangin' Bruschetta	Argentine Salmon
TUESDAY	Huevos Tacos	Slammin' Turkey Sammy	Devilish Deviled Eggs with Watermelon	Steak Chimichurri
WEDNESDAY	Maple Pecan Porridge	BBQ Steak Salad	Organic Jerky (purchased)	Lemon Lamb Chop
THURSDAY	The California Poach	Quick and Easy Fish Tacos	Super Mommy Mix	Veggie Pasta
FRIDAY	Lori and Jamie's Feel-Good Muffin	Chicken Burrito Bowl	Cheese Plate	Baked Trout
SATURDAY	Apple Zucchini Flap Jacks with Turkey Bacon	Chicken Chop	Fruity Gazpacho	Thai Steak
SUNDAY	Baby Booster Smoothie	Chicken Artichoke Pizza	Awesome Artichoke	The Ultimate Turkey Burger

Meal Plan 2 Weeks 2, 6, 10

	BREAKFAST	LUNCH	SNACK	DINNER
MONDAY	Hot Mama Smoothie	Chicken Chop	Veggies and Dip	Peach Pork Chop with Fennel Salad
TUESDAY	B4 Power Parfait	Summer Shrimp Salad	Cottage Cheese and Peaches	The Ultimate Turkey Burger
WEDNESDAY	The California Poach	Chicken Burrito Bowl	Hummus and Pita Chips (purchased)	Veggie Pasta
THURSDAY	Baby Booster Smoothie	Slaw Salad	Red Ants on a Log	Thai Steak
FRIDAY	Feta Frittata	Chicken Parmesan Orzo Salad	Chocolate Cherry Smoothie	Lemon Lamb Chop
SATURDAY	Apple Zucchini Flap Jacks with Turkey Bacon	Chicken Artichoke Pizza	Super Mommy Mix	Baked Trout
SUNDAY	Breakfast Bowl	Slammin' Turkey Sammy	Fruity Gazpacho	Steak Chimichurri

Meal Plan 3 Weeks 3, 7, 11

	BREAKFAST	LUNCH	SNACK	DINNER
MONDAY	Maple Pecan Porridge	Quick and Easy Fish Tacos	Beat-the-Bloat Baked Potato	Argentine Salmon
TUESDAY	The California Poach	Chicken Chop	Organic Jerky (purchased)	Veggie Pie
WEDNESDAY	Hot Mama Smoothie	Slaw Salad	Cottage Cheese and Peaches	Peach Pork Chop with Fennel Salad
THURSDAY	Breakfast Bowl	Mediterranean Chicken Sandwich	Bangin' Bruschetta	Thai Steak
FRIDAY	Feta Frittata	Summer Shrimp Salad	Super Mommy Mix	Mussels Marinara
SATURDAY	Lori and Jaime's Feel-Good Muffin	BBQ Steak Salad	Cheese Plate	Veggie Pasta
SUNDAY	Apple Zucchini Flap Jacks with Turkey Bacon	Slammin' Turkey Sammy	Chocolate Cherry Smoothie	Lemon Lamb Chop

Meal Plan 4 Weeks 4, 8, 12

	BREAKFAST	LUNCH	SNACK	DINNER
MONDAY	Bad A$$ Breakfast Burrito	Chicken Parmesan Orzo Salad	Cottage Cheese and Peaches	Veggie Pie
TUESDAY	Lori and Jaime's Feel-Good Muffin	Chicken Burrito Bowl	Super Mommy Mix	Peach Pork Chop with Fennel Salad
WEDNESDAY	Apple Zucchini Flap Jacks with Turkey Bacon	Quick and Easy Fish Tacos	Devilish Deviled Eggs with Watermelon	Lemon Lamb Chop
THURSDAY	Huevos Tacos	Chicken Artichoke Pizza	Hummus and Pita Chips (purchased)	Steak Chimichurri
FRIDAY	B4 Power Parfait	Slammin' Turkey Sammy	Veggies and Dip	Mussels Marinara
SATURDAY	Hot Mama Smoothie	BBQ Steak Salad	Beat-the-Bloat Baked Potato	Baked Trout
SUNDAY	Feta Frittata	Slaw Salad	Organic Jerky (purchased)	Argentine Salmon

FIRST TRIMESTER FITNESS

Now you may be wondering, "What about that slammin' mama body Jillian promised?" Fitness is where this happens! This is not the time to worry about looking hot, however. (You probably do anyway, by the way—you have that pregnancy glow, even if you feel sick and bloated!) However, fitness now and throughout your pregnancy will do so many great things for you that it is totally worth the investment of time and energy. You will get through all of it more easily, you will feel strong, it may help prevent any possibility of gestational diabetes,[57] and when it's all over, you will have a much swifter transition back to your prepregnancy state (or even better).

You already know the Fitness Rules of Thumb we covered in Chapter 3, and all of those rules still apply. However, for the first trimester, we are going to customize even more precisely based on what you need and what you can do right now. We'll start with some fitness solutions for some common first trimester issues, go through

Andy Says . . .

Our esteemed pregnancy personal trainer, Andrea Orbeck, otherwise known as Andy, has this advice for exercise during the first trimester:

The first trimester is the time to maintain and solidify the form and skill you will need in the latter trimesters, when the maintenance of strength is so necessary for the rapid spinal and physiological changes caused by a growing fetus. Deadlifts and rows are super important now. You will lose your posture faster than at any other time in your life while pregnant, so building postural strength in the first trimester is crucial to maintaining it later. Also, it might seem there is no point in working your abs right now because you are going to "lose" them during pregnancy, but core conditioning builds you a muscular "corset" that literally supports the lumbar, which is the hinge we use all day, every day. Add a 20-pound baby strapped to you in a carrier, and your back will thank you for preparing for what feels like a Navy SEALs weight vest!

In other words, exercising now is incredibly functional for the pregnant woman! The moves in the exercise program for this trimester set a thorough foundation to build the necessary strength. Just remember to take your time, breathe, and modify any position that feels uncomfortable.

the do's and don'ts, caveats and recommendations that specifically apply to this trimester, and finally give you a comprehensive workout program.

First Trimester Fitness Do's and Don'ts

The great thing about the first 3 months is that there are minimal restrictions and guidelines (beyond the Fitness Rules of Thumb), compared to the second and third trimesters. The most important "do" I can tell you now is to shoot for consistency and *keep exercising!*

At this point, you can still do many of the same things you were doing prior to being pregnant. Remember the Golden Rule: If you feel up to it, you can maintain the same level of fitness you currently have, but do not push the "up" button on intensity. Pregnancy is not the time to prove a point, train for a marathon, win a weight lifting competition, or beat your PR at CrossFit.

That said, you might be feeling a little crappier in this trimester than you will be later, especially in the glorious feel-good second trimester. Obstacles to training in this month are not necessarily physical restrictions and limitations, but more as a result of pregnancy symptoms of exhaustion, nausea, and so forth. Let's take a look at what might hold you back and how best to navigate it.

If you are puking

Also known as morning sickness, which is ironically not at all relegated to the mornings, this one just sucks. So bad. If you get hit, hang in there—it does eventually pass. When you are going through morning sickness, however, it can stop you in your tracks. Exercise will likely be the *last* thing you want to do. Remember that little personal anecdote I shared with you about Heidi's fitness regimen—the part where she called me an insensitive ass when I asked her if she wanted to work out? Yeah, she wasn't feeling it very often in those first couple of months.

So . . . yes, tackle the nausea first, if you can. Try some of the suggestions from earlier in this chapter. Another option is to track when you are nauseated and schedule your workouts around it. Most women who struggle with morning sickness say it "comes and goes" throughout the day. See if you can pinpoint the times it's "gone" and then get your sweat on.

If you are simply ill all the time, so be it. No guilt. Andy, our very own pregnancy fitness expert, experienced this herself. The mere thought of exercising seemed impossible to her. "Imagine you have the stomach flu and I just told you to go work out," she said to me one day. "Imagine all you can do is sleep and puke foam. Could you do it?!" My abashed answer was no.

So while we must encourage you to try, and I can tell you it's one of the best things for you and your baby, if you can't, you simply can't. Don't feel bad—know that by the end of your third month, you'll have your energy back and you'll be raring to go. (Spoiler alert: The second trimester rocks.)

If you are dead tired

For many women, the utter exhaustion is shocking and in some cases debilitating. Oddly, the best way to combat this fatigue is to exercise. It helps you sleep better and releases all the feel-good brain chemicals and energy-boosting hormones to help get you through the day. So, while this might seem completely counterintuitive as a remedy for fatigue, do your best to move your body three to five times a week for 30 to 60 minutes. It really will help.

One of the ways I would coax Heidi into working out on her off days (until we got Andy on board as her trainer) was by saying, "Let's just go for 15 minutes. If after 15 minutes you want to leave, we will leave." Nine times out of ten, once she started, she was able to complete a full 30 minutes.

If you have back pain, indigestion, or low blood pressure (or all of these!)

The hormones estrogen, progesterone, and relaxin have already begun to do their job of softening your cartilage, relaxing the muscles and ligaments, and loosening your joints in preparation for birth. Relaxin can also affect arteries, veins, and many muscles in the digestive tract. All of this can result in back pain, indigestion, and low blood pressure.

The best ways to help manage the above are as follows:

- **Incorporate strength training** into your regimen and make core strength a primary focus at this time (great exercises for this will be incorporated into the workouts that follow).

- **Don't lift weights that are too heavy.** If you feel any pain or discomfort, back off. This isn't the time for heavy deadlifts or back squats.

- **Decrease your range of motion.** If you feel pain or discomfort, avoid squatting below parallel or doing deep lunges off a platform.

- **Stop eating at least 60 minutes before you work out** to help avoid cramps and indigestion.

- **Avoid workouts that make you get up and down a lot,** to manage dizziness and light-headedness.

If you feel breathless

Your diaphragm and rib cage raise up during pregnancy, and progesterone adapts the way your body absorbs oxygen into the blood stream, all for the sake of your little one. For this reason, you will likely huff and puff more than usual when you exercise. What used to feel like a 7 on your RPE (rate of perceived exertion) scale now feels like a 10. This does not mean you have suddenly become horrifically out of shape, so don't be discouraged. This is all completely normal. But do slow down a bit if you are hyperventilating or overly winded.

I know for those of you who are very active, this can be a bit discouraging. Heidi found that part a bit shocking, having been an athlete her entire life and then suddenly getting winded walking up the stairs. Try to remember, if you are feeling this way, that it's only temporary and it's totally normal. *Listen to your body!* Slow down if you need to slow down.

If for some reason the condition becomes extreme, contact your doctor, especially if you experience any of the following:

Irregular heartbeat or palpitations

Severe breathlessness, fainting, or feeling faint

Chest pain

Difficulty breathing when lying down

The Yeah Baby! First Trimester Workouts

Ready to get started? The following are four workouts Andy and I have created for you to utilize over your first trimester, complete with an exercise index that describes and illustrates each move for you. We have already taken into account all the Fitness Rules of Thumb and first trimester specifics, to take all the guesswork out of your workouts for you.

Each workout is roughly 30 minutes. I recommend the following schedule:

- Workout 1 on Mondays and Thursdays for weeks 1, 2, 5, 6, 9, 10
- Workout 2 on Tuesdays and Fridays for weeks 1, 2, 5, 6, 9, 10

Andy Says . . .

It's totally normal to feel breathless during exercise when you are pregnant. Your total blood volume is increasing, and your cardiac output will ultimately increase by 40 percent. You will also make 2 percent more red blood cells, to carry more oxygen around your body . . . so pace yourself!

- Workout 3 on Mondays and Thursdays for weeks 3, 4, 7, 8, 11, 12
- Workout 4 on Tuesdays and Fridays for weeks 3, 4, 7, 8, 11, 12

These workouts are designed by muscle splits with "push muscles" (chest, shoulders, biceps, triceps) on Mondays and Thursdays, and "pull muscles" (back, biceps, hamstrings, glutes) on Tuesdays and Fridays.

If you are feeling up to it, add a straight cardio session on one of your off-days, like Wednesday, Saturday, or Sunday. This will be a great way to keep your mood boosted.

ABOUT KEGELS AND MULA BANDHA

Most women have heard about Kegels—those "private part" exercises that contract and relax the muscles used to hold and release urine. It has been said that Kegels can help not just with age-related incontinence but with labor, delivery, and pregnancy and postpartum complications like uterine prolapse and postpartum incontinence.

However, this is a bit of an exaggeration. Dr. Suzanne says that the entire pelvic floor is involved in the pregnancy and birth process, and without strengthening the entire area—not just the limited area you work while doing Kegels—you won't do yourself all that much good. Kegels are still relevant, and we still include them in the workouts in this book, but know that they are not the whole story. For that reason, Dr. Suzanne suggested that we offer an option when we include Kegels in our exercise plan: the mula bandha.

Mula bandha is a somewhat esoteric yoga practice, but if you are an advanced practitioner of yoga, you may have heard of it and may already know how to do it. The benefit to mula bandha is that unlike Kegels, it activates the entire pelvic floor. It is used to retain energy during yogic breathing, but it can also benefit those muscles you will need during pregnancy and delivery.

A qualified yoga teacher can instruct you on how to do mula bandha correctly. It can be difficult to learn how to feel your pelvic floor muscles, and it takes some practice. However, here are the basics, if you want to try it on your own:[58]

1. Sit on the floor in a cross-legged position. Close your eyes, relax your body and breath, and pay attention to the feeling of your breath expanding your rib cage

Keep in mind, these workouts are simply a staple. Feel free to take prenatal yoga classes, prenatal Pilates, or any other class or workout that adheres to the guidelines laid out for this particular trimester.

I also highly recommend Andrea Orbeck's *Pregnancy Sculpt* DVDs. Why not get the best pregnancy trainer right in your own living room? Remember, she trained Heidi throughout most of her pregnancy. She is one of the foremost experts in the field of prenatal fitness, and I can't say enough good things about her programs.

as you think about releasing tension from your entire abdominal area. Then, begin by slowly squeezing the entire perineal region—front, center, and back. Think about pulling it inward and upward as you breathe steadily and smoothly. When you have contracted as much as you can, slowly release. This will help you get used to how it feels to contract that area. Repeat this five times. As you get more advanced, gradually increase your reps until you are doing 20 in one sitting.

2. The next step is to contract and hold the perineal muscles. Continue to breathe smoothly. Notice how you are contracting the area around the anus, then think about contracting the area around your cervix, and then add a Kegel, contracting the muscles around your urethra. Continue to tighten each area as you focus on it, then slowly release the entire contraction as you continue to breathe.

3. Next, begin to coordinate this entire pelvic floor contraction with your breath, contracting on a slow inhale and releasing on a slow exhale. Work on making both the contraction and the breath smooth and steady.

4. Finally, practice this complex contraction without affecting your breath at all. This is the advanced practice.

Don't worry if you don't get it right away. It really does take practice because we aren't used to feeling, let alone paying attention to, those muscles. But the more you work on it, the more you can gain conscious control over them. This can make a real difference not only in how comfortable your pregnancy is, but also on your labor and, finally, on preventing future complications from pregnancy and delivery, like urinary incontinence and organ prolapse.

First Trimester WORKOUT GUIDELINES

Here are some basic rules for your workouts during this trimester:

- Based on the indicated warmup exercise, be sure to go at the pace, incline, or resistance that brings you to a 12 on the RPE scale. (For a reminder about what RPE is, see page 89.)

- For all unilateral exercises (exercises that you do on both sides, first on one side, then the other), do the first set on the right and the second set on the left side every time.

- For exercises that incorporate weights, go as heavy as you can lift safely and with good form and without pain.

- Modify the exercise if it's too hard.

- If at any point you feel you have exceeded a 14 on your RPE scale, pause and rest between exercises.

- Remember not to get overheated. A good sweat is fine. Verge of heatstroke? Not fine.

- During the cooldown, go slowly into the stretch. Don't force it and don't bounce in the stretch. This is no time for an injury.

Workout 1

Please refer to Appendix B, starting on page 296, for photos of all the exercises.

1. When an exercise has "Alternating" in the title, the reps listed are total reps for both sides inclusive.

2. When an exercise is pictured with weights, they are optional. If you use them, go light—between 2 and 8 pounds—depending on your strength and comfort level.

To begin: Warm up with a 5-minute jog or incline walk on the treadmill at RPE 12.

CIRCUIT 1	CIRCUIT 2	CIRCUIT 3	CIRCUIT 4	COOLDOWN
1. Pushups: 15 reps 2. Chest Fly Bridges: 15 reps 3. Pilates Roll-Backs: 15 reps 4. Alternating Knee Switches: 16 reps *Rest 30 seconds, then repeat Circuit 1.*	1. Side Plank: 30 seconds each side 2. Uneven Table Hold: 20 seconds each side 3. Modified Hollow Man Hold:* 30 seconds 4. Incline Triceps Push-ups: 15 reps *Rest 30 seconds, then repeat Circuit 2.*	1. Squats with Goblet Hold: 15 reps 2. Alternating Backward Lunges with Lateral Raises: 20 reps 3. Alternating Side Lunges with Anterior Raises: 20 reps 4. Triceps Kickbacks in Crescent Pose: 15 reps *Rest 30 seconds, then repeat Circuit 3.*	1. Standing Oblique Crunches: 15 reps each side 2. Alternating Standing Toe Tap Crunches: 16 reps 3. Sumo Squats with Shoulder Presses: 15 reps 4. Mula Bandha or Kegels: 10 reps *Rest 30 seconds, then repeat Circuit 4.*	1. Chest Stretch: 30 seconds 2. Triceps Stretch: 30 seconds each side 3. Psoas Stretch: 30 seconds each side 4. Butterfly Stretch: 30 seconds each side 5. Side Lying Quad Stretch: 30 seconds each side

Workout 2

To begin: Warm up with 5 minutes on the recumbent or stationary bike (use enough resistance to get you to RPE 12).

CIRCUIT 1	CIRCUIT 2	CIRCUIT 3	CIRCUIT 4	COOLDOWN
1. Squats with Wide Rows: 15 reps 2. Stiff Leg Deadlifts to Upright Rows: 15 reps 3. Good Mornings with Arms Crossed on Chest: 15 reps 4. Sumo Squats with Rotator Cuff Flys: 15 reps *Rest 30 seconds, then repeat Circuit 1.*	1. Alternating Forward Lunges with Hammer Curls: 16 reps 2. Alternating Crossover Lunges with Reverse Curls: 16 reps 3. Alternating Curtsy Lunges with Biceps Curls: 16 reps 4. Modified Skater Lunges: 16 reps *Rest 30 seconds, then repeat Circuit 2.*	1. Alternating Renegade Rows: 10 reps 2. Pelvic Thrusts on Physio Ball: 15 reps 3. Bent Leg Donkey Kicks: 10 reps each side 4. Alternating Low Rows in Table: 20 reps *Rest 30 seconds, then repeat Circuit 3.*	1. Alternating Hamstring Curls in Ab Hold: 20 reps 2. Crunches: 20 reps 3. Side Lying Leg Circles: 20 reps each side 4. Mula Bandha or Kegels: 10 reps *Rest 30 seconds, then repeat Circuit 4.*	1. Pigeon Stretch: 30 seconds each side 2. Mermaid Stretch: 30 seconds each side 3. Cat Cow Stretch: 30 seconds 4. Side Lying Quad Stretch: 30 seconds each leg 5. Thoracic Rotation Stretch with One Leg Extended: 30 seconds each side

Motivation from Andy!

Deadlifts are crucial! The American Academy of Orthopedic Surgeons found that initially, you will be lifting a 7- to 10-pound baby up to 50 times a day! This back strength will come in incredibly handy.

Workout 3

To begin: Warm up with a 5-minute climb on the step mill or stairmaster at RPE 12.

CIRCUIT 1	CIRCUIT 2	CIRCUIT 3	CIRCUIT 4	COOLDOWN
1. Triceps Dips: 15 reps 2. Sumo Squats with Shoulder Presses: 15 reps 3. Triceps Kickbacks in Crescent Pose: 15 reps 4. Alternating Standing Toe Tap Crunches: 16 reps *Rest 30 seconds, then repeat Circuit 1.*	1. Alternating Stepups: 20 reps 2. Alternating Backward Lunges with Lateral Raises: 16 reps 3. Alternating Side Lunges with Anterior Raises: 16 reps 4. Alternating Surrender Lunges with Shoulder Presses: 16 reps *Rest 30 seconds, then repeat Circuit 2.*	1. Pushups: 15 reps 2. Walking Plank: 10 reps 3. Head Bangers on Physio Ball: 15 reps 4. Side Plank: 30 seconds each side *Rest 30 seconds, then repeat Circuit 3.*	1. Camel Sitdowns: 16 reps 2. Chest Presses on Physio Ball: 15 reps 3. Plank to Wide Child's Pose:* 10 reps 4. Mula Bandha or Kegels: 10 reps *Rest 30 seconds, then repeat Circuit 4.*	1. Calf Stretch: 30 seconds each side 2. Center Splits Oblique Stretch: 30 seconds each side 3. Chest Stretch: 30 seconds 4. Shoulder Stretch: 30 seconds each side 5. Triceps Stretch: 30 seconds each side

Workout 4

To begin: Warm up with a 1,000-meter row on a rowing machine at RPE 12.

CIRCUIT 1	CIRCUIT 2	CIRCUIT 3	CIRCUIT 4	COOLDOWN
1. Alternating Renegade Rows: 16 reps 2. Alternating Reverse Flys in Plank: 16 reps 3. Pelvic Thrusts on Physio Ball: 20 reps 4. Side Crunches: 15 reps each side *Rest 30 seconds, then repeat Circuit 1.*	1. Good Mornings with Arms Crossed on Chest: 10 reps 2. Bridges: 15 reps 3. Alternating Bicycle Crunches: 20 reps 4. Bear Crawls: 4 rotations *Rest 30 seconds, then repeat Circuit 2.*	1. Medium Grip Rows in Crescent Pose: 15 reps 2. Stiff Leg Deadlifts with Low Rows: 15 reps 3. Stationary Lunges with Hammer Curls and Pelvic Tilts: 15 reps 4. Squats with Serving Biceps: 15 reps *Rest 30 seconds, then repeat Circuit 3.*	1. Alternating Forward Lunges with Hammer Curls: 20 reps 2. Sumo Squats with Rotator Cuff Flys: 15 reps 3. Squats with Wide Rows: 10 reps 4. Mula Bandha or Kegels: 10 reps *Rest 30 seconds, then repeat Circuit 4.*	1. Hip Rotation Stretch (both legs bent to rotate): 30 seconds each side 2. Figure 4 Glute Stretch: 30 seconds each side 3. Arm Biceps Stretch: 30 seconds each side 4. Sitting Trapezius Stretch: 30 seconds each side 5. Wide Child's Pose: 30 seconds

Alright, you got this. I'm here for you. And the second trimester is right around the corner! The pregnancy honeymoon period awaits!

CHAPTER 6

YOUR SECOND TRIMESTER:
Nestling In
(or Boobalicious Momnesia)

The second trimester was as uneventful as pregnancy got for us, and I've heard this is pretty common. A few of the issues from the first 3 months carried over, but very few. Heidi was still emotional, which graduated into bad dreams during the second trimester. (More about that in a minute.) Her superhuman sense of smell and cravings still lingered, but the exhaustion, brief bouts of nausea, and other unpleasant first trimester stuff mostly subsided.

Perhaps *my* favorite part of this trimester was the double D bra cup. You would have thought Heidi would have enjoyed this aspect of her pregnancy more, but she was pretty blasé. I, however, compensated for her lack of enthusiasm with sheer bliss. (A tiny bit of jealousy, but mostly it was pure elation on my part. I mean, *wow!*) I'm not sure, I could be wrong, but it's *possible* she didn't enjoy this because her boobs were incredibly tender and sore. She also did not enjoy fishing crumbs out of her cleavage for months on end. Overall, the boobs got a big thumbs-up from me.

Some women say they feel awesome in their second trimester, with no symptoms and tons of energy. However, for Heidi, just as the nausea left her, that's when the heartburn began—so consistently that, at a certain point, I began to feel like my only purpose in life was to be a Tums dispenser. Our interactions often went something like this:

ME: Babe, I know why you are having this heartburn. I just read about the physiological process behind it. You see, when . . .

HEIDI: Did I *ask you* for an explanation?

ME: (Silently holding out a Tums as a peace offering, then slinking back to my corner, where I waited until I was summoned to provide another backrub.)

My ill-advised advice-giving hit its peak the night I made fun of her restless leg syndrome. *Big* mistake. *Huge.* I mistakenly inquired about what constituted a "syndrome" and then joked, "Now you're just making shit up. I bet we can walk that off." I slept on the couch that night.

So . . . take it from me, restless legs is a very real thing, and the sufferers of it find it extremely annoying. (To all spouses or partners reading this book: Just say no to giving advice. It never works out the way you would hope. And here's another tidbit of hard-won wisdom: Do not question. Anything. Just nod supportively and listen.)

We'd heard about "mommy brain," and although this doesn't hit some until the postpartum period, second trimester was when it hit Heidi. She became a bit more spacey and forgetful. Heidi would walk into a room with her sunglasses on her head and ask me if I had seen her sunglasses. She would swipe her driver license to pay for groceries, and when she did remember to pay with her credit card, she would leave it behind. She would get out of her car at the valet and take off with the keys. She would get up and get ready for work, only to realize it was Saturday. And she wasn't the only one! We've both noticed how the brain ceases to function with the sharpness and clarity it once did, both BK and AK ("before kids" and "after kids"). Maybe it is the simple proximity to children, because it seems to have hit me, too!

But I think perhaps the biggest thing in the second trimester for Heidi was the emotions. I remember one weekend when she was about 22 weeks, and we found ourselves in wine country with some of our closest friends for my birthday. Being pregnant and all, Heidi seemed like the obvious designated driver. (I didn't realize at the time that this assumption was not appreciated in the least.) Our buddies and I were pleasantly buzzed, singing along to "Call Me Maybe" (yes, that happened, thankfully not recorded by anyone), while Heidi, the "chauffeur," whisked us all around from winery to winery.

Yeah Baby! REMEDY Heartburn

As your belly starts to change shape to accommodate a new life, it is pretty common to experience some gastrointestinal discomfort, especially heartburn. This can become extremely uncomfortable when everything you eat seems to cause that burning acidy-upchuck feeling. Apart from keeping Tums in your purse, you can also add more fiber and digestive enzymes, which can make a big difference. Try black beans, celery, papaya, and oatmeal. You can also try herbal tea. Both ginger and chamomile tea are known for calming heartburn. You may also find that you need to eat smaller meals more often, rather than a few larger ones. This can be difficult if you are ravenous, but your stomach will thank you. Also back off the spicy foods and citrus juices, as those can both aggravate heartburn.

Well, after about 3 hours of this fun and frivolity, Heidi pulled the car over to the side of the road, smashed the power button on the radio, swiveled around to face everyone—and there was Linda Blair again.

"Shut up!!!" she barked. "Will all you drunken idiots just shut the F#$% UP?!!!"

Needless to say, no one made a peep the rest of the trip.

Admittedly, a trip to the wine country while pregnant was probably not the best idea, and even when you aren't pregnant, it's not that fun to hang around sober with a bunch of tipsy people. But the mood swings were not relegated to this one experience.

During Heidi's pregnancy, we actually traveled quite a bit. We went to Japan for my work, Paris for New Year's Eve, Aspen for Thanksgiving. Looking back on this now, I think we were trying to get all the travel and freedom out of our systems, knowing that we were going to be "grounded" for some time after the kids arrived. However, as in wine country, the idea of this wonderful "freedom" sometimes didn't match the reality.

One of the harder things about Heidi's pregnancy was how isolated it made her feel. She couldn't ski in Aspen while we were all on the slopes. She couldn't indulge in the sushi in Japan, or the cheese plates in Paris. No champagne on New Year's Eve, not to mention no wine on that notorious wine country venture. The truth is, no matter what you do, many aspects of your life are on hold for a while, and that can exacerbate the moodiness that comes with your new hormonal fluctuations. You may not feel like yourself anymore, and while it's not one of the obvious "symptoms" everyone talks about, loneliness can be insidious and pervasive at this time. I wish more people would talk about this, so women would understand that it's important to reach out for help if they feel isolated.

I've often wondered if her loneliness, which went predominantly unacknowledged, was what led to her bad dreams (a common affliction in the second trimester—those feelings have to come out somehow). During this time, Heidi would often wake up in tears, having dreamed that I had cheated on her. Didn't matter with whom—although apparently it was with anyone and everyone! The checkout girl or even the checkout guy at the grocery store, our veterinarian (who was about 70 years old)—you name it, in Heidi's dreams, I apparently slept with them all. No matter how often I reassured her and reiterated that it was a *dream*, and that I had never and would never cheat on her, it felt real enough to her that she would remain pissed at me the entire day. (I was iced out for most of the second trimester over this, to be honest.)

Her sensitivity and vulnerability definitely was the biggest challenge of the second trimester. Other than her heartburn and restless legs, Heidi escaped many of the other outward symptoms some women experience during the second trimester, except one that initially scared the crap out of us: Heidi momentarily thought she had bum cancer.

Yes, bum cancer. And so I lived the scene straight out of the movie *This Is 40*, only with my 31-year-old partner. Boy, that was fun for me to try to offer an opinion about! Thank God for Google. By the way, "hemorrhoids" is a really unpleasant word, and I highly recommend calling them "bum bumps" instead. Much less jarring. (And also extremely common during pregnancy!)

I can think of just one more, quite remarkable change in the second trimester:

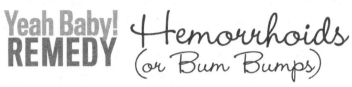

Hemorrhoids are an unpleasant, sometimes startling, but all-too-common symptom of pregnancy that often occurs in the second trimester. If you've never felt those "bum bumps" before, you might be shocked at how they could suddenly emerge from your nether region. Don't worry, this is a relatively harmless if uncomfortable problem that should subside after pregnancy. In the meantime, a natural hemorrhoid cream can help, as well as an Epsom salt bath. (Add 1 cup Epsom salt per 6 inches of warm bathwater. Submerge bum for 20 minutes every 3 to 4 hours if possible.)

And be sure to add more fiber so that what comes out down there is softer and less painful. Prunes, lentils, peas, sun-dried tomatoes, artichokes, broccoli, chia seeds, hemp seeds, carrots, whole grains, berries, oatmeal, and organic air-popped popcorn can all add more fiber to your diet. Drinking more water can make a big difference. Also, more extra virgin olive oil on your salads can help with this issue.

You can also drink these two concoctions, which are thought to ease hemorrhoid discomfort: To a glass of water, add 1 tablespoon of raw apple cider vinegar and drink it (for external hemorrhoids, you can also apply the vinegar topically, with cotton balls). Or put a cup of water in a shaker or jar with a lid, then add a few slices of fresh ginger, the juice from one fresh lemon, and a few fresh mint leaves. Shake it up, strain it, and drink it down to feel better fast. (Note that these are folk remedies—no studies prove these work, but a lot of people say they work, so try them if you like that sort of thing.)

If your hemorrhoids are particularly uncomfortable, you can also buy an inflatable donut pad to sit on, especially if your work requires you to sit at a computer for long hours each day.

If your hemorrhoids are severe and don't improve with other therapies, your doctor can write you a prescription for stronger medicine, and they can also be treated with surgery if all else fails. However, most hemorrhoids will get much better on their own after birth.

Heidi started to snore with the intensity and the ferocity of a chain saw. By month six, I almost bought her a CPAP machine—I couldn't believe my precious little Heidi could saw logs like that. The walls would shake. The pets would startle out of a dead sleep. Honestly, it was pretty impressive. Apparently, the reason is pregnancy-related swelling of the nasal passages,[1] but I wasn't about to offer up that fascinating factoid. (Be warned: If your significant other is even half the jerk I am, it's likely he or she will whip out the phone and record your cataclysmic snores. Protect yourself! Grab a shot of them on the toilet early on to use for leverage, when they are still unsuspecting. This will be your insurance policy—you'll be safe no matter what embarrassing moments of your pregnancy might get recorded for posterity!)

Now let's look at what you need to know during this exciting trimester and what you can learn from your doctor.

QUICK LIST: WHAT TO ASK YOUR DOCTOR IN THE SECOND TRIMESTER

You'll see your doctor every 4 weeks during this stage of pregnancy. While these visits can be inconvenient to schedule, the ritual becomes very reassuring and gives you a chance to ask any questions you have as your pregnancy proceeds.

- Most visits will begin with a hop on the scale, a blood pressure test, and a pee strip. And you'll likely get to hear the baby's heartbeat every time, too! Ask if you have any concerns.

- Your physician will recommend a number of tests, including a triple or quad screen at around 15 weeks and an ultrasound around weeks 18 to 20,[2] where you should be able to learn your baby's gender, if you choose. Before your first ultrasound, be sure to tell your physician whether you want to know the gender of your baby—no fun finding out when you want to be surprised!

- If you have no family history or other risk factors for diabetes, ask whether you need a glucose tolerance test. Your doctor may or may not automatically do this test around week 24 to check for gestational diabetes,[3] but if you do not have any risk factors for diabetes, you may not need it.[4] (See "A Deeper Look at Tests: Second Trimester" on page 163.)

- Definitely mention any swelling, vaginal bleeding or spotting, or any other symptoms that concern you.

- Ask for recommendations on doulas, lactation consultants, and childbirth, parenting, and breastfeeding classes.

SHOULD YOU USE A DOULA?

Should you hire a doula to be with you throughout labor, delivery, and the early postpartum period? While there are many delivery decisions you may not make until later, you should interview and hire a doula by about your 20th week of pregnancy, according to Dr. Suzanne Gilberg-Lenz, the fantastic and multitalented ob-gyn on our dream team of experts. Doulas and labor assistants are not trained to deliver babies, but they stay with you throughout labor, offering support and help. Doulas are trained to know what you need and to get you through the experience more easily. Some research has suggested that mothers who have doulas or labor assistants have shorter labors, shorter hospital stays after the birth, and a 10 percent lower rate of C-section births.

A doula can also provide you with peace of mind. She can help you develop your birth plan, ease your worries and fears, aid you in adjusting your or the baby's posi-

Heidi Says . . .

The second trimester for me was somewhere between "Oh my gosh I'm pregnant" and "When is this going to be over?" It was like a waiting period where nothing incredible was happening. I felt almost normal, except for a few notable discomforts. Like heartburn. Day and night, heartburn. Left side, right side, standing up, sitting up: heartburn. I hesitated to take Tums at first because I wanted to be completely drug-free, but in the end I caved . . . and in the end, I still had heartburn. Sleeping was becoming a bit rough, as restless legs kicked in about this time as well. Normally I can shake this with a few pushups or jumping jacks or boxing punches for 30 seconds, but these were beyond normal restless legs. I just had to get up until it stopped.

Around the end of the second trimester was also when regular exercise became a little more challenging. Intense yoga classes had to be curtailed, and the Up Dog pose was no longer a reality for me. For some reason, I couldn't get myself to do prenatal yoga. I thought I would be bored. I know some people swear by it, though. I stuck to jogging and resistance training with Andy.

I also refused to buy new pants. Instead, I stuck to wearing leggings, a Bellaband, or Jillian's pants. I did, however, have to get fitted for a new bra. Being pregnant isn't totally comfortable, but it's even more uncomfortable when you are told that by the end, you will be a double D and you have to wear a not-so-flattering grandma bra! (No offense, mom.) I never thought that would be me. Jillian, however, did not seem to mind at all.

tion, support you throughout labor, and even help with lactation after the baby is born (lactation consultants also provide this service separately).

On the other hand, a doula is an additional cost that you might prefer to spend elsewhere, and some families may find a third-party involvement intrusive. If that whole midwife way of thinking is not what you are about, you probably don't need one.

Our doula was a really cool chick named Lori Bregman whom Heidi loved. (Check out her great book, *The Mindful Mom-to-Be!*) However, despite the fact that we had a great doula, Heidi still had a long labor that ended in a C-section. Doulas are not miracle workers, but they are an incredible source of support and information, which can help you emotionally through the process, no matter what happens.

If you have the money and you are so inclined, here are a few tips to help you find the right doula/labor assistant around the 6th month of your pregnancy:

- **Education and experience.** This is by far the most important component in hiring a doula. You can always go with an obstetrical nurse or a DONA (Doulas of North America)- or CAPPA (Childbirth and Postpartum Professional Association)-certified doula. Check their credentials and be sure to obtain references to gauge their experience and the quality of their work.

- **Personality and preference.** Like any profession, different professionals have different opinions. When you are interviewing prospective doulas, be sure you like them! Do they make you feel at ease? Are they like-minded? What are their thoughts on birth environment, pain medication, and other essential issues? How do they work with the birth partner? Feel free to ask them to describe a recent birth—what were some pain-relief methods they used? Were there any special situations that they helped manage?

- **Cost and availability.** Cost will range with regard to the service, so see if they offer what you need at a price you can afford. Some doulas will offer a flat fee for predetermined services. I have seen the price range from hundreds to thousands of dollars, depending on the individual, the city you live in, and the services you require from them. Student doulas currently pursuing certification will have the knowledge but must be at a certain number of births before being officially certified—you could offer your birth as a training session, if cost is an issue. Some insurance will cover a portion of the cost as well, so be sure to discuss it with your healthcare provider and your insurance representative.

Also keep in mind that a good doula will likely have many clients! Be sure yours has availability around the time that you anticipate giving birth. Ask your ob-gyn if he or she recommends someone. Word of mouth is also a great source of information—ask friends and friends of friends for recommendations of good people they felt comfortable with. You could also check the online directories at the certifying organizations, DONA and CAPPA, at dona.org and cappa.net.

DEVELOPMENT IN THE SECOND TRIMESTER: WEEKS 13 TO 16

When they hit the second trimester, many women finally start to get a sense that they're really, truly pregnant (as opposed to just being constantly nauseated and sleepy all the time), which is pretty damn cool.

As your doctor's visits become more frequent, you'll have some decisions to make about which tests you want to take or don't want to take. Mostly, the second trimester is just about getting plenty of rest, eating well, and keeping active—and wrapping your head around the idea of becoming a parent.

What's Happening to Me?

In the beginning of the second trimester, your placenta has developed and is now producing hormones to maintain the pregnancy as well as provide your baby with everything it needs—oxygen, nutrients, and waste disposal.[5] Your body is gradually making adjustments, but beyond the placenta growth, nothing too radical happens

 TRUE or FALSE Avoid spicy foods, as they can trigger early labor.

False! There are countless old wives' tales about all the wacky food combinations pregnant women crave, and if you sift through the anecdotes long enough, it seems some cultures believe spicy foods can trigger labor and so they should be avoided. Admittedly, Heidi did swallow a frickin' bottle of hot sauce out of desperation when she was 7 days past her due date. No luck. And beyond this personal anecdote, there is also no scientific evidence to back up that notion, so if you are a hot sauce fanatic, feel free to enjoy. That said, as your baby grows, there is less room for normal stomach acids to circulate, which leaves some women more sensitive to heartburn in the later stages of pregnancy (like Heidi). If that's your situation, by all means, ease up on your spice intake and see if your symptoms subside.[6]

to your body between weeks 13 and 16. At week 16, you can usually find out the sex of your baby, if you so choose!

What's Going On in There?

In this second trimester, your embryo-turned-fetus is now looking more like a baby. Your baby's tooth buds appear, and the miniscule fingers are able to clench into a fist.[8] In the 14th week, your baby will have a layer of soft hair, called *lanugo*. This peach fuzz protects your baby's skin in the watery womb. The thyroid gland matures and begins to produce thyroid hormones.[9] At week 15, hair emerges on the eyebrows and the head, and the skeletal and muscular system gets into full swing, allowing your baby to make some movements.[10] By week 16, your baby will be able to hold his head up and develop enough muscles to make facial expressions like squinting and frowning.[11] Your baby might even start making sucking motions with its mouth.[12]

DEVELOPMENT IN THE SECOND TRIMESTER: WEEKS 17 TO 20

Now the second trimester is under way, and while you are probably having some symptoms, most people are feeling pretty good about now. Take a good look in the mirror—I bet you are glowing.

What's Happening to Me?

This month, your doctor will schedule an ultrasound to check the baby's development and growth and screen for birth defects.[13] As you enter the 20th week, you may begin to feel movement. Those little flutters and flips are barely noticeable at first, but don't worry—soon you will be feeling kicks and hiccups. While you are only about halfway through your pregnancy, your body begins prepping for delivery day by day by increasing bloodflow to the breasts and amping up the size of the glands to support milk production. This means you might grow one or two cup sizes and need to wear more supportive bras, depending upon how much your breasts had grown already in the first trimester.[14]

By the end of this month, your baby will weigh around 11 ounces and measure 6.3 inches, taking up more room in your belly and putting pressure on your lungs, stomach, bladder, and kidneys. Be prepared to make frequent trips to the bathroom, and, like Heidi, don't be surprised if a walk up the stairs leaves you winded![15]

What's Going On in There?

Your baby's ears have been slowly migrating these past few weeks, from their initial alien-like location toward the top of the head to their final position on the sides. The bones of the middle ear and the nerve endings start to take shape, allowing your baby to hear sounds in the next few weeks.[16] The eyes also settle into their final spot, facing forward, with retinas and eyelids. Bones begin to harden, specifically leg bones and the clavicles.[17] In the 19th week, your baby's skin gets an additional coating

 TRUE or FALSE Cocoa butter will prevent stretch marks.

Sadly, false. Many women experience stretch marks during pregnancy, and unfortunately, massaging cocoa butter onto your belly isn't a reliable means to avoid them (although it does feel and smell delicious). That said, cocoa butter is a terrific moisturizer, so feel free to slather the stuff all over your body if it helps you feel more comfortable. A healthy diet, like our *Yeah Baby!* nutrition plan, can also help maintain collagen and possibly prevent or lessen the severity of stretch marks,[18] but unfortunately, the tendency for them also has a genetic component, so while you can mitigate them, you may not be able to forgo them entirely. I like to think of them as badges of honor that you made a frickin' kid.

called *vernix caseosa*—a white, waxy substance that acts like Chapstick to protect that delicate newborn skin. Your baby gets additional protection with the development of brown fat, which provides warmth and some cushioning after birth.[19] When you reach the halfway mark, at week 20, your baby's skin will thicken and develop layers while hair and nails continue to grow.[20]

DEVELOPMENT IN THE SECOND TRIMESTER: WEEKS 21 TO 24

You are probably showing pretty obviously by now, even if it is your first pregnancy. If you haven't already gone shopping for maternity clothes, this is probably the time.

What's Happening to Me?

Between weeks 21 and 24, if you are already at high risk of gestational diabetes (such as if you are overweight or prediabetic), you will probably be screened for gestational diabetes at this time (normal-risk women are typically screened between weeks 24 to 28).[21] You'll be asked to guzzle a disgustingly sugary drink and then your blood will be drawn about an hour afterward to see how high your glucose levels rise. If you end up with high glucose levels, you will need to come back for a fasting glucose test followed by another disgustingly sugary drink, and blood draws at 1, 2, and 3 hours afterward. Those results will determine if you have gestational diabetes.[22] (See more in "A Deeper Look at Tests: Second Trimester" on page 163.) A diagnosis of gestational diabetes doesn't mean you will have diabetes for the rest of your life, but it does mean you will need to take care of your blood sugar levels for the remaining weeks of your pregnancy.[23] Dr. Suzanne says this also means you have a greater risk of developing diabetes later in life, so if this is you, stay vigilant about your health habits!

By 24 weeks, your baby will begin to sleep and wake on a regular schedule, and

TRUE or FALSE

It's best to avoid sex during pregnancy; orgasms can cause miscarriage.

Happily, false! In fact, as long as your pregnancy remains complication-free, you and your partner can enjoy sex as frequently as you desire. Go ahead and get it on! Many women say that they feel particularly sexy and vital during the second trimester, and they enjoy sex as their bodies are changing. Orgasms do cause uterine contractions, but they are different from the type of contraction experienced in labor. As far as choosing the best position, know that your baby is well cushioned inside your body, so let comfort dictate what positions you use, and you can reaffirm to your significant other that he will not be stabbing your unborn infant with his "manhood." (This is a very real concern for some men!)

However, remember that STDs are still a concern and can pose serious health risks for you and your baby. If you're single and/or you don't have the full assurance that your partner is STD-free, be sure to use condoms and practice safe sex![24]

you may notice the rhythm of the movements. You also might start to feel some contractions—don't worry, this doesn't mean you are going into labor. Your uterus is simply doing some rehearsals for the big day. These practice contractions, or Braxton Hicks contractions, are painless, but you may feel a bit of squeezing. If you feel painful, strong, regular contractions, call your doctor.

What's Going On in There?

Up to this point, your baby was completely reliant on you for supporting all bodily functions. By week 21, your baby's systems begin to take over and function on their own. (How cool is that!?) For example, your baby's intestines absorb sugars from the amniotic fluid and pass it through their digestive system. The liver and spleen produce blood cells until the bone marrow is ready to take over the job (which won't actually happen until the third trimester).[25] In week 22, taste buds form on your baby's tongue, and the neural connections that will enable a sense of touch begin to form. Little tiny testes begin to descend in boys, while girls will have their uterus, ovaries, and vagina in place.[26] (All of the egg cells your daughter will ever have will be in her ovaries by the time she's born—these can number in the millions, although only about 400 will be released during her entire reproductive life.[27]) By week 24, your baby forms the tiny swirls of footprints and fingerprints.

A Deeper Look at Tests: Second Trimester

Sometimes it can feel as though all your doctors' visits in the second trimester are about tests. Some of these tests can sound a bit scary—but they are just precautionary. Taking these tests gives you and your doctor information—that's it. If they come back positive, you can be prepared and give your baby the healthiest start possible. If they come back negative, all the better! Here is a closer look at the most common tests in the second trimester.

- **Glucose screening test:** Between weeks 24 and 28, your healthcare provider will measure the level of glucose in your blood.[28] Typically, you will consume a specific sugary drink called Glucola, at your doctor's office, and then 1 hour later, your healthcare provider will take a blood sample to look for high blood sugar levels. If your levels are normal, you will not require another test. If they are elevated (between 130 and 140 mg/dL), your doctor may suggest a glucose tolerance test.[29]

- **Glucose tolerance test:** If your glucose screening test reveals higher than normal blood sugar levels, your doctor is likely to order a glucose tolerance test

Dr. V. Says . . .

Dr. Katja Van Herle is our supertalented endocrinologist. That means she knows a lot about gestational diabetes and other hormone-driven disorders. Here's what she has to say about those disgusting sugary drinks that are part of the glucose tolerance test for gestational diabetes.

Some of my patients don't want to take the glucose drink typically used for the glucose tolerance test, and understandably so. It contains glucose, but also artificial ingredients, including colorings and flavorings, and fizz. It is like a supersweet soda. I tell my clients who are opposed to this that what we need is 75 grams of carbohydrates for the glucose tolerance test. I have a lot of patients who will bring in agave or honey. They have a nutritionist calculate out exactly how much glucose is in the natural sweetener they brought, and they take that instead. This is completely fine. Glucose is glucose, whether it comes from cane sugar, agave, honey, beet sugar, or something else. While 90 percent of my patients don't want to bother with trying to figure this out and just drink the provided drink, it is always fine with me if they want to BYOG (Bring Your Own Glucose!).

Dr. Suzanne Says . . .

Dr. Suzanne Gilberg-Lenz, our resident ob-gyn, has an opinion about those vile sugary drinks, too.

I agree that Glucola is a disgustingly sugary drink with artificial ingredients. I let my patients use 8 ounces of orange juice and a banana as an alternative to the screening test when they would normally need 50 grams Glucola for the glucose screening test.

to look for gestational diabetes, which is diabetes brought on by pregnancy that can lead to complications in mom and baby. Done at 26 to 28 weeks of pregnancy, a glucose tolerance test just gives your doctor a more detailed look at how well your body processes sugar.

Your doctor will give you instructions about what you should eat for the few days leading up to the test. You will then have to fast for 14 hours before the actual test. On the day of the test, you'll get a blood test to determine your fasting blood glucose level. You will then drink a sugary drink (or your own more natural source of glucose—see the box above) and your blood will be tested once an hour for 3 hours to see how your body processes the sugar.[30] If only one of your readings comes back abnormal, your doctor may talk to you about changing your diet and then retest you later in pregnancy. If two or more of the readings come back abnormal, you will be diagnosed with gestational diabetes, and your provider will move forward with a treatment plan.[31]

- **Second trimester screen:** To screen for genetic conditions, chromosomal abnormalities, or birth defects, your doctor may order screening tests in the second trimester. Combined with the first trimester screening, the second trimester screen is more effective; nearly all cases of Down syndrome are identified when a healthcare professional uses both the first and second trimester screen. The second trimester screen may include the triple screen or quad screen (see below).[32] If you test positive for any of these screens, you will be sent for an amniocentesis, where a doctor tests the amniotic fluid surrounding your baby for genetic conditions.

- **Triple screen:** Also called the triple test, the triple screen measures levels of three substances in your blood to check for increased risk of genetic disorders such as trisomy 21 (Down syndrome) and trisomy 18 (Edwards syndrome), as well as neural tube defects such as anencephaly or spina bifida. Results may also tell you if you're having twins (or triplets!). The three substances the test measures are alpha-fetoprotein (AFP), a protein produced by the fetus; human chorionic gonadotropin (HCG), a hormone produced by the placenta; and estriol, an estrogen produced by both the fetus and placenta. The triple screen is a screening test only—not a diagnostic test—meaning it just identifies an increased risk for a genetic disorder or neural tube defect. There are many false positives, so a positive result does not necessarily mean your baby has one of the conditions the test screens for. If your test reveals increased risk, your doctor may suggest a follow-up diagnostic test. Healthcare professionals should offer all pregnant women the triple screen between 15 and 20 weeks of pregnancy, but it is especially recommended for women who will be 35 or older at the time of delivery, those who have a family history of birth defects, women who have used harmful drugs or medication during pregnancy, those with diabetes, or women who suffered a viral infection or exposure to high levels of radiation while pregnant.[33]

- **Quad screen:** The quad screen is similar to the triple screen in that it measures AFP, HCG, and estriol. In addition, it looks at levels of inhibin-A, a

TRUE or FALSE When you're pregnant, sleeping on your left side is best.

True, but not until later in your pregnancy. In late pregnancy, doctors usually advise women to try sleeping on their left sides to increase bloodflow to the baby and mother's kidneys. But does altering your sleeping habits beforehand make a difference? According to one study that followed 500 women during their healthy pregnancies, there seemed to be some correlation between the mothers' preferred sleeping positions and where the placenta grew in the uterus. However, if you don't normally sleep on your left side and you don't find it comfortable, trying to control that pattern during pregnancy may result in a less than satisfying night's sleep, so don't stress too much if you find your body doesn't cooperate. A lot of pillows can help you get comfortable, and that's more important than strict left-side sleeping. Getting good-quality sleep is what's most vital.[34, 35, 36] That being said, Dr. Suzanne says that after about 22 weeks don't sleep on your back because that can restrict bloodflow to the uterus and placenta.

protein produced by the placenta and ovaries. The quad test is more likely to identify pregnancies at risk for Down syndrome than the triple screen, and it is also less likely to yield false positives. As with the triple screen, healthcare professionals should offer all pregnant women the quad screen between 15 and 20 weeks of pregnancy, but it is specifically recommended for women who will be 35 or older at the time of delivery, those who have a family history of birth defects, women who have used harmful drugs or medication during pregnancy, those with diabetes, or women who suffered viral infection or exposure to high levels of radiation while pregnant.[37]

- **MSAFP:** MSAFP is a screening test done between the 14th and 22nd weeks of pregnancy that looks at the amount of AFP in the mother's blood. It is often part of the triple screen or quad screen test that determines whether or not further diagnostic tests are necessary. Healthcare providers should offer all pregnant women the MSAFP screening test, but it is especially recommended for women who will be 35 years of age or older at the time of delivery, those who have a family history of birth defects, women who have diabetes, or those who were exposed to harmful medications or drugs during pregnancy. If levels of AFP are too high, it may signal that the baby has a neural tube defect such as anencephaly or spina bifida or that there is a problem with the baby's esophagus or abdomen. (But inaccurate pregnancy dating can also cause elevated levels of AFP.) Low AFP levels may mean the baby has a chromosomal abnormality, such as trisomy 21 (Down syndrome) or trisomy 18 (Edwards syndrome).

  The MSAFP screening test has a high rate of false positives; there are about 25 to 50 abnormal results for every 1,000 pregnancies tested, but only

TRUE or FALSE Eating vegetables and other healthy foods ensures your baby will like them, too.

True! Take advantage of those newly formed taste buds. Numerous research studies have confirmed that babies exposed to the flavor of specific foods before birth show greater acceptance of those same foods later in life. Load up on the healthy stuff while you're pregnant if you want to improve the odds of your child having healthy eating habits down the road.[38] Yep, good parenting has already begun!

1 in 16 to 1 in 33 will actually have a baby affected with a chromosomal problem or neural tube defect.[39]

- **Rh antibodies:** If your first trimester Rh factor test revealed you are Rh negative, your healthcare provider will test you for Rh antibodies between pregnancy weeks 28 and 29. If the test reveals you indeed have Rh antibodies, you may require special care. If the test finds you do not have Rh antibodies, your healthcare provider will give you an Rh immunoglobulin shot to prevent you from making Rh antibodies for the remainder of your pregnancy.[40]

- **Chorionic villus sampling (CVS):** This test should be offered to all pregnant moms who are over 35.

- **Ultrasound:** An ultrasound is a procedure that uses high-frequency sound waves to create a picture (sonogram) of the baby and placenta. There are different types of ultrasound procedures, and your healthcare professional may use a different type depending on where you are in your pregnancy and the reason for the exam. There is no standard recommended number of ultrasounds, and the average number differs among providers. Your healthcare provider should order one only if there is a medical reason for it.

  You may get an ultrasound at any point in your pregnancy. In the early second trimester (or at the end of the first trimester), medical reasons for an ultrasound include to diagnose fetal malformation (done at 11 to 13 weeks to look for characteristics of Down syndrome and anywhere from 18 to 21 weeks to look for congenital malformations); to look for structural abnormalities; to confirm a multiples pregnancy; to look for high or low levels of amniotic fluid; to confirm intrauterine death; and to verify dates and growth (it can also be used later, in the third trimester, to verify fetal position and to evaluate the baby's overall well-being). An ultrasound technician may also be able to determine your baby's gender at the 16- to 20-week ultrasound, but the position of the fetus sometimes complicates things and makes it difficult to tell the gender.[41]

SECOND TRIMESTER NUTRITION

"Looks like we made it . . . " Most of you are probably too young for that song—a Barry Manilow classic, circa 1977. I was only 3 years old myself, but my mom was a fan and still is, and I think this is an apropos lyric for the second trimester when it comes to eating because . . . glory hallelujah, you don't feel like throwing up anymore! In fact, you might even feel . . . could it be . . . *hungry?*

As I mentioned, for most women, the second trimester usually is the easiest of the pregnancy. Going into weeks 13 to 24, perhaps a few new issues have cropped up. You may have started to notice heartburn (this one sucks), muscle cramps, indigestion, gas, stretch marks, hemorrhoids (this one ain't so fun either), or hyperpigmentation of the skin. This trimester is a time of rapid brain growth and weight gain for baby, and it's also when serious pregnancy complications, such as gestational diabetes and preeclampsia, may appear. To help get you through some of these discomforts, I've highlighted below some specific nutritional do's and don'ts to help you combat some common symptoms that might come up during this time. (Remember that the nutrition Rules of Thumb *always* apply.)

Second Trimester Don'ts

- **Don't: Eat any of the chemicals or crap** we covered in the Rules of Thumb nutrition chapter.

- **Don't: Eat or drink right before bed** to avoid exacerbating any potential heartburn.

- **Don't: Eat tomato sauce, citrus, or spicy foods** if you suffer from heartburn. As space in your stomach decreases due to the growing baby, stomach acid can back up into the esophagus. These foods can increase stomach acid production, making the situation worse.

- **Don't: Eat estrogenic foods** (soy, flax) if you have melasma or hyperpigmentation of your skin (brown spots, sometimes called the mask of pregnancy because they tend to occur on your face). This condition is caused by fluctuating hormone levels, and estrogenic foods like soy and flax can further disrupt hormone levels.

Second Trimester Do's

Now let's talk about the good stuff since you might finally feel like actually eating and savoring your food. What you eat now continues to impact your growing baby, so make good decisions, but by all means, enjoy that healthy food!

- **Do: Drink water.** Water and other noncaffeinated fluids help with everything from bloat and headaches to constipation and fatigue to reducing swelling and water retention. (Talk to your doctor if fluid retention is excessive—that's one symptom of preeclampsia.) Drinking fluids between meals instead of with them may help prevent heartburn.[42]

- **Do: Eat slowly and take a little stroll,** if possible, if you are struggling with heartburn. At the very least, make sure to sit or stand immediately after eating.

- **Do: Eat high-enzyme foods** like papaya and pineapple for gas or indigestion.

- **Do: Eat foods high in probiotics** like kefir and yogurt to help with gas and indigestion.

- **Do: Eat foods high in fiber,** both soluble (dissolves into a gel in the digestive tract) and insoluble (is not changed through the digestive process), to help manage constipation and heartburn and alleviate hemorrhoids. Even more importantly, fiber helps lower your risk of gestational diabetes, which tends to occur in the second trimester, and could help prevent large birth weight caused by high blood sugar, which can necessitate a higher-risk C-section. Interestingly, it also prevents low blood sugar, which can lead to seizures, and could even prevent type 2 diabetes later in life.[43]

- **Do: Make sure you get your omega-3s,** from sources like grass-fed beef and wild salmon. Your baby's brain growth accelerates during the second trimester, and these healthy fats help promote healthy brain and eye development. They may also help your baby attain a healthy weight and improve insulin sensitivity.[44] They may help your "mommy brain," too—women's brain cells tend to shrink during pregnancy, possibly because low supplies of essential fatty acids require the body to shuttle some of those valuable brain fats to your baby,[45] so replenish them now to keep your own brain well supplied. Omega-3s may also help lower your risk of pregnancy-induced hypertension and preterm birth. Good sources include supplements, many varieties of fish, krill oil, and walnuts.

Cheryl Says . . .

Our dietitian, Cheryl Forberg, says that we need both insoluble and soluble fiber in our diets to keep our gastrointestinal systems moving comfortably and to feed the good bacteria in our guts. For insoluble fiber, she recommends fruit, vegetables, dried beans, wheat bran, seeds, popcorn, brown rice, and whole grain products such as bread, cereal, and pasta. For soluble fiber, she recommends apples, oranges, pears, peaches, grapes, prunes, vegetables, seeds, oat bran, dried beans, oatmeal, barley, and rye. (Yes, some foods have both types.)

- **Do: Eat collagen-boosting foods** to help fend off stretch marks. You may still get them (thanks, genetics!), but foods containing omega-3s, vitamin C, lycopene, vitamin A, vitamin E, selenium, zinc, healthy fats, and gelatin could all help make them less severe. Shoot for more watermelon, tomatoes, coconut oil, olive oil, berries, melons, carrots, peaches, shrimp, egg yolk, turkey, and salmon.

- **Do: Eat foods that are high in magnesium** and natural stool softeners to help with constipation and hemorrhoids. Apricots, peaches, plums, grapes, figs, and prunes are all good choices. Blackstrap molasses, avocados, yogurt, bananas, nuts, and seeds will also help a lot. Magnesium also helps ward off preeclampsia.

- **Do: Up your olive oil** to help ease constipation symptoms.

- **Do: Be diligent about protein consumption.** Protein helps boost tissue growth (muscle and organ development) for your baby. Eggs, beef, lamb, pork, chicken, and wild-caught (low-mercury) seafood are all fine options. Low-fat dairy protein and legumes like lentils and beans are good vegetarian sources.

- **Do: Eat iron-rich foods.** A 2013 review of 44 studies on maternal iron supplementation published in the *British Medical Journal* found that it substantially improved birth weight, which may improve survival rates. Iron supplementation also lowered risks of preterm birth and its medical complications, including cerebral palsy, as well as suspected long-term complications such as hypertension, diabetes, and heart disease.[46] Our dietitian, Cheryl, says the best way to get iron into your body is with iron-rich food, so get more iron from grass-fed beef, organic turkey, organic chicken, wild salmon, organic eggs, quinoa, spinach, cashews, white beans, dark chocolate (yeah!), tempeh, prune juice (also good for constipation), and stewed tomatoes.[47] (Remember: The iron from nonmeat sources is not as readily available to the body as iron from meat is unless it's accompanied by a food high in vitamin C. For example, adding tomato sauce, which is abundant in C, to a cup of white beans increases the iron absorption from the beans *and* tomatoes.)

- **Do: Remember other core vitamins, minerals, and nutrients.** All the basics are still extremely important to your baby's bone, brain, nerve, eye, and overall development, but here is what becomes really important in the second trimester. (See "First Trimester Nutrition" on page 131 or the nutrition Rule of Thumb chapter on page 42 for more specific food options.)

  - **Calcium and vitamin D** help prevent maternal bone loss while building your baby's bones and reduce your risk of pregnancy-induced hypertension.

  - **Folic acid** helps keep levels of the amino acid homocysteine low during the second and third trimesters, when they tend to rise. High homocysteine in pregnancy can harm the health of the placenta and has been linked to preeclampsia, preterm birth, fetal growth retardation, and recurrent pregnancy loss.[48] Again, this is in your prenatal vitamin.

- ■ **Potassium** helps prevent gestational diabetes.
- ■ **Iodine** helps supplement the small amount of thyroid hormone the baby is producing in the second trimester. Thyroid hormone and iodine strongly influence brain development. To meet your own and the baby's requirement, you need to take 50 percent more than normal.[49]

● **Do: Eat foods rich with manganese** for your baby's cartilage and bone development. Manganese is not generally in prenatal vitamins, but I have worked it into the Yeah Baby! meal plan. A few foods rich in manganese are pecans, walnuts, oatmeal, brown rice, pineapple, spinach, and almonds. You could also give birch water a try.

The Yeah Baby!
SECOND TRIMESTER MEAL PLANS

Now that you are at the second trimester mark, we are going to switch up some things, nutritionally. While the first trimester meal plan is great, this one adds some specific nutritional components that are relevant to your baby's development right now. You will recognize many of these recipes, but you'll also get a few cool new ones, not just for broadening your nutrient intake but to keep things interesting. You may also notice that the same recipes taste different this trimester than they did last trimester—chalk it up to your continuously changing sense of taste and smell.

Again, note that each of the four meal plans in this chapter is to be used at different weeks during your pregnancy, so you never do an identical meal plan for 2 weeks in a row. No boredom, plenty of variety. For example, the first meal plan is for weeks 13, 17, and 21. You don't have to follow this exactly, however. If you really like the second meal plan, for example, then you can enjoy it more often. It's all good.

Also, as with the first trimester meal plan, you certainly don't have to adhere rigorously to this outline, but it's here for you when you need it. You can always try new things, go out to eat, etc., but if you rely on this plan and come back to it frequently, you will reap all the great nutritional benefits.

You can find complete recipes for everything in this meal plan in Appendix A, beginning on page 271.

Meal Plan 1 Weeks 13, 17, 21

	BREAKFAST	LUNCH	SNACK	DINNER
MONDAY	B4 Power Parfait	Slammin' Turkey Sammy	Bangin' Bruschetta	Lemon Lamb Chop
TUESDAY	Huevos Tacos	Mediterranean Chicken Sandwich	Devilish Deviled Eggs and Watermelon	Veggie Pasta
WEDNESDAY	Maple Pecan Porridge	Quick and Easy Fish Tacos	Organic Jerky (purchased)	Argentine Salmon
THURSDAY	The California Poach	BBQ Steak Salad	Super Mommy Mix	Steak Chimichurri
FRIDAY	Baby Booster Smoothie	Chicken Burrito Bowl	Cheese Plate	Thai Steak
SATURDAY	Apple Zucchini Flap Jacks with Turkey Bacon	Chicken Artichoke Pizza	Fruity Gazpacho	Baked Trout
SUNDAY	Lori and Jaime's Feel-Good Muffin	Chicken Chop	Beat-the-Bloat Baked Potato	The Ultimate Turkey Burger

Meal Plan 2 Weeks 14, 18, 22

	BREAKFAST	LUNCH	SNACK	DINNER
MONDAY	Maple Pecan Porridge	Slaw Salad	Red Ants on a Log	Lemon Lamb Chop
TUESDAY	Breakfast Bowl	Chicken Chop	Bangin' Bruschetta	Veggie Pie
WEDNESDAY	Hot Mama Smoothie	Quick and Easy Fish Tacos	Super Mommy Mix	Thai Steak
THURSDAY	Feta Frittata	Mediterranean Chicken Sandwich	Cottage Cheese and Peaches	Peach Pork Chop with Fennel Salad
FRIDAY	The California Poach	Summer Shrimp Salad	Organic Jerky (purchased)	Veggie Pasta
SATURDAY	Apple Zucchini Flap Jacks with Turkey Bacon	BBQ Steak Salad	Veggies and Dip	Mussels Marinara
SUNDAY	Lori and Jaime's Feel-Good Muffin	Slammin' Turkey Sammy	Awesome Artichoke	Argentine Salmon

Meal Plan 3 Weeks 15, 19, 23

	BREAKFAST	LUNCH	SNACK	DINNER
MONDAY	Bad A$$ Breakfast Burrito	Summer Shrimp Salad	Devilish Deviled Eggs with Watermelon	Veggie Pie
TUESDAY	Lori and Jaime's Feel-Good Muffin	Quick and Easy Fish Tacos	Beat-the-Bloat Baked Potato	Steak Chimichurri
WEDNESDAY	Apple Zucchini Flap Jacks with Turkey Bacon	Chicken Burrito Bowl	Super Mommy Mix	Lemon Lamb Chop
THURSDAY	Huevos Tacos	BBQ Steak Salad	Cheese Plate	Peach Pork Chop with Fennel Salad
FRIDAY	B4 Power Parfait	Chicken Chop	Hummus and Pita Chips (purchased)	Mussels Marinara
SATURDAY	Hot Mama Smoothie	Chicken Artichoke Pizza	Organic Jerky (purchased)	Baked Trout
SUNDAY	Feta Frittata	Slaw Salad	The PBB	Argentine Salmon

Meal Plan 4 Weeks 16, 20, 24

	BREAKFAST	LUNCH	SNACK	DINNER
MONDAY	Baby Booster Smoothie	Summer Shrimp Salad	Hummus and Pita Chips (purchased)	Peach Pork Chop with Fennel Salad
TUESDAY	B4 Power Parfait	Chicken Chop	Cottage Cheese and Peaches	Lemon Lamb Chop
WEDNESDAY	The California Poach	Chicken Parmesan Orzo Salad	Red Ants on a Log	The Ultimate Turkey Burger
THURSDAY	Hot Mama Smoothie	Chicken Artichoke Pizza	Super Mommy Mix	Thai Steak
FRIDAY	Feta Frittata	Chicken Burrito Bowl	Chocolate Cherry Smoothie	Veggie Pasta
SATURDAY	Apple Zucchini Flap Jacks with Turkey Bacon	Slammin' Turkey Sammy	Awesome Artichoke	Baked Trout
SUNDAY	Bad A$$ Breakfast Burrito	Slaw Salad	Cheese Plate	Steak Chimichurri

SECOND TRIMESTER FITNESS

As you progress through your second trimester, you may notice that while you potentially have more energy to train, some of the exercises you have been doing feel different and may gradually become more difficult or uncomfortable. To accommodate what is happening in your hot mama body right now, I have designed a second trimester fitness program.

Of course, our Fitness Rules of Thumb are our golden rules. They all still apply, but I also want you to think of our trimester rules as cumulative. Everything that applied in your first trimester, such as managing possible breathlessness, feeling light-headed, and so on, still applies in the second. In this section, we'll cover the successive additions of fitness recommendations and caveats that specifically apply to your second trimester. The four new workouts in this trimester also take all of this new information into account for you.

We've talked about how the second trimester is the "easiest"—I've even heard it called the "honeymoon phase" of pregnancy. You probably have more energy, your belly isn't big enough to get in the way much yet, and exercise may feel easier now overall. You may even feel like you can do it all. However, the feelings of being winded and light-headed tend to increase when training during these months, so remember to go slow and be careful. Don't overexert yourself or put yourself in a position where you could fall and injure yourself. Don't get up or down too quickly.

We have two specific additional issues to take into account for the second trimester exercise regimen. Let's go over them before we get to the workouts:

Second Trimester Issue 1: Back Pain

Your tiny little human is starting to become *not quite so tiny*. Your belly is starting to "show," which is all very exciting! On a physical level, however, this growth definitely shifts your center of gravity and throws your body out of alignment.

As your uterus grows, it pulls your pelvis forward, creating a condition called *lordosis*—a fancy way of saying you have a low back curve that's creating a "swayback." Lordosis can make you compensate by letting your shoulders slump forward and your neck jut out—which results in pain. Sometimes lots of pain—low back pain, neck pain, pain between your shoulder blades. (Remember my "thumbs of steel" that I developed during the first trimester? It was all in the name of combating lordosis.)

If you are plagued with back and neck pain, don't panic. Lordosis is temporary, and you can do many things to ease this condition: Proper stretching of the neck and chest helps, as does proper strengthening of the upper and midback, pelvic floor muscles, and core. Knowing lordosis is a common issue, I've built these exercises into the Yeah Baby! workouts.

Second Trimester Issue 2: Balance

As many as two-thirds of pregnancy falls occur during the second trimester. Indeed, with your center of gravity being thrown off, which is compounded by postural changes, you can develop a bit of instability and lack of balance. In other words, this would not be the best time to do anything on the BOSU ball.

One theory about these falls is that, although your center of gravity is shifting forward, your mind-body connection is still working off your prepregnancy neural pathways or "muscle memory," holding your body in ways that are no longer correct for your new shape. That's why these workouts do everything possible to keep you as fit and stable as possible, so you can stay safe.

A few pointers:

- Wear comfortable and stable shoes. Remember our conversation in the fitness Rules of Thumb chapter about proper gear? This is not the time to experiment with the "five finger" shoe trend. Stability is key now.

POSTURE CHECK ALERTS!

Bringing body awareness into your daily routine will make a big difference in how much pain you experience as your center of gravity shifts to accommodate your baby. In addition to your second trimester workouts, I want you to set your watch or phone alarm to go off every hour as a reminder to:

- Stand up tall.
- Tuck your chin back and in toward your collar bone.
- Squeeze your bum and tuck in your tailbone.
- Pull your belly button and your shoulder blades in toward your spine.

Also, whenever you are exercising or just going about your day, remember to:

- Avoid lifting heavy weight over your head, which compresses your spine.
- Avoid torso rotation as much as possible.

I know this sequence can feel tedious, but trust me—after a couple of weeks, adjusting your body this way will become second nature and the hourly reminder will no longer be necessary. This set of adjustments is also a great thing to do throughout your life to help you perform better and avoid chronic pain, both during pregnancy and beyond!

- Keep your body on a stable platform and avoid fitness equipment designed to challenge your balance. No glides, BOSU balls, sand bells, active motion bars, or anything designed to challenge your stabilizing muscles at this time. These tools are fine for when you are not pregnant, but not recommended during your second and third trimesters.

- Prenatal classes that help with posture and core strength are fine. Those prenatal yoga, Pilates, or barre classes are also good workouts to try out. Just be sure your teacher has actually been trained in pregnancy fitness.

A Note about Abdominal Separation, or Diastasis Recti

Before we start working out, I want to mention one more potential issue. This may not happen to you, and it may not happen until your third trimester (it can happen any time in the second half of your pregnancy), but the separation of the muscles in your abdominal wall (also called *diastasis recti*) is a common symptom of pregnancy or postpartum, occurring in up to two-thirds of pregnancies,[50] and it can be the bane of your existence—or a minor issue that causes you no concern.

What happens in this condition is that as the uterus stretches with pregnancy, the muscles of the abdominal wall can become separated, so that only a little connective tissue holds the muscles together. This can cause tissue to bulge out or can make your skin bulge out in a weird shape in the middle of your torso. You may not even notice this has happened until after you give birth and your stomach is shrinking back down into a strange poochy shape; you might have already noticed it because it can cause back pain or urine leakage and could even end up causing a hernia. The reason I mention it now is that if you have this, you will have to be more careful when you work out. I also mention it because good core strength now could help to prevent this from happening later. This condition is more likely to occur in women who are out of shape to begin with, have had multiple pregnancies, are over 35, or are pregnant with multiples, but it could potentially happen to anyone.

If you end up with this issue, don't panic. This is not a permanent condition. It can be healed. Your abdominal muscles will not be forever compromised. It does not cause a permanent belly bulge. That said, if you do sustain abdominal separation, you must be careful during your pregnancy not to exacerbate it. After you have given birth and your doctor has cleared you for exercise, our trainer, Andy, has some exercises that can gradually and safely help you restore your core strength and stabilization and bring the muscles of your abdominal wall back together after your peanut is born. (We'll talk about those in Chapter 9.)

Speak with your doctor about following the exercises below. Unless cleared by your doctor, if you have diastasis recti, you will want to avoid the following types of movements, starting now:

- Heavy lifting

- Straining, as with intense coughing, without abdominal support (if you need to cough, wrap your arms around your belly and hug your midsection to provide support)

- Torso rotation

- Movements that stretch or strain the abdominal wall, obliques, and transverse abdominals, such as Cat Cow, Up Dog, side bends, back bends, front planks, bicycles, double leg extension, and so on.

Note: I have put an * by all exercises in the second and third trimester workouts that could be aggravating for diastasis recti, so you know to avoid them unless your doctor clears you to perform them.

It's important to check for a diastasis before beginning these workouts or any

MATERNAL SUPINE HYPERTENSION

Maternal supine hypertension sounds intimidating, but this is really just a fancy way of saying, "Don't lie on your back." Many doctors caution pregnant women to avoid lying flat on their backs in the second and third trimester. This is because, in theory, the uterus has grown large enough to potentially decrease bloodflow by putting pressure on the main vein (*inferior vena cava*) that returns blood from your lower extremities to your heart, resulting in "maternal supine hypertension." This tendency can also potentially affect the flow of blood and nutrients to your baby.

While there've been many studies on this, none are very conclusive. So, if you wake up and find yourself sleeping on your back, or you just bought this book in the 5th month of your pregnancy and you've been doing the savasana with your in-home yoga DVD, don't panic. Many women have been doing this for centuries. Heidi would often wake up flat on her back in the middle of the night. She'd simply roll over and switch to her side and go back to sleep (snoring away!). Several years later, she and our son are fine.

That said, we always want to be smart and safe and err on the side of caution. You can simply modify any exercise in which you're on your back by propping your torso up on a pillow or by going up on your forearms to a 45-degree angle.

And trust me—you would know if you are putting pressure on the vena cava long before it could pose problems. It would be very uncomfortable. Should you feel dizzy and/or faint, simply raise your torso up and rest—and definitely talk it over with your doctor, just to be 100 percent safe.

Motivation from Andy!

Did you know that the symphysis pubic *(aka your hip bones) can widen as much as 12 mm during pregnancy? This can be part of the reason for hip discomfort and is one very important reason why lumbar strength and stability is so important when you are pregnant!*

other prenatal workout program after the 4th month of your pregnancy. You want to be aware of the condition and avoid anything that could make it worse, as mentioned above. To see if you have this on your own, try this easy at-home check. If you think you have it based on this test, talk to your doctor about precautions, specifically regarding exercise:

- First, lie on your back with your knees bent, soles of your feet on the floor, ankles directly under your knees.

- Relax your abs and place one hand at the base of your head to support your neck. Then lift your head up a few inches off the floor.

- Take your other hand, point your fingers down toward your toes, and starting at your belly button, run your fingertips vertically along your centerline toward your head (the midsection of your abdomen).

You are looking to see if there is a gap between the muscles. Even without this condition, many pregnant women may notice a little bit of separation. Think of each fingertip as a centimeter. Anything over one fingertip will require caution and strict adherence to the guidelines I outlined above.

The Yeah Baby! Second Trimester Workouts

The following are four workouts I have created for you to utilize over your second trimester, complete with an exercise index that describes and illustrates each move for you. As promised, all of the guesswork has been taken out for you.

Each workout is roughly 30 minutes. I recommend the following schedule:

Workout 5 on Mondays and Thursdays for weeks 13, 14, 17, 18, 21, 22

Workout 6 on Tuesdays and Fridays for weeks 13, 14, 17, 18, 21, 22

Workout 7 on Mondays and Thursdays for weeks 15, 16, 19, 20, 23, 24

Workout 8 on Tuesdays and Fridays for weeks 15, 16, 19, 20, 23, 24

Like the last set of workouts, these workouts are also designed by muscle splits with "push muscles" (chest, shoulders, biceps, triceps) on Mondays and Thursdays and "pull muscles" (back, biceps, hamstrings, glutes) on Tuesdays and Fridays. Also like the first trimester, if you are feeling up to it, feel free to add in a straight cardio session on one of your off-days, like Wednesday, Saturday, or Sunday.

Each exercise will offer modifications so you can make the workouts easier if you need to. You can also continue to take prenatal yoga classes, prenatal Pilates, or any other class or workout that adheres to the guidelines laid out for this particular trimester.

And remember, if the exercise is marked with a *, skip it if you have diastasis recti, unless your doctor gives you the thumbs-up to perform it.

Second Trimester
WORKOUT GUIDELINES

Here are some basic things for you to remember during this trimester:

- Repeat each circuit one time before moving on to the next circuit.

- Based on the indicated warmup exercise, be sure to go at the pace, incline, or resistance that brings you to a 12 on the RPE scale. You can always refer back to the RPE scale on page 89 if you need a reminder about what this is (because mommy brain).

- For all unilateral exercises, do the first set on the right and the second set on the left side.

- For exercises that incorporate weights, go as heavy as you can lift safely and with good form.

- Modify the exercise if it's too hard.

- If at any point you feel you have exceeded a 14 on your RPE scale, pause and rest between exercises.

- During the cooldown, go slowly into the stretch. Don't force it and don't bounce in the stretch.

- And don't forget about Andy's *Pregnancy Sculpt* DVDs, too! It's always refreshing and good for your body to change things up, as long as you do it safely.

Please refer to Appendix B, starting on page 296, for photos of all the exercises.

Workout 5

To begin: Warm up with a 5-minute jog or incline walk on the treadmill at RPE 12.

CIRCUIT 1	CIRCUIT 2	CIRCUIT 3	CIRCUIT 4	COOLDOWN
1. Incline Push-ups: 15 reps (on bench or back of couch)	1. Diamond Pushups on Knees:* 15 reps	1. Walking Plank:* 10 reps	1. Alternating Heel Drops:* 16 reps	1. Chest Stretch: 30 seconds
2. Alternating Stepups: 20 reps	2. Triceps Dips: 15 reps	**BELLY ALERT**: *Drop to knees and slightly walk out on hands, then back to feet.*	2. Side Lying Inner Thigh Raises: 15 reps each side	2. Triceps Stretch: 30 seconds each side
3. Squats with Goblet Hold: 15 reps	3. Chair Squats with Anterior Raises: 15 reps	2. Modified Side Plank: 30 seconds	3. Boat Extensions with Forearms on Ground:* 15 reps	3. Side Lying Quad Stretch: 30 seconds each side
4. Sumo Squats with Shoulder Presses: 16 reps	4. Alternating Backward Lunges with Lateral Raises: 15 reps each side	3. Pilates Roll-backs: 10 reps	**BELLY ALERT:** *Keep knees bent, especially if your lower back is achy.*	4. Butterfly Stretch: 30 seconds each side
Rest 30 seconds, then repeat Circuit 1.	*Rest 30 seconds, then repeat Circuit 2.*	4. Side Lying Triceps Presses: 10 reps each side	4. Mula Bandha or Kegels: 10 reps	5. Shoulder Stretch: 30 seconds each side
		Rest 30 seconds, then repeat Circuit 3.	*Rest 30 seconds, then repeat Circuit 4.*	

BELLY ALERT!

In the second trimester workout plan, note **BELLY ALERT** modifications—if your belly or your boobs are already in the way, making some of these exercises awkward, or if you are having other issues like rotator cuff or balance issues, our trainer Andrea Orbeck, otherwise known as Andy, will advise you how you can modify them. If your belly isn't a problem yet and you aren't having any of these other issues, you can ignore these modifications for now, but definitely take heed if/when any of these issues occur.

Workout 6

To begin: Warm up with 5 minutes on the recumbent or stationary bike (use enough resistance to get you to RPE 12).

CIRCUIT 1	CIRCUIT 2	CIRCUIT 3	CIRCUIT 4	COOLDOWN
1. Crescent Pose with Wide Rows: 15 reps	1. Squats with Biceps Curls: 15 reps	1. Side Lying Leg Abductions: 15 reps each side	1. Mountain Climbers:* 16 reps	1. Pigeon Stretch: 30 seconds each side
2. Stiff Leg Deadlifts with Low Rows: 15 reps	2. Alternating Forward Lunges with Hammer Curls: 16 reps	2. Bent Leg Donkey Kicks:* 15 reps each side	**BELLY ALERT:** *Step into position instead of jumping.*	2. Calf Stretch: 30 seconds each side
3. Alternating Side Lunges with Serving Biceps: 16 reps	3. Alternating Curtsy Lunges with Biceps Curls:* 16 reps	**BELLY ALERT:** *If you have rotator cuff issues, do this from the elbows.*	2. Pelvic Thrusts on Physio Ball: 20 reps	3. Cat Cow Stretch: 30 seconds
4. Alternating Renegade Rows: 10 reps	**BELLY ALERT:** *If balance is an issue, use a chair for support.*	3. Fire Hydrants:* 15 reps each side	3. Modified Back Extensions on Knees: 20 reps	4. Hamstring Stretch: 30 seconds each side
Rest 30 seconds, then repeat Circuit 1.	4. Alternating Crossover Lunges with Reverse Curls:* 16 reps	**BELLY ALERT:** *If you have rotator cuff issues, do this from the elbows.*	4. Mula Bandha or Kegels: 10 reps	5. Mermaid Stretch: 30 seconds each side
	BELLY ALERT: *If balance is an issue, use a chair for support.*	4. Alternating Reverse Flys in Table: 16 reps	*Rest 30 seconds, then repeat Circuit 4.*	
	Rest 30 seconds, then repeat Circuit 2.	*Rest 30 seconds, then repeat Circuit 3.*		

EQUIPMENT

As in the other trimesters, we are predominantly using your body weight and a pair of light dumbbells, with one exception. We have incorporated a physio ball into the exercises for this trimester. You can buy one online or at any sporting goods store for around $15.

Workout 7

To begin: Warm up with a 5-minute climb on the step mill or stair master at RPE 12.

CIRCUIT 1	CIRCUIT 2	CIRCUIT 3	CIRCUIT 4	COOLDOWN
1. Triangle Presses:* 10 reps each side	1. Incline Push-ups: 15 reps	1. Modified Side Plank: 20 seconds each side	1. Camel Sitdowns: 15 reps	1. Side Lying Quad Stretch: 30 seconds each side
BELLY ALERT:	2. Alternating Backward Lunges with Lateral Raises: 16 reps	2. Walking Plank (modified on knees):* 10 reps	2. Uneven Table Hold: 20 seconds each side	2. Center Splits Oblique Stretch: 30 seconds each side
Do this from your knees.	3. Alternating Sumo Touch Downs:* 16 reps	3. Chest Presses on Physio Ball: 10 reps	3. Plank:* 30 second hold	3. Chest Stretch: 30 seconds
2. Side Squats with Military Presses: 15 reps	**BELLY ALERT:**	4. Plank to Wide Child's Pose:* 10 reps	**BELLY ALERT**:	4. Shoulder Stretch: 30 seconds each side
3. Chair Squats with Anterior Raises: 15 reps	*Lean slightly at the bottom of the squat.*	**BELLY ALERT:**	*Drop down to your knees to decrease the intensity if needed.*	5. Triceps Stretch: 30 seconds each side
4. Leaning Oblique Crunches with Alternating Leg Lifts:* 15 reps	4. Alternating Surrender Lunges with Shoulder Presses: 16 reps	*Do this from the elbows.*	4. Mula Bandha or Kegels: 10 reps	
BELLY ALERT:	*Rest 30 seconds, then repeat Circuit 2.*	*Rest 30 seconds, then repeat Circuit 3.*	*Rest 30 seconds, then repeat Circuit 4.*	
Drop your hands to your sides instead of putting them behind your head, and don't go down as far.				
Rest 30 seconds, then repeat Circuit 1.				

Andy Says . . .

Breathe during your reps! As your uterus grows bigger, your diaphragm will get compressed, making it seem difficult to breathe deeply. However, you are actually breathing more air, so keep at it! Your deep breathing really is helping.

Workout 8

Tuesdays and Fridays for Weeks 15, 16, 19, 20, 23, 24

To begin: Warm up with a 1,000-meter row on a rowing machine at RPE 12.

CIRCUIT 1	CIRCUIT 2	CIRCUIT 3	CIRCUIT 4	COOLDOWN
1. Medium Grip Rows in Crescent Pose: 15 reps	1. Good Mornings with Arms Crossed on Chest: 10 reps	1. Bent Leg Donkey Kicks:* 15 reps each side	1. Bridges: 15 reps	1. Mermaid Stretch: 30 seconds each side
2. Sumo Squats with Rotator Cuff Flys: 15 reps	2. Stiff Leg Deadlifts to Upright Rows: 15 reps	**BELLY ALERT:** *Do this from your elbows.*	2. Boat Extensions with Forearms on Ground:* 15 reps	2. Pigeon Stretch: 30 seconds each side
3. Squats with Biceps Curls: 15 reps	3. Alternating Side Lunges with Serving Biceps: 16 reps	2. Alternating Reverse Flys in Table: 16 reps	**BELLY ALERT:** *Keep your legs bent.*	3. Arm Biceps Stretch: 30 seconds each side
4. Stationary Lunges with Biceps Drags: 15 reps	4. Alternating Stepups: 16 reps	3. Mermaids: 15 reps each side	3. Alternating Heel Drops:* 16 reps	4. Sitting Trapezius Stretch: 30 seconds each side
Rest 30 seconds, then repeat Circuit 1.	*Rest 30 seconds, then repeat Circuit 2.*	4. Fire Hydrants:* 15 reps each side	**BELLY ALERT:** *Do this from your elbows.*	5. Wide Child's Pose: 30 seconds
		Rest 30 seconds, then repeat Circuit 3.	4. Mula Bandha or Kegels: 10 reps	
			Rest 30 seconds, then repeat Circuit 4.	

Okay, my lovelies. Onward! The third trimester awaits.

Motivation from Andy!

Your rotator cuff muscles provide stability to your shoulder and crucial strength when your bundle of joy feels like a 15-pound medicine ball that you are required to hold for hours at a time. So keep those shoulders strong!

CHAPTER 7

YOUR THIRD TRIMESTER:
The Homestretch
(or the Insomniac Pee Machine)

Wow, third trimester already? How did that happen? Didn't that second trimester just fly by? Well, maybe it did and maybe it didn't, but this is where you are now, on the homestretch, and I probably don't have to tell you that at this point in your pregnancy, the symptoms can really start to pile up. The issues Heidi struggled with in her second trimester carried into the third and got moderately exacerbated. Then a few new ones got sprinkled into the mix. The restless leg syndrome was still there, as was the heartburn, snoring, back pain, "bum bumps," double D cup, memory blackouts, nightmares of my apparent ongoing infidelity, and so on.

In the third trimester, God/Mother Nature/The Universe really pushed the "Up" button for Heidi. She may have struggled a bit more during months 7 to 9 than the average bear. She is pint-size (5 feet 2 inches, and when not pregnant, 100 pounds soaking wet) and happened to be carrying a mammoth-size boy in her stomach (unbeknownst to us at the time). And this ginormous child was banging into everything from her ribs to her bladder.

Around this time, I stopped laughing and poking fun, and I genuinely began to wish that pregnancy was a team sport. While we've all heard couples use PC lingo like "We're pregnant!"—this is simply bullshit. *You* are pregnant; your partner is on the sidelines, maybe feeling a bit helpless, definitely trying to be understanding and supportive, but absolutely *not* feeling everything you're experiencing. I really did wish I could have shared some of that physical burden. Little did I know at the time that my role as well-meaning-but-totally-clueless bystander was only a gentle precursor to what was soon to come in the delivery room—but we'll get to that a bit later.

Throughout most of the third trimester, Heidi was exhausted but couldn't sleep well, for a myriad of reasons. No matter how many wedge pillows we shoved under her tummy, legs, or back, she couldn't get comfortable. When she did sleep, her bladder would wake her every hour on the hour.

But it wasn't just sleeping that was uncomfortable—it was pretty much everything. Sitting for too long hurt. Lying down for too long hurt. Standing for too long hurt. By the middle of month 8, Heidi was ready to have our precious bundle out of her belly. By month 9, the real absurdity began.

Heidi tried everything to get our son out—or, rather, "naturally induce labor." From acupuncture to the "big O," nothing worked. She ate every hot sauce under the sun, which the bum bumps did *not* appreciate. She read about a certain kind of salad dressing that supposedly induced labor and ate it like she would never eat a salad again.

Nothing worked. The kid did not come out—but everything else did. Judging from the intensity and ferocity of her subsequent diarrhea attack after that salad binge, I am guessing that "special" dressing may have had castor oil in it.

Next, Heidi read online that stairclimbing and jogging had worked for other women. You can't imagine the death stares I got while coaching a very pregnant Heidi to do sprints and stair intervals in an attempt to "bounce" our son out of her uterus.

Learn from our mistakes. Fact is, you won't get the kid out of there this way or by any other mystical means. If the baby does not come out by 2 weeks past your due date (assuming there are no other complications), your doctor will induce you— which is exactly what ended up happening with Heidi. I'll tell you the rest of that story when we move on to Chapter 8, Labor and Delivery.

Now, let's get into *your* third trimester and discuss how we can make it as comfortable as possible.

QUICK LIST: WHAT TO ASK YOUR DOCTOR IN THE THIRD TRIMESTER

During this final stage of pregnancy, you'll see your doctor at least every week. Your baby is considered full-term at the end of week 38. Here are some things to ask, relevant to the homestretch.

- Ask for advice for soothing aches, pains, and bodily discomfort like heartburn, hemorrhoids, urine leakage, or pelvic pain.

- Talk about the difference between normal Braxton Hicks contractions and the real thing. Find out whom you can call, especially after hours, for advice on whether you are really in labor and whether it's time to head to the birth center or hospital.

- If your baby remains in a head-up (breech) position, ask for advice about encouraging the baby to turn head down. Gentle inversions—with your buttocks elevated—may give the baby more room to turn. Dr. Suzanne says there is also a procedure called external cephalic version that can be done at about

37 weeks to turn the baby around manually. If your healthcare provider is familiar with or practices integrative medicine, he or she might also recommend acupuncture, chiropractic, or hypnotherapy.

- As your due date nears, ask what you can do to prepare for delivery.

- Ask about specific exercises that can help prepare your body for delivery. Although we do cover much of that in our exercise plan, it can't hurt to get your doctor's feedback as well.

- If your physician recommends bed rest for any reason, ask why. There are some good reasons, including high blood pressure. However, some doctors may be overly careful, so ask lots of questions to make sure it's warranted.

- If you are considering banking your baby's cord blood, talk to your healthcare provider about the pros and cons to help you make your decision. See page 218 for more info on what this is.

Heidi Says . . .

By this time, I was in full nesting mode—buying baby clothes, arranging the nursery, and dreaming of meeting the little one. I was also part of a one-sided boxing match, or so it seemed. The little guy was punching me and kicking me from the inside so hard that I actually ended up with bruises on my stomach! Around this time, he also decided to lodge his foot in my back rib cage, where it stayed for the remaining duration of the pregnancy. I remember sitting at Jillian's birthday party dinner in Napa, trying to get him to move with no luck whatsoever. No amount of pushing, prodding, or jumping would move him. He would stay in that position until delivery.

The heartburn was still very much a reality and getting worse by the day. Sleep-ing became almost impossible when combined with the never-ending urge to pee. I suppose my body was preparing me for the many sleepless nights to come. At least, that's how I rationalized it.

I also began to balloon in places that I didn't know I could balloon: my toes, my legs, my fingers. Everything was swelling near the end. I never felt more unattractive in my life. When the acupuncturist told me I was carrying a 9-pound baby, no one believed him but me. With the 41 pounds of weight gain and the legs and elbows poking me from every angle, I knew this was not going to be a petite child. I did, however, know that I wanted him out! And with the delivery date come and gone, I felt like it was literally never going to happen.

DEVELOPMENT IN THE THIRD TRIMESTER: WEEKS 25 TO 30

The third trimester can sneak up on you. There you are, happily going through the second trimester feeling like your due date is ages away, and then suddenly, boom, it's almost time for the big day. This can have many different, simultaneous effects on you. You might be excited, impatient, and terrified, all at the same time. You may feel as though you aren't mentally prepared for any of it. (None of us really are, by the way. Totally normal. I just kept thinking, we are walking in as a couple and out as a "family"—holy crap.) So, let this chapter help ease you into that state of full preparedness, if you are not in that headspace already.

What's Happening to Me?

You are two-thirds of the way to delivery day! Somewhere between weeks 28 and 34, your doctor will check if the baby is headfirst or breech (bottom or feet first). If the baby is breech, don't worry—many babies flip into the correct position on their own.[1] In fact, Dr. Suzanne says she doesn't check until 34 weeks because by that time, approximately 96 percent of babies are in the right position, and if they aren't, there is still enough time to try to get the baby turned around.

During the 29th week you should be feeling frequent movement, such as kicks and jabs,[2] and you might even feel hiccups or rhythmic twitches.[3] According to research into baby movements, most babies move about 30 times every hour.[4] Although each baby seems to have his or her own schedule, many tend to be most active right after you decide to try to go to sleep. This is likely due to fluctuations in your blood sugar level at this time.[5] (If you don't feel movement at least 10 times in 2 hours, this is probably nothing to worry about, but contact your doctor just to be safe.[6])

Our son seemed to never rest in this trimester. He would pummel away at Heidi's rib cage nonstop. The only thing that seemed to quiet him temporarily was when I played Coldplay for him through Heidi's Belly Buds (tummy headphones to play music to your little one—see page 323 of the Products and Resources section). If all else fails, give those a try.

Any back pain and bodily discomfort you notice now is, in all likelihood, a result of the extra weight you are carrying around, as well as relaxin, the hormone that loosens up your ligaments to make room for the baby's passage. Your uterus alone has grown from a mere 2 ounces before pregnancy to 2.5 pounds at the time of birth—and that doesn't even include the weight of the baby inside of it.[7] To alleviate back pain, sleep on your left side and keep moving during the day as much as possible. Gentle physical activity such as yoga and water exercise can help take the pressure off your back muscles. Massage and acupuncture also helped Heidi so much with this, and Dr. Suzanne confirms that pregnancy massage and acupuncture as well as physical therapy can help a lot with back pain.

Also, remember that blood test to measure Rh factor, a substance found in red blood cells? As we discussed earlier, if you don't have Rh in your blood, but your baby does, it increases the odd of health problems such as jaundice and anemia. If so, you may require a shot of Rh in week 28 and again after delivery.[8] Your doctor can advise you about this.

What's Going On in There?

Your fetus is now really looking like a little human. The ears have developed enough at this point that the baby might hear the sound of your voice.[9] Your baby now needs

TRUE or FALSE
Pregnant women shouldn't fly during their third trimester.

Depends. Only you and your doctor can make this decision because individual needs vary. If you are on bed rest or have a medical condition that could make flying more dangerous, your doctor may advise against it. In most cases, however, healthy pregnant women can fly, and the process of flying is not any more likely to induce labor than anything else you might do, according to the American College of Obstetrics and Gynecology.[10] For that reason, most domestic carriers will allow passengers to fly up to their 36th week without restriction or a note from your doctor. Dr. Suzanne adds that if you do plan to travel by air while pregnant, it is important to stay hydrated and pee often, or you are likely to get edema (swelling), especially in your legs and feet. Consider wearing support stockings to decrease the risk of edema and of deep vein thrombosis, which would be unusual but possible. Also, she cautions not to fly anywhere you don't want to have your baby after approximately 34 weeks, and she doesn't advise it after that time unless you can be comfortable. For example, if you can afford business or first class, you will have more room. If you can book an aisle seat, you will have an easier time stretching out your legs or getting up when you need to if you are in the air for more than a couple of hours. If you can drive instead of fly, you have the luxury of stopping more often to stretch. Cramped quarters and airplane restrooms are pretty miserable in your third trimester! Also, avoid carbonated beverages and other gas-producing foods so you don't risk feeling bloated or having indigestion on the plane.[11]

Dr. Suzanne Says . . .

Although you might have heard that you need to feel constant movement or you need to worry about your baby, this isn't true. Most moms start to feel their babies move between 18 and 25 weeks, and a kick-count test is a good way to quantify that movement and let your doctor know how often you are feeling it, but it won't work at all times. We don't all feel every movement—there is a "white noise" effect in which you become used to the feeling and don't notice it. Also if the placenta is more to the front of your uterus or you tend to be awake when the baby is sleeping, you may not feel movement very often. This is no cause for alarm. Instead, stimulate the fetus before you do a kick-count test. Shake your belly, lie on your side, or eat or drink something. After that, you should feel 8 to 10 movements over the next hour or two, and that can be reassuring. If you don't feel movement, if the movement seems to decrease noticeably at a time when your baby is typically active, or if you are concerned for any other reason, call your doctor, who can check that everything is proceeding normally.

to focus on developing lungs and an immune system so he can survive outside the womb—he also needs to put on some fat to help cushion the bumpy exit during delivery. By week 28, the eyelids are partially open with tiny eyelashes. In the 29th week, the bones are fully developed,[12] which means you might really start to feel the jabbing and poking inside the womb.[13] In the 30th week, your baby will fully open his eyes[14] and begin breathing regularly with the diaphragm.

DEVELOPMENT IN THE THIRD TRIMESTER: WEEKS 31 TO 34

Maybe you are counting the days to your due date by now, but you still have a way to go. You are getting larger and larger and probably having more discomfort now, but trust me, you look absolutely amazing.

What's Happening to Me?

Even if you've never experienced it before, it's likely you'll experience heartburn as the baby takes up more space in your abdomen. Avoid common heartburn triggers like carbonated drinks, caffeine, chocolate, citrus, tomatoes, mustard, vinegar, breath mints, spicy foods, and fried foods. You can also try sleeping with your upper body elevated. I gave you some heartburn remedies in the previous chapter on page 152, so check that out if you are only now experiencing it.

Hemorrhoids are also common during this trimester, as the weight of the baby presses down on your pelvis. To soothe the itch or pain, naturopathic physicians recommend topical aloe vera gel or witch hazel.[15] (I talked about other remedies for this in the previous chapter on page 154.)

At this point, your milk glands will start producing colostrum—a thin precursor to milk that will supply nutrients and calories to your baby until your milk comes in. Your breasts might start leaking this fluid early, so be ready with nursing pads to avoid embarrassing stains on your shirt.[16] This happened to Heidi a couple of times. Once, she made me swap shirts with her, logic being "you're not pregnant." I of course felt like this would make even less sense, but nevertheless I didn't argue and made damn sure after that to keep those nursing pads handy.

Now is also a good time to start planning your delivery, packing your hospital bag, and washing your baby's first outfit! Keep in mind that every delivery is different and they don't always go as planned. Be prepared to scrap those plans and go with the flow once the big day arrives. We will get into this in more detail in the next chapter.

What's Going On in There?

In these weeks, your baby is rapidly developing all the systems it needs to function on its own, including the central nervous system and digestive tract. For example, your baby will urinate several cups a day into the amniotic fluid at week 31.[17] While the lungs aren't fully formed yet, in week 32, the baby will practice breathing, and his eyes can open and close with plenty of eyelashes, eyebrows, and even hair on the

TRUE or FALSE If you're "carrying high," you're carrying a girl; if you're "carrying low," it's a boy.

Uh, no. This particular wives' tale is completely crazy. How your body looks during pregnancy is a result of so many factors *not* related to your baby's gender—like your body shape, the position of the baby, your muscle tone, and the amount of weight you've gained during pregnancy.[18] Everybody likes to think they can predict a baby's sex based on weird things like this, but no. There is no correlation. You're just as likely to get it right by asking the Magic Eight Ball.

head.[22] At this point, toenails are visible, and the soft peach fuzz, or lanugo, that covered the skin starts to fall off while the Chapstick-like coating, or *vernix caseosa*, gets thicker.[23] In the 33rd week, the pupils can dilate and constrict, allowing your baby to detect light.[24] In fact, your baby will already experience rapid eye movement during sleep—your little one could be having his or her very first dreams![25]

Your baby's brain has also made great strides, with billions of neurons developed and connected that allow it to listen to and feel its surroundings in your womb.[26] At this point, the lungs are almost completely developed.[27] By the 34th week, fingernails have grown long enough to reach the fingertips.[28] And while many of the bones have hardened, the bones that make up the skull are positioned in such a way that they can move as they pass through the birth canal—your baby's head may look lumpy shortly after birth, but it will eventually settle into a normal shape.[29]

DEVELOPMENT IN THE THIRD TRIMESTER: WEEKS 35 TO 40 OR DELIVERY

Now you really are almost there. You may be feeling nervous, excited, overwhelmed, or all the feelings you've ever had, all at once. Totally normal. The birth is imminent, and you're about to be a mama, Mama! Let me be the first to congratulate you! Now, let's get you to the big day feeling as good as possible.

What's Happening to Me?

As you near your due date, your doctor will want to see you every week to check your cervix for dilation.

You may also feel the baby drop lower into your pelvis, which not only relieves some pressure on your stomach (and makes eating a bit easier), but also means the baby is preparing for its exit.[30] By week 37, the mucus plug that was dutifully protecting your baby inside the womb might dislodge. The thick, yellowish or bloody mass will fall out anywhere from hours to weeks before labor. Also, by week 39 your amniotic sac might rupture—this is the "I think my water just broke!" moment, and it can result in a gush of fluid or just a tiny trickle. Either way, you should let your doctor know if this happens, or if you see any discharge you think could be amniotic fluid, because in some cases this means labor needs to begin soon.[31]

At week 39, it might be hard to tell the difference between Braxton Hicks contractions and the real thing, as these "false" contractions can actually be quite painful. The difference is that Braxton Hicks do not increase in frequency, while true contractions occur at a steady, regular frequency and amp up in strength as they progress.[32] If your body is preparing for labor, your cervix may already be 2 to 3 centimeters dilated, even if you are not experiencing contractions.

What's Going On in There?

Your baby has been steadily gaining fat and now looks pretty much like a chubby newborn. As the baby grows, you may notice movement slowing down. Don't panic—it's just getting too crowded in there for womb gymnastics. But you should still feel some movements, like kicks and twitches.[33] Most babies naturally turn from a head-up to a head-down position as the due date nears, somewhere around weeks 33 to 36. Somewhere between weeks 37 and 40, your baby will drop lower into your pelvis as your body prepares for labor and delivery.[34]

By week 37, your baby is now considered full-term and ready to survive outside your womb—although it's better to wait until 39 weeks to deliver to allow further final developments of the lungs, brain, and liver.[35] The eyes are developed enough that your baby will turn toward a bright light held up to your belly.[36] In preparation for the big day, your baby's head will descend all the way into your pelvis.[37] Your baby will also start to create his or her first poop (lucky for you, the first of many)—a dark, sticky substance called meconium that is made up of dead skin cells, leftover lanugo hair, cells shed by the intestines, and other waste that has accumulated in your baby's intestines.[38] For some reason, I was not fully prepped on the aesthetic of meconium, and when our son crapped tar, I nearly passed out. Obviously, I found out very quickly that it's perfectly normal. So, consider yourself prepped. That first poop

BIRTH PLAN

A birth plan is basically a written-down plan for how you would like things to go during your labor and delivery. This can be as simple or as detailed as you like, and there is no particular required format for it, but the purpose is to think about and plan for things that you can't just decide on at the last minute when you are already in labor. In Chapter 8, the labor and delivery chapter, I will go into much greater detail about all of these items, so as you work on your birth plan, please read that chapter and refer to it often. Your birth plan could be half a page or a multipage document, although if it is longer than one page, be forewarned that your healthcare providers may not have time to read it—brief is better. You could also make a succinct version for your doctor and a longer version for yourself and family members. Once you have it, make copies and give them to everyone involved: your doctor, your midwife, your doula, your partner, your family members, and anyone else who will be participating in the process. Just to get you started, here are some of the things you will want to include in your birth plan.

1. **Where you would like to have your baby.** In a hospital, a birthing center, at home? Look into the options, make the appropriate arrangements, and write it down in your birth plan.

2. **Whom you would like to deliver your baby.** A doctor? A midwife? Both at different stages? Have you hired a doula who will be in the room with you? Put this in your birth plan.

3. **How you feel about medical intervention, like epidurals and C-sections.** Have it on record if you don't mind these interventions or even want them, or if you are opposed unless they become medically necessary. But keep in mind that sometimes a C-section might become necessary. Flexibility is important on this one. I'll talk a lot more about this in Chapter 8.

4. **What to take to the hospital.** Make your packing list. Your hospital bag should be ready, and be sure to get an infant car seat installed in the car you will come back home in with your baby. It's much easier to figure that out now rather than later.

5. **Who else you want to be present before and/or during the birth.** Just your partner? Just your best friend? Just your mom? Or the whole gang? Put this on record.

6. **Anything else important to you.** This is the time to start thinking about this, deciding between things that matter and things that don't, and putting it all together.

is something else—get ready! (This won't be one of the photos you want to post on Facebook.)

A DEEPER LOOK AT TESTS: THIRD TRIMESTER

By now, you're an old pro at tests—you've likely come to see them as more of an ally than a foe, and giving a little blood from a finger stick probably feels like nothing to you at this point. Now that you can feel the baby move, you may also be more anxious for extra information about how he or she is doing. Here are a few tests your doctor might order if he or she feels they are warranted. They can give your doctor more insight—and you peace of mind.

- **Nonstress test:** A fetal nonstress test is so named because it places no stress on the baby. A doctor may perform a nonstress test after 28 weeks of pregnancy to assess the baby's health by looking at movement, heart rate, and reactivity of the heart rate to movement. Reasons for a nonstress test include

 TRUE or FALSE Pregnant women should avoid carrying heavy items.

Not necessarily true in every case, but go easy. If you follow the plot line on old television shows, the minute a woman reveals she is pregnant, she is no longer able to lift a finger, for fear it will harm the baby. That scenario is clearly overly dramatic, but with all the natural changes that occur in your body, from loosening joints to over-stretched muscles that are prone to cramping, the reality is that when it comes to lifting heavy objects, you are the one who is more at risk of injury. Your baby is nicely cushioned in there, but you could easily strain your back or otherwise hurt yourself, adding to your list of uncomfortable symptoms.

By the third trimester, you may find it hard to lift anything with that baby bump in the way, anyway. If you are already used to lifting things, such as doing that regularly at a job, then you may be just fine, but always follow the advice of your doctor—when in doubt, it's a good idea to ask for help from others. If you must lift something heavy, always make sure to follow healthy lifting practices by bending at your knees (not your waist), keeping your back straight, and pushing up with your legs.[39]

being overdue, decreased fetal movements, suspicion the placenta may not be functioning properly, or a high-risk pregnancy.[40]

- **Biophysical profile:** The biophysical profile involves an ultrasound examination coupled with a nonstress test. Its goal is to monitor the overall health of the baby by looking at his or her movement, muscle tone, breathing, heart rate, and amount of amniotic fluid to help determine whether or not the baby should be delivered early.[41]

- **Group B strep:** Group B strep (GBS) is a strain of bacteria that lives in the vagina and rectum. This is not an STD, and about 25 to 30 percent of women have it as a naturally occurring bacteria, with no symptoms. However, it is dangerous for a newborn, so you will want to wipe it out before giving birth. To test for it, your physician will do a swab of your "privates" somewhere between 33 and 36 weeks to check for the presence of this bacteria. If you do have it, antibiotics will get rid of it simply and safely,[42] protecting the baby. Just be sure to counteract the negative internal effects of antibiotics (like gut bacteria imbalance, stomach discomfort, and yeast infections) with foods rich in probiotics like kefir and yogurt. Consider a probiotic supplement as well.

- **Ultrasound:** As we talked about in the second trimester, an ultrasound is a procedure that uses high-frequency sound waves to create a picture (sonogram) of the baby and placenta. There are different types of ultrasound procedures, and your healthcare professional may use a different type depending on where you are in your pregnancy and the reason for the exam. There is no standard recommended number of ultrasounds, and the average number differs among providers. Your healthcare provider should order one only if there is a medical reason for it. In the third trimester, your provider may use ultrasound to check on the location of the placenta, look at the baby's position and movements, assess fetal growth or amniotic fluid status, or look for any pelvic or uterine abnormalities. A provider may also use a 4D ultrasound to get a detailed look at your baby's face and movements prior to delivery, if that is necessary for any reason.[43]

THIRD TRIMESTER NUTRITION

It's the final countdown. Yep, you're almost there, and it's more important than ever that you keep your good nutrition habits going. In fact, this is a time to step it up. Your body will go through a lot of changes during this time, and it's likely you will feel and notice all of them. You want to be as well nourished as possible when you go through labor and delivery! And while stretch marks, constipation, heartburn, hemorrhoids, and all that lovely stuff may continue or even increase at this time, good third trimester nutrition can mitigate some of those uncomfortable symptoms as well as support your baby's tremendous growth during this time.

The third trimester meal plan and eating strategy incorporate all the tips and tricks from the second and the first trimesters, but with a few extra ones to support you and baby through all the aforementioned. Remember, once again, that all the nutrition Rules of Thumb still apply. First, here are your third trimester do's and don'ts.

Third Trimester Don'ts

- **Don't: Eat any of the chemicals or crap** we covered in the Rules of Thumb nutrition chapter.
- **Don't: Consume high quantities of sodium.** This is always important, but even more so in the third trimester, to help reduce bloat and high blood pressure that is probably most noticeable right now.
- **Don't: Consume processed high-sugar foods,** to help keep blood sugar stable and blood pressure at healthy levels and to tame that awful heartburn.

Third Trimester Do's

- **Do: Be sure to eat every 3 to 4 hours** to stabilize blood sugar and try to avoid constant snacking throughout the day to keep insulin levels from surging. If your heartburn is severe, then it is okay to break up your meals and eat every 2 or 3 hours, but be sure to avoid those high-sugar foods as mentioned above.

 TRUE or FALSE Eating pineapples when you're overdue can help induce labor.

Worth a shot! Fresh pineapple contains the enzyme bromelain, which is an important ingredient in meat tenderizers because it helps break down proteins. Plenty of anecdotal evidence supports the idea that eating fresh pineapple can hasten labor if you're overdue, but there's no medical evidence to back up that claim.[44, 45] But honestly, who cares if it *really* works? Fresh pineapple is delicious and can quell heartburn because its enzymes speed digestion, so if it helps you feel like you're doing something productive, go for it.

- **Do: Get protein in every meal** and every snack to help stabilize blood sugar.

- **Do: Consume foods that are rich in potassium and magnesium** to help lower blood pressure and prevent preeclampsia. Spinach, sunflower seeds, beans, potatoes, and bananas are all good sources.

- **Do: Consume foods high in tryptophan** like turkey, walnuts, and safe cheeses to help you sleep and to calm restless legs. Melatonin boosters such as cherries, bananas, and oats help with this as well.

- **Do: Consume foods high in chromium** to help balance blood sugar and diminish sugar cravings. Broccoli, barley, tomatoes, black pepper, and cinnamon all fit the bill, if they don't give you heartburn.

- **Do: Continue to get your choline** because a 2013 study revealed that large amounts of the nutrient are needed in the third trimester to support fetal development, particularly brain growth. Choline is used to make a substance that is an integral part of every cell membrane, and this study found that pregnant women's bodies used more choline than normal to produce it.[46] Choline also prevents birth defects by lowering levels of homocysteine, an amino acid linked to congenital heart defects and spina bifida. Whole eggs are a great source.

- **Do: Remember all of your key vitamins, minerals, and nutrients!** We've been over this a ton, but all of these are still very important to your baby's bone, brain, nerve, eye, and overall development. Stay the course, Mama—you're almost there.

- **Do: Eat foods high in bioflavonoids** (aka super antioxidants) to help strengthen arterial walls and prevent varicose veins. These also help with preventing hyperpigmentation and stretch marks. Ironically, most of the foods that help with hyperpigmentation of the skin ("mask of pregnancy") are themselves hyperpigmented, or very rich in colors! Garlic, spinach, broccoli, berries, and red bell peppers are good choices.

- **Do: Eat dried cranberries** or put some straight (unsweetened) cranberry juice in with your water. You're peeing a lot due to the extra pressure on your bladder, which can lower the "force" of your stream. The lack of intensity can prevent your body from pushing out all the bad bacteria, and you may become more prone to urinary tract and bladder infections during this trimester. Cranberries are great for dispelling and combating bad bacteria in your urinary tract.

- **Do: Continue getting your omega-3s** to feed your baby's brain growth. A 2008 Canadian study found that intake of omega-3 fatty acids, specifically

DHA, during the last 3 months of pregnancy significantly improved an infant's visual acuity and cognitive and motor development at 6 and 11 months.[47] EPA and DHA are always important, both for you and baby, but it's time to really up the stores as you'll need plenty to help you counterbalance baby blues. Get that salmon in there! Also note that while these omega-3s are great, junky saturated fats in the third trimester are not great. According to a 2014 Yale University animal study, mice mothers fed a high-fat diet during the last months of pregnancy had babies who faced an increased risk of being overweight throughout their lives because of changes to their metabolism in utero.[48]

- **Do: Get your vitamin D.** Be sure to spend time out in the sun for 15 minutes during nonpeak hours without sunscreen. Talk with your doctor about supplementation, and look for vitamin D in portobello mushrooms, eggs, and fortified foods like coconut milk, almond milk, and dairy milk.

- **Do: Get some vitamin K.** Vitamin K can help prevent excessive bleeding at childbirth because of its role in blood clotting, and babies who are vitamin K deficient are at risk of a brain bleed. Vitamin K in your diet will also help supply vitamin K to your baby through your breast milk, so keep it up after the birth.[49] Good sources are parsley, collard greens, turnip greens, spinach, kale, broccoli, carrot juice, pumpkin, or blueberries.[50, 51]

The Yeah Baby!
THIRD TRIMESTER MEAL PLAN

You are now a pro at following the meal plans, and this one will look a lot like the others, but with some new elements specifically geared toward your third trimester nutritional needs. Don't give in to unhealthy cravings now, thinking your baby has developed enough and that poor food choices don't matter. They continue to matter as long as you are breastfeeding and, in reality, as long as you are parenting! So get those habits solidified now, and your baby will reap the benefits for a lifetime.

As usual, each of the four meal plans in this chapter is to be used at different weeks during your pregnancy, as indicated. For example, the first meal plan in this third trimester is for weeks 25, 29, 33, and 37. Also remember that you can vary these plans and mix them up, favoring the recipes you like the most, if you choose.

You can find the complete recipes for everything in this meal plan in Appendix A, beginning on page 271.

Meal Plan 1 Weeks 25, 29, 33, 37

	BREAKFAST	LUNCH	SNACK	DINNER
MONDAY	Baby Booster Smoothie	Summer Shrimp Salad	Organic Jerky (purchased)	Veggie Pie
TUESDAY	The California Poach	Chicken Parmesan Orzo Salad	Super Mommy Mix	Baked Trout
WEDNESDAY	Maple Pecan Porridge	Chicken Chop	Devilish Deviled Eggs with Watermelon	Mussels Marinara
THURSDAY	Huevos Tacos	Slammin' Turkey Sammy	The PBB	Thai Steak
FRIDAY	B4 Power Parfait	Mediterranean Chicken Sandwich	Hummus and Pita Chips (purchased)	Veggie Pasta
SATURDAY	Feta Frittata	Slammin' Turkey Sammy	Veggies and Dip	Peach Pork Chop with Fennel Salad
SUNDAY	Bad A$$ Breakfast Burrito	Chicken Artichoke Pizza	Cottage Cheese and Peaches	Lemon Lamb Chop

Meal Plan 2 Weeks 26, 30, 34, 38

	BREAKFAST	LUNCH	SNACK	DINNER
MONDAY	Lori and Jamie's Feel-Good Muffin	Slaw Salad	Bangin' Bruschetta	Steak Chimichurri
TUESDAY	Breakfast Bowl	Quick and Easy Fish Tacos	Veggies and Dip	Peach Pork Chop with Fennel Salad
WEDNESDAY	Apple Zucchini Flap Jacks with Turkey Bacon	BBQ Steak Salad	Hummus and Pita Chips (purchased)	Veggie Pasta
THURSDAY	Hot Mama Smoothie	Chicken Chop	Devilish Deviled Eggs with Watermelon	Lemon Lamb Chop
FRIDAY	B4 Power Parfait	Summer Shrimp Salad	Organic Jerky (purchased)	Argentine Salmon
SATURDAY	Huevos Tacos	Chicken Burrito Bowl	Chocolate Cherry Smoothie	Baked Trout
SUNDAY	Feta Frittata	Chicken Parmesan Orzo Salad	Awesome Artichoke	Thai Steak

Meal Plan 3 Weeks 27, 31, 35, 39

	BREAKFAST	LUNCH	SNACK	DINNER
MONDAY	B4 Power Parfait	Summer Shrimp Salad	Cheese Plate	Lemon Lamb Chop
TUESDAY	Lori and Jamie's Feel-Good Muffin	Chicken Burrito Bowl	Chocolate Cherry Smoothie	Argentine Salmon
WEDNESDAY	Breakfast Bowl	Mediterranean Chicken Sand-wich	Bangin' Bruschetta	Veggie Pie
THURSDAY	The California Poach	Quick and Easy Fish Tacos	Fruity Gazpacho	Thai Steak
FRIDAY	Hot Mama Smoothie	Chicken Chop	Veggies and Dip	Mussels Marinara
SATURDAY	Bad A$$ Break-fast Burrito	Slaw Salad	Hummus and Pita Chips (purchased)	The Ultimate Turkey Burger
SUNDAY	Apple Zucchini Flapjacks with Turkey Bacon	Slammin' Turkey Sammy	Devilish Deviled Eggs with Watermelon	Baked Trout

Meal Plan 4 Weeks 28, 32, 36, 40

	BREAKFAST	LUNCH	SNACK	DINNER
MONDAY	Feta Frittata	Chicken Artichoke Pizza	Chocolate Cherry Smoothie	The Ultimate Turkey Burger
TUESDAY	Breakfast Bowl	Summer Shrimp Salad	Veggies and Dip	Steak Chimichurri
WEDNESDAY	Apple Zucchini Flap Jacks with Turkey Bacon	BBQ Steak Salad	The PBB	Veggie Pasta
THURSDAY	Baby Booster Smoothie	Chicken Burrito Bowl	Super Mommy Mix	Mussels Marinara
FRIDAY	Bad A$$ Break-fast Burrito	Chicken Parme-san Orzo Salad	Bangin' Bruschetta	Lemon Lamb Chop
SATURDAY	Maple Pecan Porridge	Slammin' Turkey Sammy	Cottage Cheese and Peaches	Argentine Salmon
SUNDAY	Lori and Jamie's Feel-Good Muffin	Slaw Salad	Cheese Plate	Peach Pork Chop with Fennel Salad

THIRD TRIMESTER FITNESS

Work out? Now? With that giant belly? You bet your baby bump! If you keep exercising all the way up to your baby's birth date, you will reap benefits galore, and an easier labor is just the beginning. Remember that your exercise now will make your baby fitter and smarter later, so keep it up. Of course, be careful, making allowances for your burgeoning belly and boobs, your increasingly challenged balance, and of course the extra weight you are carrying. With all that in mind, I bring you your third trimester workouts!

As always, our Fitness Rules of Thumb are our golden rules, and all the caveats and guidelines from the previous two trimesters apply. Heartburn, back pain, lack of balance, and breathlessness will be at their height during this trimester, so it's crucial that you adhere to all the guidelines we've covered previously for safety and comfort.

Not to worry, though. As always, I will give you four new workouts that comply with all restrictions, fitness requirements, and guidelines. The same workout schedule will apply, as outlined below. Unlike the last trimester, when we had special Belly Alert modifications for those whose bellies were already getting in the way, this trimester we *assume* your belly is totally *out there,* and these exercises make allowances for that.

But first, let's talk about the final fitness concerns and restrictions for the third trimester in particular. During the third trimester is when we show the most restraint with fitness—no, you are not crippled, but your body *has* changed and still will change so much and so rapidly in preparation for birth over the next few weeks that it can be easy to overdo it without realizing your new limitations.

That said, staying active now is crucial. Just in case you need more convincing, exercise during the third trimester also helps you avoid gaining too much weight in the final weeks. It reduces the risk of gestational diabetes and aids in a speedy postpartum recovery. Plus, the third trimester is when the fetus gains most of its fat tissue. Studies have found that exercising mommies give birth to babies with an average of 41 grams less body fat mass than babies born from mommies who exercised the least, and that will benefit your baby later.

Here are a few specific additional issues we must take into account for your third trimester exercise regimen.

Third Trimester Issue 1: Abdominal Separation/Diastasis Recti

I already mentioned this in the last chapter, but women are most prone to developing separated abdominal muscles around week 28 and beyond, as the baby's size grows and stretches the abdominal wall. That's why, during the third trimester, you're better off using a very elevated platform for all pushups, planks, and prone position exercises. This elevation helps to minimize pressure to your abdominal wall, which could help prevent abdominal separation, but will also help minimize discomfort if you already have it; the core strengthening these exercises accomplish will also help your abdominal wall seal back up again more quickly after birth. Like the second trimester workouts, any starred move (*) should be cleared by your doctor or avoided if you know you already have this condition.

Third Trimester Issue 2: Overexertion

I have stressed repeatedly that you should not overdo it. Now, I'm going to recommend no more than four workouts a week—and I flat-out draw the line at five. Too much is simply too much. Rest is crucial for you and your little one. Plus, injuries can occur when we are tired and run-down.

Third Trimester Issue 3: Back Safety

Do not do any exercises that twist or compress your abdomen or spine. That means avoiding crunches, overhead presses, overhead squats, back squats, twisting yoga poses (side bends are okay), or exercises with torso rotation. We want to avoid any chance that you could pull a muscle and/or strain your lower back.

Yes, I have seen women doing all of these exercises practically minutes before delivery, and I'm not saying that if you do them, you will absolutely 100 percent get injured . . . but why take a risk? Even if you're a well-conditioned athlete, I wouldn't recommend it. These exercises dramatically increase your chances of pulling a muscle

Motivation from Andy

I know you feel huge and I know you are in the homestretch, but try to continue movement all the way through your third trimester (with your doctor's permission, of course). Some of the best outcomes associated with exercise during pregnancy occur when activity continues as late into the pregnancy as possible. Besides, since you have been exercising throughout the first and second trimesters and growing your bundle of joy at the same time, you have way more conditioning than you might think. Enjoy your superhuman vigor!

or straining your lower back, and that could really make delivery painful. Hormones make you super flexible right now, which means you can get injured more easily. We can get you or keep you in great shape without taking that risk.

In addition, do not use heavy weights or jerking motions like cleans, for the same reason. Yes, I have seen women back-squatting 100 pounds in their third trimester—but that certainly doesn't mean I would recommend it. Remember, this is not about proving a point—it's about being smart and playing it safe.

You are not relegated to a pair of 3-pound dumbbells, however. Exceptions include exercises that don't compress the spine, such as incline chest presses, lat pulls, rows, leg extensions, and arm exercises. All of these can and should be safely performed with weights. Just remember, moderation is key. No personal records, please.

THE YEAH BABY! THIRD TRIMESTER WORKOUTS

I've created the following four workouts for you to use in your third trimester, complete with an exercise index that illustrates each move for you. Each workout is roughly 30 minutes, and again, I take out all the guesswork, giving you the exercises that are safe for you to do right now. I recommend the following schedule:

Workout 9 on Mondays and Thursdays for weeks 25, 26, 29, 30, 33, 34, 37, 38

Workout 10 on Tuesdays and Fridays for weeks 25, 26, 29, 30, 33, 34, 37, 38

Workout 11 on Mondays and Thursdays for weeks 27, 28, 31, 32, 35, 36, 39, 40

Workout 12 on Tuesdays and Fridays for weeks 27, 28, 31, 32, 35, 36, 39, 40

Like the last two sets of workouts, these workouts are once again designed by muscle splits with "push muscles" (chest, shoulders, biceps, triceps) on Mondays and Thursdays and "pull muscles" (back, biceps, hamstrings, glutes) on Tuesdays and Fridays.

If you are feeling great and you have lots of extra energy, you can add one straight cardio session on one of your off-days, such as Wednesday, Saturday, or Sunday. If not, four workouts a week is more than enough. In fact, I think four is an ideal number to aid in rest and workout recovery.

Don't forget, you can also continue to take prenatal yoga classes, prenatal Pilates, or any other class or workout that adheres to the guidelines laid out for this particular trimester.

And don't forget to check out Andrea Orbeck's *Pregnancy Sculpt* DVDs.

Third Trimester WORKOUT GUIDELINES

Here are the basic things to keep in mind during this trimester:

- Repeat each circuit one time before moving on to the next circuit.

- Based on the indicated warmup exercise, be sure to go at the pace, incline, or resistance that brings you to a 12 on the RPE scale. What was a 12 to you 2 months ago may not be a 12 to you during this trimester, so if you find you are getting the same exertion from a lower level of warmup, that's just fine. Also, you can always refer back to the RPE scale on page 89 to remind you what RPE 12 should feel like.

- For all unilateral exercises, do the first set on the right and the second set on the left side.

- For exercises that incorporate weights, go as heavy as you can lift safely and with good form.

- Modify the exercise if it's too hard.

- If at any point you feel you have exceeded a 14 on your RPE scale, pause and rest between exercises.

- During the cooldown, go slowly into the stretch. Don't force it and don't bounce in the stretch.

You can find photos for all the exercises in Appendix B, starting on page 296.

Motivation from Andy!

Doing glute work can go beyond function. It's amazing how it can boost your self-esteem when your body resembles a fertility doll. I recall a time when I was in my third trimester, and a car drove by as my back was turned. Somebody whistled at me out the car window, and despite the shock on their faces when I turned around, I still took that as incentive to maintain the butt and leg work!

Workout 9

To begin: Warm up with a 5-minute jog or incline walk on the treadmill at RPE 12.

CIRCUIT 1	CIRCUIT 2	CIRCUIT 3	CIRCUIT 4	COOLDOWN
1. Chest Presses on Physio Ball: 12 reps 2. Chest Fly Bridges: 16 reps 3. Supported Side Angles: 20 seconds each side 4. Wall Squats on Physio Ball: 15 reps *Rest 30 seconds, then repeat Circuit 1.*	1. Squats with Goblet Hold: 12 reps 2. Triceps Dips: 12 reps 3. Chair Squats with Anterior Raises: 12 reps 4. Triceps Kickbacks in Crescent Pose: 12 reps *Rest 30 seconds, then repeat Circuit 2.*	1. Woodpecker Pushups: 12 reps 2. Goddess Squats: 20 reps **EASY DOES IT:** *Skip this exercise if your baby is in breech position or if you have hemorrhoids.* 3. Uneven Table Hold: 20 seconds each side 4. Side Lying Inner Thigh Raises: 15 reps each side *Rest 30 seconds, then repeat Circuit 3.*	1. Modified Boat Poses:* 20 seconds **BELLY ALERT:** *Keep your knees bent.* 2. Side Lying Leg Circles: 15 reps each side 3. Bent Leg Donkey Kicks: 15 reps each side 4. Mula Bandha or Kegels: 10 reps *Rest 30 seconds, then repeat Circuit 4.*	1. Chest Stretch: 30 seconds 2. Triceps Stretch: 30 seconds each side 3. Side Lying Quad Stretch: 30 seconds each side 4. Center Splits Oblique Stretch: 30 seconds each side 5. Shoulder Stretch: 30 seconds each side

EASY DOES IT!

In the Third Trimester Workout plan, note Easy Does It modifications—if an exercise feels too difficult or awkward for you right now, these modifications will help you complete the exercises successfully and without injury, courtesy of our pregnancy fitness expert, Andrea Orbeck.

Workout 10

To begin: Warm up with 5 minutes on the recumbent or stationary bike (use enough resistance to get you to RPE 12).

CIRCUIT 1	CIRCUIT 2	CIRCUIT 3	CIRCUIT 4	COOLDOWN
1. Single Arm Braced Wide Rows in Half Squat: 12 reps each side	1. Stationary Lunges with Hammer Curls and Pelvic Tilts: 12 reps	1. Alternating Low Rows in Table: 10 reps	1. Side Lying Leg Abductions: 10 reps each side	1. Pigeon Stretch: 30 seconds each side
2. Biceps Curls: 15 reps	2. Hammer Curls: 15 reps	2. Bent Leg Donkey Kicks: 12 reps each side	2. Clams: 15 reps each side	2. Mermaid Stretch: 30 seconds each side
3. Standing Oblique Crunches:* 12 reps each side	3. Lat Pullovers on Physio Ball: 12 reps	**BELLY ALERT:** *Do this from your elbows.*	3. Modified Back Extensions on Knees: 10 reps	3. Calf Stretch: 30 seconds each side
EASY DOES IT: *Instead try leg lifts with a slight lean.*	4. Pelvic Thrusts on Physio Ball: 12 reps	3. Fire Hydrants: 12 reps	4. Mula Bandha or Kegels: 10 reps	4. Hamstring Stretch: 30 seconds each side
4. Sumo Squats with Rotator Cuff Flys: 12 reps	*Rest 30 seconds, then repeat Circuit 2.*	**BELLY ALERT:** *Do this from your elbows.*	*Rest 30 seconds, then repeat Circuit 4.*	5. Thoracic Rotation Stretch with One Leg Extended: 30 seconds
Rest 30 seconds, then repeat Circuit 1.		4. Alternating Reverse Flys in Table: 15 reps		
		Rest 30 seconds, then repeat Circuit 3.		

Workout 11

To begin: Warm up with a 5-minute climb on the step mill or stair master at RPE 12.

CIRCUIT 1	CIRCUIT 2	CIRCUIT 3	CIRCUIT 4	COOLDOWN
1. Leg Presses on Physio Ball: 12 reps	1. Supported Side Angle: 20 seconds each side	1. Sumo Squats with Shoulder Presses: 12 reps	1. Camel Sit-downs: 15 reps	1. Side Lying Quad Stretch: 30 seconds each side
2. Wall Squats on Physio Ball: 12 reps	2. Triceps Kick-backs in Crescent Pose: 15 reps	2. Side Lying Inner Thigh Raises: 12 reps	2. Alternating Heel Drops:* 12 reps	2. Butterfly Stretch: 30 seconds each side
3. Head Bangers on Physio Ball: 12 reps	3. Incline Push-ups: 12 reps	3. Elevated Heel Slides: 12 reps	**BELLY ALERT:** *Do this from your elbows.*	3. Chest Stretch: 30 seconds
4. Chair Squats with Anterior Raises: 12 reps	4. Triceps Dips: 12 reps	4. Modified Side Plank: 20 seconds	3. Goddess Squats: 20 reps	4. Shoulder Stretch: 30 seconds each side
Rest 30 seconds, then repeat Circuit 1.	*Rest 30 seconds, then repeat Circuit 2.*	*Rest 30 seconds, then repeat Circuit 3.*	**EASY DOES IT:** *Skip this exercise if your baby is in breech position or if you have hemorrhoids.*	5. Triceps Stretch: 30 seconds each side
			4. Mula Bandha or Kegels: 10 reps	
			Rest 30 seconds, then repeat Circuit 4.	

Workout 12

To begin: Warm up with a 1,000-meter row on a rowing machine at RPE 12.

CIRCUIT 1	CIRCUIT 2	CIRCUIT 3	CIRCUIT 4	COOLDOWN
1. Good Mornings with Arms Crossed on Chest: 12 reps 2. Sumo Squats with Rotator Cuff Flys: 12 reps 3. Alternating Forward Lunges with Hammer Curls: 12 reps 4. Hammer Curls: 15 reps *Rest 30 seconds, then repeat Circuit 1.*	1. Braced Single Arm Medium Grip Rows: 10 reps each side 2. Squats with Serving Biceps: 12 reps 3. Alternating Stepups: 12 reps **BELLY ALERT:** *If you have balance issues, lower the height of the step.* 4. Alternating Reverse Flys in Table: 16 reps *Rest 30 seconds, then repeat Circuit 2.*	1. Bent Leg Donkey Kicks: 12 reps each side **BELLY ALERT:** *Do this from your elbows.* 2. Alternating Low Rows in Table: 12 reps 3. Fire Hydrants: 12 reps **BELLY ALERT:** *Do this from your elbows.* 4. Side Lying Leg Abductions: 15 reps each side *Rest 30 seconds, then repeat Circuit 3.*	1. Heel Slides: 12 reps 2. Boat Extensions with Forearms on Ground:* 15 reps 3. Modified Back Extensions on Knees: 12 reps 4. Mula Bandha or Kegels: 10 reps *Rest 30 seconds, then repeat Circuit 4.*	1. Thoracic Rotation Stretch with One Leg Extended: 30 seconds each side 2. Pigeon Stretch: 30 seconds each side 3. Arm Biceps Stretch: 30 seconds each side 4. Sitting Trapezius Stretch: 30 seconds each side 5. Wide Child's Poses: 30 seconds

All right! Who's excited?! This girl! And hopefully you are, too, because you are about to meet your child for the first time, my friend. I'm getting chills. For real. Your little soul mate is about to be born and placed in your arms for your first embrace. Truly awesome.

For me, meeting my son and daughter for the first time were the two most magical, memorable moments of my life. I am so, so happy for you. And speaking of this special delivery, that is coming up next. Let's make sure it goes as smoothly for you and your child as possible.

PART 3
The Yeah Baby!
FAMILY

CHAPTER 8

LABOR AND DELIVERY:
And So It Begins (or the Plan That Went Out the Window)

et the guilt begin . . .

Strangely, it seems like the moment you begin forming your birth plan, the guilt starts. Maybe you've already been experiencing this over the past 40 weeks in one way or another—guilt about the look you got when you had that half glass of champagne at Sunday brunch with your pals, guilt based on the passive-aggressive comments you received when you took a few sips of a latte at the office ("Are you allowed to have that?"), guilt following the lecture on your lack of gratitude when you expressed some anxiety about the ways in which your life would change post-baby, guilt about worrying in any way, shape, or form about whether or not you will get your prebaby waistline or perky breasts back.

But this guilt trip thing really kicks into high gear at delivery time—and, in my opinion, there is a reason for this—it is preparation for all the judgmental, insecure, holier-than-thou assholes you will encounter during motherhood (doesn't that sound like fun?). Delivery is definitely where the whole "a good mommy is a good martyr" thing begins, and I am here to say in print: That sucks and it is also totally unfair. And yet, for most mothers, it is part of their reality.

First on deck is the guilt that comes from the question, spoken or unspoken: "Are you woman enough to get through childbirth 'naturally'—no drugs and no Caesarean section, heaven forbid?! If you really loved your baby, you wouldn't be selfish. You'd tolerate the pain. After all, your mother did, and her mother did, and all the women in the videos you watched did, and all the friends of the family did" . . . blah blah blah blah.

Hear me on this: You are *never* going to win in the eyes of others. Knowing this going in, I urge you to let the haters be damned. The way to win is to *do what is best for you*. When you are okay, your children will be okay—I guarantee it. There have been a gazillion kids born out of medicated births and C-sections who are happy, healthy, strong, and wonderful, and there are also plenty who were born "naturally"

213

that have experienced all the issues you worry an epidural could create. No matter how it goes for you, chances are very high that your baby will be just fine.

But wait, you say. You have a plan, and so you know how it's all going to go. You've got it all documented to be sure everyone is in compliance, and you have spent months researching and preparing so you'll be ready for the big day. Everyone has been given a copy of your birth plan and understands his or her duties.

Can you hear that? That's me laughing out loud.

No, I'm not laughing at you. After all, I *suggested* you make that birth plan in the last chapter. But if you think that a birth plan is any sort of guarantee about how things will go, I have to tell it to you straight: A birth plan is just a piece of paper, and a plan is just a guideline when it comes to labor and delivery. It is certainly no guarantee, and it definitely shouldn't be the reason for any sort of disappointment or feelings of inferiority or failure on your part. It's just a plan, that's all. And you know what they say about the best-laid plans.

Okay, I will concede that it's totally possible (although not probable) that things really will go exactly according to your birth plan. Let me just say this: Do all your homework and make all your plans—and then be prepared to throw all of it out the window, because the fact is, *you just never know how it's going to go,* and the other fact is, *you yourself are about to enter an event over which you have very little control.*

Birth is a mysterious, beautiful, terrifying, unpredictable process. And honestly, you and your midwife, doctor, nurses, doula, or whoever else is in the room as it is all happening are just facilitators to something very primal that is going to progress in its own unique way. You can *hope* you will be able to follow your birth plan, but if you can't, then I suggest you just go with it. Parenting requires flexibility, so you might as well start now! Also, I hope you will open your mind to a willingness to participate in those aspects of modern technology that can help make childbirth happen more safely, if that becomes necessary. True, for some women, those babies practically slide right out, but most of the time, it is a little more involved.

Heidi was probably a lot like you. She spent months watching documentaries on everything from home birth to water birth to natural childbirth and more. She poured over books and blogs on how to feel your most "at one" with the baby. She anguished over what would be the healthiest and most peaceful way to bring him into this world.

I remember watching these videos with certain unnamed celebrities subtly laying on the guilt trips, passing judgment on women who choose anything other than "drug-free vaginal birth." I couldn't help thinking how unfair it was to put this kind of pressure on women. Only in America do we say "natural childbirth," implying that anything other than an unmedicated vaginal birth is "unnatural."

Hello—in other parts of the world, an epidural or a C-section is called modern medicine!

All I had to do was look at Heidi to see the size of her belly in comparison to her tiny hips, and I knew (or at least had a very strong feeling) that "natural childbirth" was not going to be in the cards for her. I tried for months to get her to release any guilt and stay open to whatever needed to happen. She ignored me, per usual. She would say things like:

"My mom had twins with no epidural."

Or, "I read that babies born vaginally also receive an early dose of good bacteria as they travel through their mother's birth canal, which may boost their immune systems and protect their intestinal tracts—so a C-section is out of the question."

Or, "I read that if I have an epidural during pregnancy, our son could have trouble 'latching on' during breastfeeding."

This went on and on, and everything she said was true, technically, but somehow she had used those facts about other people to create guilt and shame in herself at the very idea that she might not be able to do all those things that *other* people did. Somehow, Heidi had gotten it in her head that if she really wanted to be a good mom, she would suffer through the pain—no matter how bad or long it persisted—in order to bring our son into the world "naturally." To me, this sounded as difficult as removing one's wisdom teeth without anesthesia, if not worse! I thought it sheer madness. But I wasn't the one physically going through the actual birth, so I felt I didn't have much say in the matter. I made my case for a more open-minded game plan, and then I acquiesced to her wishes.

Well, the big day came, and big surprise, our baby did not come "naturally." At this point, Heidi was a week past her due date. Our doctor had first tried "stripping the membrane" (a procedure to separate the amniotic sac from the wall of the uterus to induce labor), and when that didn't work, 24 hours later, our doctor deemed it best to induce labor. We went into the hospital at about midnight. Heidi was 1 centimeter dilated and had been for about 2 weeks. The doctor gave her Pitocin to begin inducing contractions, and a prostaglandin drug to "ripen" her cervix, that is, to help her dilate. We began waiting for it to work.

At this point, there is no more food, just liquids—hot, frozen, or otherwise. The contractions were not comfortable, to say the least, so any hope of sleeping while she waited to dilate was off the table.

Flash forward to 8 hours later: Heidi had dilated only 1 more centimeter. She was at 2. She had 5 centimeters to go before she would even be done with active labor and go into transition. She wouldn't be able to actually push out the baby until she was at 10 centimeters. The extremely slow progression was making this natural childbirth scenario seem improbable, but what do I know, right?

Our doctor came to check on her, and seeing that she hadn't progressed much overnight, she manually broke her water in order to help "move things along," which is not the most comfortable thing in the world, either. Poor Heidi. I was dying inside for her, but trying to keep a cool façade.

Flash forward to 13 hours later: The Pitocin drip had been doubled in dosage. She was hungry and exhausted from the pain and lack of sleep. Dilation: 3 centimeters.

Now, I don't want to scare you at all—but it would be a huge lie to say she wasn't in pain. She was in tears and hurting so much that when I begged her to let them give her an epidural to manage the pain, she acquiesced.

So they did. And the relief came. Not completely, but enough.

Flash forward to 27 hours later: Heidi was dilated to only 4 centimeters. It was 3 a.m.—*the next day*. She still hadn't slept or eaten. She had a catheter in her nether region, an epidural catheter in her spine, and an IV in her hand. She began to run a fever at this point. Our son's heartbeat started to sound "irregular."

I couldn't stand it anymore. The whole "I am woman hear me roar" thing had gone far enough. I called our ob-gyn at 3 a.m. and said, "Get over here and cut this kid out of her now, or I'm going to MacGyver this myself with an X-Acto knife and some Xanax!"

She came immediately.

Heidi was so depleted at this point that she had no strength to fight me. I believe, deep down, she really wanted someone to tell her it was okay to give in.

Fifteen minutes later, our 9-pound, perfectly healthy son was born via C-section. He had no issues taking the boob or "latching on." He is perfectly healthy to this day. The epidural did no damage to him.

The lesson here? Our son was 9 pounds! His shoulders were simply too broad to get past Heidi's hips, rendering him unable to "drop" and therefore Heidi unable to dilate. All those good intentions and best-laid plans went out the window, but it didn't matter anymore because we had our healthy son.

We were happier than we'd ever been in our lives. Our son was here. Heidi was safe, out of pain, and intoxicated with oxytocin and maternal bliss!

I'm *not* telling you our story to scare you. I am not telling you because I am an advocate of drugs and C-sections—unless they become necessary. I respect anyone's birth plan, as long as you feel it's right for you at *every stage* of your delivery—and as long as it is flexible and in keeping with the reality of the situation.

I *am* telling you this in the event you have been shamed or guilted into a birth plan that might not actually be the best for you, a birth plan that scares you or stresses you out unnecessarily. I am also telling you this, as a friend, to give you permission ahead of time to amend any plan at any point if you need or want to.

Heidi Says . . .

Have a plan, they said. Always have a birth plan. I challenge that. At this point, I say don't bother with a plan because it will never go the way you think! No amount of staring at YouTube videos, no number of Google searches, will ever be like your individual birth experience. Everyone is different, and mine couldn't have gone more off course.

I had an amazing doula who worked on my birth plan with me, and I had decided on a natural childbirth. If my mom could deliver two at the same time with no drugs, then I could do it, too. Or so I thought.

When the due date had come and gone and a week had gone by and the baby seemed to be in no rush, I was induced. I remember going in that night around midnight. I was so excited that I was finally going to have my baby! But it was slow-going. They tried multiple methods to get labor started, but nothing was working. The doctor came in and broke my water, which is maybe one of the weirdest feelings I've ever experienced. I really wanted to see at least some sort of progress after this—anything at all—but I seemed to be stuck at 3 centimeters, even after a very kind nurse tried to stretch my cervix.

This is where it gets a little foggy. I defer to Jillian on this one because she was alert and fed! I think that after about 13 hours, I finally gave in and got an epi-dural. I will be honest—it hurt! However, after just a little time, the pain and pressure did subside quite a bit.

Then came the oxygen, then came the fever, then came the increased heart rate. Down went the Pitocin, and eventually, after what felt like an eternity, the doctor (and Jillian) decided it was time for a C-section. At this point, I was just ready.

What happened next was a bit of a whirlwind—I remember being in a really cold room, with my arms strapped down. I remember going in and out of sleep. I remember a sheet tented over me so that Jillian and I would both be spared the view that inevitably accompanies a C-section. I remember being asked if I felt anything and saying something about how it felt like they wiped me with some gauze. Then I remember everyone gasping and saying things like, "Oh my god, that's a big baby!" and "Wow, he's huge!"

Then I remember Jillian bringing him to me so that I could see his precious little face. They wanted me to hold him, but I was still so out of it that I wasn't able to. Jillian went with him, and he grasped her finger with his tiny hands while he was being cleaned up, and then he came back to me for his first meal.

I have never been more amazed at what my body was capable of than I was when I saw that little being that I grew in my tummy.

Ultimately, the more physically and emotionally comfortable you are and the more safe you feel, the better the delivery will go for both you and the baby. Labor and delivery is very personal and should be planned in lockstep with a medical professional you have researched, feel comfortable with, and trust implicitly.

Now let's talk about a few factors to consider and discuss with your partner and your doctor to make sure you get as informed as possible.

WHO'S ON FIRST? DOCTOR OR MIDWIFE?

Some people wouldn't want anybody but a full-fledged medical doctor to deliver their baby, but others would rather have midwives, who are thoroughly trained to manage labor and deliver babies. Although midwives are not medical doctors, some are professional nurses. Midwives must be licensed in all 50 states, and although they often work in birthing centers or can be hired to manage home births, many also have hospital privileges. This is largely a matter of preference, so talk to people and do some research to determine what you would prefer. You can find out a lot more about midwives from the American College of Nurse-Midwives: midwife.org/find-a-midwife. This Web site has a feature that lets you search for qualified midwives based

SHOULD YOU BANK YOUR BABY'S CORD BLOOD?

The blood in your baby's umbilical cord may be the last thing on your mind right now, but you should know that you have the option to bank it, if you arrange for this in advance (not while you are in labor!). Our resident ob-gyn, Dr. Suzanne, says that using cord blood is mostly experimental, and there is some fear-based marketing around it to get people to pay to bank it—which is expensive. It can cost $1,500 initially, and then $150 a year for storage (you can sometimes find discount deals or payment plans).

On the other hand, it can be used in a few very specific situations, if your child needs it, such as if he ever contracts leukemia. However, it is most useful if another sibling (current or future) needs it. Dr. Gordon, our pediatrician, always recommends it because he says we have no idea whom it could benefit over the next half-century or more.

If you think you probably won't need it and you don't want to do this or can't afford it, you can also consider donating your cord blood. Dr. Suzanne says this is a great way to advance science and make cord blood available to many more people in the future.

on your location. Also check out Citizens for Midwifery: cfmidwifery.org/find/ for more information.

We chose to work with a doctor (and as you may recall, we also chose a doula).

BIRTHING ENVIRONMENT

Okay, so where are you going to have your peanut? Generally, there are three choices: the hospital (which could have a birthing center inside it), a nonhospital birthing center, or home. You may also want a water birth (which could be supervised at home or may be at a birthing center, likely one that is not also a hospital).

On this issue, preferences range widely. Some women wouldn't even think of having their babies anywhere but a hospital, while others much prefer a home birth environment to feel more comfortable and in control of what happens. Nonhospital birthing centers are a compromise between the two. All of these choices have their pros and cons, so let's consider them.

Home Birth

Some women opt for a home birth because it provides, quite literally, a homey environment. Home birth offers greater privacy, intimacy, and control than a hospital or birthing center. You can have any friends or family you choose in the room during the birth; you can control the light, heat, sounds, and smells. You pick what kind of sheets you have on the bed.

However, the cons of this scenario are pretty obvious and significant. If there would be any complications, you would need to be immediately transferred to the hospital. Once there, you may not have the option of being admitted to the birthing wing before the baby is born, so you might have to deliver in the ER.

Many women choose the best of both worlds and labor at home until the last possible moment, then transition to the hospital for the remainder of labor and the delivery. Talk it all over with your doctor ahead of time, so they have an idea of your preference before they make the call that it's time to "come on in!"

Birthing Center

Birthing centers might be the perfect option for healthy women having low-risk pregnancies who absolutely object to a hospital environment but also want the benefits of technology. They are medical facilities, but they have a more homey, less medical environment. You will feel more like you are giving birth at home, but you will still get the advantage of skilled professionals helping you and a higher level of technology than you would get at a home birth. You will be more likely to have your baby delivered by a midwife. Some birthing centers are in stand-alone locations, while others are located inside hospitals, which is a nice compromise because if anything happens that requires more advanced medical intervention, you will be right there.

Birthing centers are typically equipped to give you an IV, oxygen, and some medications and have infant resuscitation equipment if that becomes necessary, but they cannot induce your labor with Pitocin and they cannot give you a C-section. You will likely be able to go to the birthing center for your prenatal health checkups, and they may also offer birthing and breastfeeding classes,[1] so by the time you give birth there, the environment will be very familiar. As I mentioned earlier, some birth centers are also located within hospitals, which can make you feel even safer.

Hospital

I am personally advocating for a hospital, because I believe strongly that all of the options above (home births, birthing centers, having a doula, even water births) can all happen at least partially at the right hospital.

Maybe you are thinking, "Wait a second. This whole book has been organic this and holistic that, and now you want me to have my kid in the coldest, most sterile institution possible?" And the answer is yes.

Well, yes and no.

Dr. Suzanne Says . . .

Although there are plenty of times when modern medicine may encourage you to do things that aren't necessary, labor and delivery is not one of those times. Forced interventions are never about making money. Although some people believe this, it is simply wrong. Obstetrics and gynecology is always a financial loss for hospitals, even when the patients get bills they feel are extremely high. Interventions are about controlling the situation and require that the patient trusts that the doctor is intervening for a good reason. This is why building your team and establishing clear and honest communication in advance with those who will be involved in your labor and delivery is so important. If a pregnant woman is birthing in an environment that is not terribly progressive, this is when a good doula in the room can be a lifesaver. However, never think that the doctors are just trying to give you an emergency C-section because they want to line their pockets. Absolutely not so.

ABOUT PLACENTA EATING/PLACENTOPHAGY

Even if you don't live in Southern California, you may have heard that some people choose to eat their own placentas—either by having them collected after birth, dried, and put into capsules, or sautéed with onions right there on the stove after a home birth. Some even say they consume it raw. Placenta sushi, anyone? (Sorry, don't retch on me!)

The placenta is a pretty unique organ—it is the only organ your body creates in adults and discards immediately after use. So it's no wonder its existence fascinates some people. But should you really eat it? Is this some weird hippie New-Age custom, or is it a legit way to stave off postpartum depression and help your milk come in, as some insist it is?

There is no actual evidence to suggest that eating the placenta has any benefits at all, and most medical experts advise against this practice. Remember, your placenta's job was to help filter pathogens (toxins, bacteria) and keep them away from your baby. Ingesting the placenta could mean you are potentially ingesting all the toxins you have been filtering. What we do know for sure is that bacteria and elements such as mercury and lead have been identified in the postterm placenta.[2] Furthermore, Dr. Suzanne advises that the person preparing it needs to be specially trained in sterile techniques to avoid cross-contamination from what is essentially human tissue. (Mad cow disease gets passed along this way, so even though we've never heard of a case of mad cow disease from placenta eating, I wouldn't want to risk it!)

For all these reasons, I strongly *discourage* this practice. However, should you choose to pursue it, please discuss your choice with a doctor you trust before moving forward, and make sure it is prepared in a safe way. Take all the necessary precautions. Your placenta is quite literally *meat,* so if you don't store and prepare it properly, you could end up eating rotten placenta, and that could cause a significant health risk to you and your baby.

And don't invite me for dinner that night . . .

The world is not black and white. Life is all about navigating the gray area. There is nothing dangerous about eating organic or avoiding drugs and procedures you absolutely don't need. However, like in Heidi's case, sometimes you do, and if you have any complications with labor and delivery, it's no time to mess around. Hospitals have made their maternity areas more and more comfortable and homey these days, so it's not like having a baby in a factory. But the bottom line is: Better safe than sorry.

Let's put things in perspective. Yes, some procedures might not be the most organic or wholesome, but your safety and the safety of your baby takes precedence over all else. Let's not forget that in the last 100 years, the infant mortality rate has gone from 150 out of 1,000 to only 8 out of 1,000, all thanks to modern medicine.

I hate to weigh in on this so strongly, and I don't want you to feel pressured to make a decision that isn't right for you. I know there are many people, including

ABOUT WATER BIRTHS

The idea of a water birth may sound bizarre to you, but it has been around for centuries in island cultures and probably also in ancient Egypt, Africa, and South America.[3] Water births enjoyed a bump of popularity in the 1970s, and some people still like the idea of easing a baby naturally from one aquatic-like environment to another before letting them hit the harsh cold air the rest of us live in. Modern advocates of this birthing method believe it facilitates a more peaceful transition from the uterus into the world for the baby and helps to manage pain and expedite labor for the mommy. Theoretically, the buoyancy of the water allows the mom to find ideal birthing positions, and the body-temperature water can help ease the pain of contractions.

Many feel it's perfectly safe as long as you immediately pull the baby out of the water right after birth. On the other hand, some doctors have advised against water births for the following reasons:

- If you decide you need an epidural, you can't have one in the pool.

- If you should poop in the water while pushing, you introduce the risk of infection for the baby into the water. (Sorry, but this happens. Don't think about it too much.)

- Water births can be difficult to monitor for complications. For example, you won't be able to monitor the baby's heart rate, or should you start bleeding during labor, it could be tough to tell.

- While very rare, in 1 out of 200 water births, the umbilical cord can snap if the baby is pulled out of the water too quickly.

- While also very rare, if your baby is exposed to air during the birth, it may override their "dive reflex" and they run a small risk of taking a breath under water.

Discuss all the pros and cons with your doctor. If you feel strongly that you'd like this option, be very open with your ob-gyn and make sure you're in agreement well in advance of the birth.

medical professionals, who advocate home births. But hear me out: If something goes wrong, you want to be fully covered with instant access to potentially lifesaving technology. In our experience with the birth of our son, we experienced fairly atypical complications that ultimately required pain medicine and a C-section. You just can't know until you're in the middle of a birth experience what will happen and what will be required.

I understand that a hospital environment can be clinical, intimidating, and impersonal. However, I believe Heidi and I were able to make the environment very comfortable by taking steps ahead of time.

We had friends and family visiting right up until the birth. We brought music, candles, and blankets from home to make things more familiar for Heidi. We both had a good bond with our doctor, and we trusted her to do what we wanted unless something was absolutely necessary (like a C-section). Ultimately, by communicating our wishes ahead of time and throughout the process, as well as preparing and having a game plan for any concerns, we were able to create a relatively pleasant environment for our son to be born in.

Also, I want to stress something important: Heidi was considered "low risk" throughout her entire pregnancy. Yet, when the day came for our son to be born, he was simply too big to be pushed out vaginally. She ended up requiring all the lifesaving benefits of modern medicine that we have come to take for granted over the last century. Shit happens—why not be prepared?

Home births and water births remain controversial—birthing centers somewhat less so. While many of you likely know many women who have experienced one of these options and were perfectly fine, I would just ask, "Why risk it?" If something happens that needs swift medical intervention, will you be able to get to the hospital in time? Is "probably" a good enough answer for you? If it is, that is totally your choice, obviously. In my opinion, safe is always better than sorry. Whatever birthing environment you end up choosing, just be sure to take into account all of the above, and consult your doctor while formulating your game plan.

INDUCING LABOR

Any doctor will tell you that spontaneous labor is the best-case scenario, and many doctors will encourage expectant mothers to wait a long time before deciding to induce labor. According to the American College of Obstetrics and Gynecology, you can wait up to 42 weeks in an otherwise low-risk, healthy pregnancy to induce labor if the cervix is not "ripe," even with a big baby. This is because this extra time allows the baby to "drop" and trigger the natural uterine contractions that do an excellent job of effacing and dilating the cervix.

Toward the end of pregnancy, most women are so ready for that little one (who is no longer quite so little) to be out that they may feel prepared to do just about anything, from stairclimbing and eating hot sauce to nipple stimulation and "getting it in" (this is how the kids say "getting it on," in case you aren't up to speed on the lingo).

While there is scant evidence to suggest any of that other than the sex part will work, I say go for it—at the very least it will make for some fun stories! But more and more often, women are choosing to schedule their labor—they have an appointment set with the hospital to be induced, if they haven't already given birth by that date. This can certainly be convenient, but as stated, spontaneous organic labor is ideal for vaginal birth due to all the reasons mentioned above. However, in some situations, inducing labor is medically required, such as the following:

- Preeclampsia or eclampsia
- Certain medical conditions (diabetes, lupus, clotting disorders, etc.)
- History of stillbirth or rapid births
- Low amniotic fluid
- Past term or "late"

This simply gives your doctor a little more control over the medical situation that exists, so everyone is ready to deal with any special situations.

There are several ways that labor can be induced.

Dr. Suzanne Says . . .

Sex actually can help initiate labor, once you are at term (but it won't induce early labor, so don't worry about that). Semen contains prostaglandins, and orgasms can cause uterine contractions, both of which can get the process going. Acupuncture may also help. However, none of these natural methods, including stripping the membrane, will put someone into labor who wasn't heading there already. Only medical induction has any real evidence to support its use, and even that must be used judiciously in a woman who appears ready to give birth. To determine who is an appropriate candidate for medical induction, doctors have a scale called the Bishop's score, by which they evaluate the condition of the cervix, so induction isn't applied randomly.

Membrane Stripping or Sweeping

This is a procedure where your doctor manually separates the amniotic sac from the cervix with a gloved hand. This triggers the release of prostaglandins that can induce labor.[4] There are no known risks or complications, but it can be uncomfortable and cause some bleeding. Heidi underwent this one. (Dr. Suzanne says this doesn't really work—and it didn't work for us either—but many doctors still practice this, so it is up to you to find out whether this is appropriate for you.)

Amniotomy, or Breaking Your Water

Your doctor will manually break your water in an attempt to stimulate the release of hormones and biochemicals that initiate and accelerate labor. This also allows your baby's head to push down against the cervix more intensely, which is the ideal way to dilate the cervix. Heidi had this one, too.

Mechanical Cervical Dilators

These are tools such as the Foley balloon or the double balloon device that are used to literally open or dilate the cervix. Some doulas or midwives do this, or even do the same thing with their hands, in situations where the mother doesn't want to use drugs to induce labor. It can work well, but it is also painful.

Pitocin Drip

This mimics oxytocin, the chemical your body naturally produces, and causes uterine contractions. It's not harmful to your baby. Generally, you start the drip on a low dose and gradually raise it over time. Pitocin can also make labor more painful because it increases the power of contractions. Again, this happened to Heidi—but it didn't work because, although it increased the contractions, our son was incapable of "dropping" in order to open the cervix effectively. After hours of this, she finally consented to an epidural.

In a perfect world, you might not need any of the above. However, as we all know, the world is not perfect. Quite honestly, based on personal observation, the downside to all the above was discomfort. As I've stated several times, my poor Heidi had pretty much all the above (except the mechanical dilator), and our little guy still had to be born via C-section. I remember our ob-gyn saying to me, after we had tried nearly everything previously mentioned above, "I have one final trick, and it never fails." Fifteen minutes later, our son was born. That's some trick!

Ultimately, communication with your doctor and preparation are key. Knowing what's going on, and why, will do so much for your peace of mind and attitude about what is happening. Just remember to stay flexible and open—you and your doctor can adjust the game plan at any time, both for pain management or complications, to make sure both you and your baby are safe and healthy. Based on our experience, I am incredibly glad we live in the age of modern medicine!

PAIN MANAGEMENT

Again, Heidi felt very strongly that she wanted our son to be born "naturally" for a variety of reasons. First, she watched all the videos of all the Hollywood celebs, from Giselle to Ricki Lake, going on and on about how blissful it was to give birth "naturally." (Um, pretty sure the birth of any human being who's been made inside of another body that grew a brand-new organ for that purpose is "natural," no matter how the child comes into the world—thank you very much.) Heidi worried that drugs in her system would have an impact on how aware she or our son would be during and after the birth. And while I'm not sure she will ever admit this, there was definitely some pressure from the outside—and inside—world.

Let's talk options for a second here.

- You can go all natural with a doula, meditation, and acupuncture. Some women have complication-free births, and this is enough.

- Conversely, if you are being induced, you have "back labor" (pain in your lower back during contractions often caused by baby's position), it's your first child, or you experience other complicating circumstances, the pain may be more significant.

When your pain is on the more significant side, you may opt (and rightfully so) for some relief. This is what you should know.

Epidural or Spinal Regional Anesthesia

Epidurals are used to help with labor pain. Spinals are primarily used for C-sections. Should you opt for an epidural, don't wait until the pain is unbearable like we did— the medication usually takes about 30 to 45 minutes to kick in. The most obvious advantage here is relief from the pain of labor, and you'll be fully cognizant for the moment when your little one is placed in your arms. There is no evidence that the *minute* amount of medication absorbed by the baby will cause him or her harm.

The disadvantage, in some cases, is that epidurals can slow down delivery because it's hard to push when you can't feel your muscles. In this instance, your doctor will dial down the dose so sensation returns and you can push more intensely to speed delivery.

One possible but uncommon side effect of an epidural is headache, but this occurs in less than 1 percent of women with a good, experienced obstetrical anesthesia team. Dr. Suzanne says that these can be relieved with a blood patch, which is a simple surgical procedure that closes up one or more holes in the tissue surrounding the spinal cord (the holes that were caused by the lumbar puncture used to administer the epidural).

Other possible side effects include a drop in blood pressure, fever, bleeding, or infection, but again these are also rare. Should you develop a fever, your doctor will likely administer IV antibiotics. To manage blood pressure, your doctor will give you intravenous fluids and, if necessary, a medication to increase blood pressure. But you may very well not need any of this.

IV Narcotics

In some cases, such as if you don't want or can't have an epidural for any reason or you need pain relief as well as rest, or if you need pain relief before it is time to get the epidural, your doctor may feel that you should have narcotics administered intravenously in small doses. This would happen earlier in labor, not close to the time of delivery, because they do cause a temporarily depressed respiratory and neurological response in the baby. While IV narcotics diminish the pain, it doesn't disappear entirely. Dr. Suzanne recommends just doing the epidural if you can, which you might need in addition anyway.

The downside to IV narcotics, besides the temporary effect on the baby, is that

Dr. Suzanne Says . . .

It is almost always better to wait for labor to begin rather than inducing labor, and there are measures we can take to help encourage labor without resorting to induction. For example, pain and anxiety can interfere with labor. More specifically, stress hormones released by the stress response (or the "fight or flight" response, caused by pain and anxiety) can prevent oxytocin release, which can hinder labor progress. When someone finally gets an epidural (relieving pain) and sleeps (relieving anxiety) and then wakes up dilated to 8 centimeters, it's not magic. It's science.

Considering all this, while women are often advised to ask potential ob-gyn doctors for their C-section rates and everyone talks about the concern over C-section rates, I suggest asking doctors for their elective induction rates. There are good reasons to induce someone, but doing it "just because" isn't great medicine, in my opinion.

you will absolutely feel drowsy and "out of it." You could also feel nauseated or dizzy. And this can all happen to the baby, too, as well as other side effects like impaired early breastfeeding, altered neurological behavior, and decreased ability to regulate body temperature. However, these last three side effects are rare, so if you do have to have IV narcotics for some reason, know that your baby will most likely be fine after the effect wears off. Also, should any of these complications occur, your doctor can administer a medication called naloxone to mitigate the effects of the opiates.

In any case, I personally would opt for just an epidural, if possible, as it affects the baby significantly less.

General Anesthesia

This is how they often did it in the "olden days," when our mothers or grandmothers were having babies and there was any sort of problem—the mother was completely unconscious and obviously could not push or participate in the birth at all. Now, however, this is rare. Dr. Suzanne says that doctors would use general anesthesia only in the case of a major emergency when there is no epidural in place and no time to place one. Because this medication does cross the placenta, doctors are hesitant to use it unless absolutely necessary—but again, if you are one of the rare cases where it *is* absolutely necessary, you need to trust your medical team.

Local Anesthesia

This is an injection that is used locally on the vaginal tissue before an episiotomy (cutting the vaginal opening to make it wider for the baby—this is no longer commonly practiced) or generally to help with vaginal pain. You may or may not need this, but it's good to know that it's a possibility. Local anesthesia options also include the pudendal block. Dr. Suzanne says that this is "old school," but some doctors still use it. This procedure applies a local anesthetic into the pudendal canal to numb the pudendal nerve, which can immediately relieve pain in the perineum, vulva, and vagina.[5]

Ultimately, you must talk with your doctor and come up with a game plan that is right for you and your baby. If you know what your options are and what could potentially happen, you won't be faced with any sudden surprises.

C-SECTION VERSUS VAGINAL BIRTH

Honestly, I hate to even write about this one. *You* really have to choose what feels right to *you* and then be willing to go the opposite way if the situation demands it. Yes, there are pros and cons to both, and in some cases, like Heidi's, you may have no choice at all. But regardless of how this one plays out, you and your baby will ultimately be just fine.

Dr. Suzanne Says . . .

When your mom was having you, she might have had an episiotomy, which is a surgical procedure that cuts the opening to the vagina to make it wider for the baby. Doctors used to believe that this would be cleaner and easier to repair than if the tissue should tear during the birth. Now, however, we know that this isn't true. While some doctors may still do this routinely, this procedure is definitely on a downtrend. Here is what Dr. Suzanne says on the subject.

Episiotomy should not be done routinely! I do it only in a few very narrow circumstances: When mom's pushing is not tolerated by the baby and the baby is in fetal distress but low enough in the birth canal to avoid a C-section; in this case an episiotomy can speed the delivery. The other situation is when there is significant concern for shoulder dystocia (this is when the baby's head gets delivered but the shoulders get stuck), or as a maneuver to relieve the shoulder dystocia while it is happening.

It is completely false that the episiotomy laceration will be cleaner and easier to repair or will heal better than spontaneously occurring perineal laceration, or tearing of tissue during birth. In fact, if the obstetrician or midwife doesn't feel confident in their repair skills, they have no business delivering a baby! The episiotomy will likely cause a larger laceration and result in more damage and pain than if things were to proceed without it.

Many women feel it would be ideal to have a vaginal birth because they worry about recovery time, scarring, a weakened core, possible infection, or other issues related to C-sections. Heidi ended up needing a C-section to deliver our son safely—but her scar is hidden and barely noticeable, and her core is stronger than ever. So either way, again, you will be fine.

That said, the negatives to a C-section are still pretty obvious.

- The recovery time is longer. It is major abdominal surgery, after all.

- It is more painful after the birth, and it is hard to sit up, stand up, and walk at first.

- Some feel that the antibiotics given to mommy and passed to baby due to the surgery can cause a gassy tummy, cradle cap (scaly, flaky skin on the baby's scalp similar to dandruff in adults—technically called *infantile seborrheic dermatitis*—that could be linked to yeast), fungal infections, and/or a compromised immune system in the baby, although this isn't proven.

While it wasn't ideal, we simply combated the antibiotics with a gentle probiotic called BioGaia that we mixed into our son's bottle. We also put a coconut oil and baking soda mixture on his head to clear up his cradle cap, which may or may not have had anything to do with the C-section (plenty of babies who are born vaginally have cradle cap).

The postsurgical recovery mixed with typical postpartum emotions and adjustments made for a rough couple of weeks for Heidi. But she and our son are both perfectly healthy, and ultimately, that's what matters.

On the other hand, some women prefer a C-section for a multitude of reasons.

- They can schedule a birth.

- It may relieve them of anxiety about having to go through labor and push out the baby.

- It may also relieve anxiety about side effects like tearing of tissue (or an episiotomy) or minor incontinence.

Dr. Suzanne Says . . .

The hot topic in the coming years will be the influence of a vaginal birth on the baby's proper microbiome development, which is absolutely influenced by the mode of delivery and can have a lasting impact on all aspects of health, including mental, digestive, and immune health. However, it is true that the mode of delivery is often not under your control, so I advise you to let it go and be flexible.

That said, there are institutions that will let you do a vaginal swab, and then swab that into the baby's nasal passages if you have had a C-section but want to give your baby the benefit of your natural bacteria. This is providing no one has an infection and everyone is healthy. I advise looking into this and asking about it if you do end up having a C-section. It can't hurt your baby, and it might give your baby some of the important benefits he or she missed out on by not having had a vaginal birth.

C-SECTION BASICS

Back in the day, C-sections left a big vertical scar on a woman's abdomen, called a midline incision, but these days, most C-sections are done through a much less obtrusive incision, horizontal and very low in the abdomen, often below the pubic hair line. This is called a bikini incision, or technically, a *Pfannenstiehl incision*.[6]

The surgeon will cut through the skin and some of the connective tissue and other areas including into the uterus, but won't cut through the muscle. Instead, the rectus abdominal muscles (your abs) will be manually separated. The tissue that was cut will be stitched up and will have to heal, but your muscles will remain intact and will need only to come back together, which will happen as you heal.

The resulting scar will be so low on your abdomen that you should be able to wear a bikini without showing your scar. A midline incision may very rarely be necessary because it makes more room to get the baby out, but chances are, you won't have that kind.

After the C-section, you will need to be gentle with yourself so you can heal. However, the sooner you get up and start walking around, the sooner the pain will abate. It will feel impossible at first, like you can't possibly even sit up, but once you do it, it gets easier quickly.

Most of these worries are unfounded, and with preparation, vaginal births are usually the least complicated. However, according to Dr. Suzanne, there are some good reasons to opt for elective C-sections, including these.

- If you have had prior pelvic trauma or fracture
- If you have had pelvic surgery that affected the bony structures or the hips
- In some cases, if you have had bladder repair surgery
- If you have chronic vulvar pain syndrome
- If you have been a victim of sexual trauma or abuse

While the surgery is more severe than a vaginal birth for mom and does present some risks for baby (like breathing issues in C-section babies because their lungs don't get the compression and fluid expulsion that happens during the trip through the birth canal[7]), it also avoids some of the complications that can occasionally happen with vaginal births, like the need for forceps or suction delivery or complications with the umbilical cord.

Of course, vaginal birth has many benefits:

- You don't have to recover from major surgery, and many women are up and about soon after the birth.

- It might sound scary, but it is actually easier for all involved.

- The baby picks up beneficial bacteria from mom while going through the birth canal. (As I mentioned, Heidi was concerned about this.)

- The breathing stimulation the baby gets from that tight squeeze can help expel fluid from the lungs and improve respiratory function immediately after birth.

The truth is, it can go well or there can be complications or downsides either way. Some vaginal births go smoothly and some don't. Some C-sections go smoothly and some don't. Ultimately, 30 percent of babies nowadays are delivered through C-section for a wide variety of reasons. While most happen due to medical necessity, it's every woman's right to choose how she wants to deliver her baby. If a C-section seems to make more sense to you, just be sure to discuss all that is involved in detail with your doctor.

FORCEPS OR VACUUM EXTRACTORS

Forceps or vacuums are used when mom is exhausted or when the baby is showing signs of stress and the medical team must accelerate the delivery. It's estimated that roughly 10 to 15 percent of all births use one or the other. Both can cause tearing to the vagina, perineum, and rectum. And both can cause some bruising to your baby's scalp. While clearly neither is ideal, in some cases it's simply a medical necessity. A local anesthetic will help you manage the pain very effectively. And fortunately, serious medical complications for you or your baby are very rare, so this fact should give you some peace of mind in the event these tools are necessary to bring your baby into the world safely.

There is one critical thing you must do ahead of time to make sure any issues with the requirement of these tools are mitigated. Be sure to discuss this with your doctor prior to your due date. It's important to know their level of proficiency and experience with forceps and vacuum extractors. If they are not very experienced, make sure they have someone who is in the delivery room to assist them.

The bottom line is that whichever way this plays out for you and your baby, be it by choice or necessity, you will both be perfectly fine.

C-Section Free Advice

Now, for my personal take on this subject matter (this is just you and me, chatting over coffee). First: In my humble opinion, *do not let your significant other "look behind the curtain" during your C-section!* I have friends who have done this. Huge mistake. They often end up passed out on the floor, and then the doctors and nurses have to deal with that. Unless your partner is a medical professional, that kind of image can be overwhelming, to say the least. Suffice it to say that plenty an operating room floor has been graced with the fainting bodies of significant others who chose to take a peek.

Also, know that you may get the shakes from the drugs. I remember it scared the hell out of Heidi, and they reassured her it was normal and that she and the baby were fine.

You will also feel pressure during the procedure. Heidi kept saying to our doctor, "I'm not numb. I still have feeling!"

"Tell me what you feel?" our doctor said.

"You're tapping me with gauze!" (Obviously after 28 hours of labor and quite a few drugs, she was not totally "with it.")

"Actually, I just cut into you," the doctor replied. In other words, the worst part was over, and she didn't even know it happened. Heidi calmed down after that.

Also, you will have gas. Crazy bum-ripping gas. Part of this is because things can get backed up from the surgery, and things aren't moving along very well in your gastrointestinal tract. That means gas can get trapped in the abdomen during the surgery and build up. I personally thought it was super cute, but Heidi did not, and it was painful for her—so I absolutely did not laugh when something accidentally "squeaked out."

Afterward, the scar will be numb. This will have no other effect on your health, but it will be numb because when they perform the surgery, some of the nerves in that area are affected. In fact, you may have less feeling over the scar for a long time, sometimes even years. Again, it's normal for that to happen, and it will have no negative effect on your health, core strength, physical abilities, or anything else. Finally, even though you didn't have a vaginal birth, there is still the possibility of incontinence if you had a very large baby or a traumatic labor. Pressure from pregnancy alone can damage the pelvic floor and urinary tract and can contribute to incontinence immediately, but this almost always resolves in 6 weeks to 6 months.

Heidi was relieved that this didn't happen to her, and I do have friends, personally, who had vaginal births and seem more likely to have this problem than those who have had C-sections. There's nothing like jumping on a trampoline at your kid's birthday at the trampoline park and peeing your pants (yes, this has happened to friends of mine). Nothing to be ashamed of, but still.

So while all this might not sound awesome, it will all pass. With a healthy diet, as much sleep as you can manage, and easing slowly back into your fitness routine, you will recover and be better than ever—with a baby onboard!

WHAT HAPPENS AFTER THE BIRTH?

Mostly, this is a time for recovery, wonderment, and mutual congratulations to all involved. You did it! You are a mom! Slowly or quickly, you will recover from birth, realize you have a baby that you are supposed to know how to care for (yikes!), and marvel at the fact that you created life. And you will marvel. Heidi would just sit

NEWBORN ANTIBIOTIC EYE TREATMENT AND VITAMIN K INJECTION

You might be surprised that your doctor wants to put eye ointment in your baby's eyes immediately after the birth. What gives? The American College of Obstetrics and Gynecology recommends that antibiotic eye ointment be administered to babies in the event that they would get an eye infection from bacteria in the vagina. On the other hand, Dr. Gordon says that the American Academy of Pediatrics has long recognized that this is unnecessary, and their official position is that zero eye care for newborns is perfectly acceptable. Dr. Gordon says that he never recommends any eye drops or eye ointments for newborns.

Vitamin K shots, says Dr. Gordon, are another matter entirely. He says he is perfectly okay with these injections, which prevent vitamin-K–dependent bleeding disorder in newborns. Vitamin K deficiency bleeding (VKDB) is rare—it happens only in about 1 in 10,000 babies—but it can cause spontaneous bruising and bleeding within the first 12 weeks. Since the vitamin K supplementation is harmless, it's probably a good idea to go ahead with this, just in case. If for any reason you are opposed to vitamin K injections, speak to your doctor about oral administration of vitamin K drops as an alternative, but do so before labor begins.

You could mention your preferences for both eye care and vitamin K treatment in your birth plan.

and stare at our son for hours because, after all, it's pretty damn amazing that she *created him.*

Dr. Suzanne tells me that some traditional cultures enforce 40 days after birth with no visitors (beyond those there to help) because the family needs that long to rest, recover, and be together. I like that. Although you may like visitors, you will also be exhausted and adjusting to your new life and your new identity as a family with a new member. This is a time to slow down and respect your own physical and emotional needs as you learn how to care for a new baby. It's a magical time, and although it is difficult (especially the sleep deprivation), it is also pretty amazing.

So let's talk about that magical time—that "fourth trimester." Now you have a family. What do you do next? Worry not. This book isn't over yet. While you are recovering in the hospital, give the next chapter a good read.

See you on the other side!

Dr. Gordon Says . . .

Minimize visitors who are not there to bring food, rub your neck, or clean your kitchen or bathroom!

CHAPTER 9

YOUR FOURTH TRIMESTER:
We Are Family (or the Dazed and Confused Dairy Dispenser)

So here we are! Now what the heck are you supposed to do?

Many books on babies are about, well ... *the babies.* Duh. However, this is not just a book about babies, as I think you've figured out by now. So even in this chapter, when that precious cargo has made it to the outside, we are going to talk about baby, but mostly I want to focus on *you.* The fact is that once you have a baby, everybody is all about the baby, and you can feel a little bit (or even a lot) like everybody forgot about you. I didn't forget about you, so let's help you through this. Because the fourth trimester can be the hardest one of all.

I didn't invent the concept of the fourth trimester, but I am definitely a believer because life doesn't just pop back to normal after labor and delivery. In fact, what you knew as normal is no longer your reality. There is a significant transition time from "pregnant person" to "parent person," both physically and emotionally, not to mention the transition for everyone in the household, from family of X number of people to family of X+1 number of people. Hence, the fourth trimester.

In looking for a standard description of the fourth trimester, I came upon an interesting definition created by lawyers in relation to pregnancy discrimination cases: "The concept of a fourth trimester, drawn from maternal nursing and midwifery, refers to the crucial 3- to 6-month period after birth when many of the physical, psychological, emotional, and social effects of pregnancy continue."[1]

Ain't it the truth. Here's another way to define it:

"WTF?!"

Your entire world gets rocked after you give birth, as you transition into the role of caretaker and provider to a helpless baby human. So many things have changed, and that's hard to conceptualize, especially while your hormones are all over the place, you are physically recovering from a major ordeal, and you aren't getting any sleep—not to mention what happens when you think about how you are now a *parent.* In my personal experience of this trimester, and in witnessing everything Heidi went through, this is a rough time for almost everyone. Sure, some women bounce right back physically and settle right in mentally, but for most, there are some major adjustments that take some time—and this is perfectly normal.

I mean, seriously, the bottom line is that you and your body have *built a frickin' human being* and then literally expelled him or her out into the world from one part of your body or another. That's major. And from that moment on, you are immediately and irrevocably charged with the most intense responsibility on the planet: protecting and sustaining said human, for the rest of your life. I remember thinking, "Are they really gonna let us leave this hospital with this baby? What the hell are we supposed to do now?" Maybe you and your significant other are having similar thoughts? Unfortunately, there is no standard baby-care manual that goes home with every new parent, and as many books as you read and as much advice as you get, you are still going to feel, sometimes, if not often, that you have no idea what you are doing.

Also normal.

Meanwhile, your body is still healing, your lifestyle has changed dramatically and you are adapting to that, and your hormones may seem like they are taking *way too*

Dr. Suzanne Says . . .

Our expert ob-gyn and integrative medicine guru Dr. Suzanne Gilberg-Lenz has this to say about recovery after childbirth:

I am a big advocate of taking the time to recover. Self-care is crucial right now. The month or so after giving birth is an important time to just be where you are. Instead of worrying about what you have to do all week, just worry about what you are going to do in the next few hours. Really dial it down. Did everyone eat? Did everyone sleep? That's all that matters. It's one day at a time.

My training in Ayurvedic medicine includes very specific instructions on care of the mom for those 40 days postpartum. Daily oil massages, specific healing foods (especially kitchari, a simple dish of mung beans and rice with digestive herbs like turmeric), and belly binding to support the healing of the abdomen are all practices I recommend. If this interests you, an Ayurvedic physician can instruct you on these and give you a personalized prescription for your own situation.

long to return your body to a prepregnancy state. Those hormones are also helping you bond with your little one and facilitate breastfeeding, but they can definitely make you feel a little crazy, weepy, joyful, angry, ecstatic, and sad, sometimes all in the span of about 5 minutes.

And then there are the *unspeakable* parts. Pregnancy and postpartum are real hot-button issues for some people, who might be terrified to speak their truths and share their stories with candor, for fear that if they admit they've experienced anything other than total and complete mind-blowing bliss they are bad moms or not "normal." Are you a "bad mother" if you worry about your waistline or your weight gain? If you don't always want to hold the baby? If you don't enjoy breastfeeding like you hoped you would? If you worry you might be all wrong for this "mother" job? If you are struck with the fear, in the wee small hours of the night, that this whole "having a baby" thing was a horrible mistake? If you sometimes feel like you would trade your loving and supportive partner for a solid 8 hours of sleep? Nope. Again,

PARTNERS IN PARENTHOOD

Not surprisingly, being the parent who was not pregnant, this fourth trimester was the hardest one for me. It can be incredibly difficult to be the partner who did not give birth when the baby has arrived and mom and baby are bonding and breastfeeding and generally have eyes only for each other.

Not to sound like a selfish ass here, but I encourage you to try to remember that if you have a partner in parenthood, he or she is likely feeling a bit misplaced and left out. Much as we try to help, we tend to get relegated to servant duty (gratefully, but still . . .). We can hold the baby, give bottles, get up when the baby cries, but a lot of what is going on during this time is about baby and mom, and that marginalizes the other partner to a large extent.

Add to that the physical reality that women who just gave birth are usually not even remotely interested in romance and getting physical, if you know what I mean, and that can put a further strain on the relationship. There we are, waiting patiently on the sidelines, but it's easy to feel like you have ceased to exist if you aren't baby or birth mommy. To be honest, even when we know the baby needs all the love, it can be hard.

So with all that in mind, I encourage you to do what you can to bring your partner into your inner circle. A little kindness and inclusion can go a long way right now, even if it's just a group hug or holding hands or holding the baby together. Do it in the name of family bonding.

all normal. Women through the ages have felt all these feelings and more, and they are a sign of only one thing: That you are human.

Some of these doubts will continue through the rest of your life (everyone has moments when they wonder if they are bad parents, even as they try their best to be good parents), but most of the extreme thoughts you may be having now come from exhaustion, stress, hormonal fluctuations, and simply adjusting to a major life change. And while you may know this in theory, part of the fourth trimester is about you getting to a place where you really accept and deeply understand that it is 100 percent okay to go through, feel, and process *anything* you need to during this intense time.

Women often hint to one another that the period postpregnancy can be challenging, but I don't think this truly prepares you for the intensity. You might think, "Lack of sleep? I can handle that." Well, it's just so much more than that. Everything gets turned inside out and upside down. Your career, your relationship with your partner, your body . . . everything.

And when it comes to you in particular, I use words like "healing" because it is true, in so many ways. Healing encapsulates the physical, emotional, mental, even spiritual changes you're faced with right now. The word isn't meant to scare you. It's meant to validate anything you may be dealing with postpartum—from postpartum depression to recovering from a C-section, diastasis recti, or an episiotomy to feeling resentful to a decrease in libido—and assure you that it's all normal and that all will be okay.

But there is a trade-off: You get to meet the love of your life. So, yeah, it's worth it.

WALK YOUR OWN PARENTING PATH

Every family is different. Some are traditional, some are nontraditional, some defy definition, and most importantly, every parent is going to make mistakes, learn from experience, and craft a unique parenting style. Every human being is going to have a certain set of priorities, tendencies, and responses, and we all parent differently. That's important to remember because during the fourth trimester, you are going to get a whole lot of advice, and it can overwhelm you and make you feel guilty, when it absolutely shouldn't.

And don't think this won't happen to you. You will get it from people passing you on the street, from strangers on the subway, from casual acquaintances who wouldn't dare criticize what you are wearing but suddenly feel like they have every right to criticize how you raise your child. You will certainly get it from your family (especially your in-laws), not to mention the checkout clerk at the grocery store, the bus or taxi driver, and those people you meet for the first time at any random social gathering. So look out! Nuggets of "advice" will be sent whizzing toward you like passive/aggressive bullets of judgment and insecurity. Unfortunately, we live in a world now that tends to lean away from empathy and compassion and toward judgment of others . . . especially mothers. Everyone will have "shoulds" for you. "You should have been watching." "You shouldn't let her play with that." "You should be sure he doesn't eat solid food until month X." (At least, that's what we hear.)

Some things you will probably actually hear, often accompanied by self-satisfied smiles and smug tones of voice:

"You will suffocate your baby putting him in the carrier that way."

"How can you dress your baby like that when it is this hot/cold outside? Aren't you afraid he's going to get hyperthermia/hypothermia???"

"You know, breastfeeding is better for babies."

"Should you really have her out of the house already?"

"I would *never* feed my child formula."

"You're not going to breastfeed right here, are you?"

"You are/aren't vaccinating, right?"

"We give our kids time-ins, not time-outs. How do *you* plan to discipline?"

"Have you got her on the waiting list for X, Y, or Z preschool yet? You'd better hurry. They fill up *years* in advance."

"Don't you think your baby is a little too fat/thin?"

"Are you already indoctrinating him/her with that blue/pink outfit?"

"If you dress your baby in green or yellow, how will anybody know if it's a boy or a girl?"

"Are you really going to feed that to your baby?"

"Shouldn't you feed him? He's crying, he must be starving!"

"Maybe you should stick a bow on her bald head."

"Shouldn't you cut his hair? He looks like a girl."

Yes, I'm serious—we or people we know have heard *every single one of these,* for real. And this kind of crap only continues to pick up speed the further you get into parenting. People judge you for what you feed your kids—or what you don't. Whether you use your TV as a babysitter when trying to get things done around the house, and how you discipline them (or how you don't). How often you leave them—gasp!—with a babysitter!? And so on.

Unsolicited parenting advice. Nobody likes to get it, but everybody (it seems) likes to give it. The only thing I can tell you is to just take it all with a grain of salt and refrain from assaulting them if you can. Remind yourself: They aren't worth the jail time. (At least, that's what I have to remind myself!)

But I also have to say that even in the face of all that advice, chances are that your worst critic will be *you*. I have watched Heidi struggle with this. She would hesitate to express any negative feelings about the parenting experience and honestly . . . still does. I also know she felt uncomfortable in her own skin for a bit. Even though she dropped down to her prebaby weight in record time (please don't hate her!), she didn't feel the same. Even though her body had just done this amazing thing, she felt unattractive, and nothing I said made her feel any differently or any better during this time. She just needed to vent and be validated.

Meanwhile, I was wondering if we were ever going to have a romantic relationship again. I was being a selfish ass, I know. However, I guarantee your significant other is wondering this, too. (We will discuss this sensitive issue more in depth starting on page 247.)

And then, of course, there is the little human . . . the one who needs you constantly, cries but can't tell you why, is always hungry and tired, and most of all, is

POOP GLOSSARY

Babies have gas. Holy mother of God, do they have gas. But that's nothing compared to the poop. The prodigious output of poop. I have now had so much experience with baby poop that I feel qualified in defining some of the most common and dramatic types, for your reference, should you need to mention them in conversation (please do this only with other mothers, who will appreciate it much more than your childless friends, I guarantee it).

- **The Blowout:** A poop explosion out the upper back of the diaper.
- **The Nuclear Nugget:** A tiny poop with an unbelievable stench, capable of crippling a thousand grown men.
- **The Poo-Mergency:** A situation in which you require immediate assistance because you have opened the diaper, but the poop has not yet stopped flowing.
- **The A-Poo-Calypse:** When your baby has diarrhea nonstop for a minimum of 24 hours, for no discernible reason.

Welcome to the joys of parenting.

really, really skilled at pooping. And you thought that new puppy you got one time was a lot of work.

I must admit, a few weeks into this fourth trimester, I was asking myself, *What happened to my awesome glamorous life? What happened to my happy wife? Holy poop, Batman—what have we done?* But as they say, it gets easier. It really does, so hang in there. As you adjust, as you slowly get used to a new sleep schedule, and as you gain more and more confidence that you really do know how to be a parent (although nobody ever totally knows), you won't feel so lost and confused. If you are struggling, let me just say this: Heidi and I are now 4 years into this parenthood thing, and it's pretty rad. We definitely have our challenges and struggles. Parenting is, without a doubt, the toughest thing either of us has ever done—but it couldn't be more worth it.

All parents make mistakes. God knows we have. No parent is perfect, and just when you think you've totally rocked any particular parenting situation (changed a diaper with one hand? Headed off a tantrum in the nick of time? Made your own baby food?), you will probably do something else totally "wrong" (forgot to bring a spit-up rag when you are wearing your first new nonmaternity shirt, forgot to pack the diaper bag, realized as soon as you got to the mall that you left the stroller at home, finally got the baby to sleep and then tripped over the changing table on the way out the door and woke him up again). The point is not to be perfect—never to be perfect. The point is to learn how to forgive yourself, learn from your mistakes, stay open to change, and be okay with your feelings (whatever they may be). *That,* my friend, is what a good parent does.

FOURTH TRIMESTER LIFESTYLE, OR THE THREE S'S: SLEEP, SUPPORT, AND SUSTENANCE

Now that we've covered some generalities about this unique trimester, let's get into some specifics. How do we get you feeling better, stronger, fitter, and more capable and in control of your body and emotions? There are some solid, proven ways to do this. You won't be able to make every lifestyle change all at once, but let this section be your guide to the transition from pregnancy person back to autonomous person. The strategies that follow will help get you out of this challenging period with your sanity, your well-being, and your relationships as strong as ever.

Sleep. No, Seriously.

I'm sure you read the first S and laughed. How the heck are you supposed to get sleep with a newborn? Fair enough—it won't be ideal, at least not for a while, but if you can learn to adjust your sleep schedule and get your sleep in less traditional ways, you will start feeling better fast. Sleep deprivation can drive anyone mad—there is a reason it has been used throughout history as a torture technique! So let's talk about how you can maximize your sleeping opportunities. Here are a few of the strategies Heidi and I employed.

Sleep When the Baby Sleeps

You've probably heard this one a million times, but have you ever actually done it? It's difficult to justify sleeping when the baby sleeps because you have that giant to-do list of things that require two hands, and you think this is your only time to do

Heidi Says . . .

The recovery from a C-section isn't glamorous in any way. Living in a three-story house and crawling up the stairs at a snail's pace made the first couple of weeks incredibly rough. I was obsessed with Phoenix (that's what we named our baby). I stared at him day and night until my neck hurt—true story. I still couldn't believe this baby came out of me. That just 2 weeks earlier, he had been growing inside me and now here he was!

Nursing was tough for me, and as much as I didn't want to give him the "evil formula" (that's what I thought about it at the time), it had to be done. He had lost 2 pounds since birth and just wasn't a happy camper because I wasn't making enough milk for him. I cherished the breastfeeding times, though—initially, these were some of my favorite moments. The pumping, however, was my least favorite part. Our original pediatrician (before we found Dr. Gordon) told me to pump every hour to increase my milk supply, which only made me want to cry. Pumping took up my entire day. I tried herbs, cookies, teas, and Guinness—everything I read

about online that was supposed to increase milk supply, but I was still lucky if I could pump out an ounce or two each time. Eventually, we had a good system down. In the end, we would do breast milk supplemented by the one formula we found that didn't make him gassy, and he would be just fine, strong and healthy. Eventually, I became okay with the fact that my body just wasn't going to produce enough milk for this enormous child.

My sister told me I barely spoke for 3 months. I really was obsessed and out of it for the entire fourth trimester. I spent almost that whole time sitting in the rocking chair, holding Phoenix and rocking and feeding, rocking and feeding, incredibly amazed by my baby but completely unable to snap back into life or be myself again after what felt to me like a somewhat traumatic birth experience. I did come out of those 3 months with approximately 3,000 photos of Phoenix that all looked pretty much the same: a sleeping baby. Then, just about at the 3-month mark, I snapped out of it and finally felt like I was back.

them. But here's a shocker: *Nothing* other than basic survival and baby care is more important than getting enough sleep—not the dishes, not the laundry, not the baby-toy clutter, and *definitely* not binge-watching your favorite TV show. Sleep, and everything else you do will get done better. When your little one goes down during the day, you need to go down, too. At first, it feels a bit odd to crash out at 1:00 in the afternoon, but it is an absolute necessity, and your body will adjust. The chores can wait. A clean house isn't nearly as crucial as your state of mind. Try to get in at least one serious nap per day during the first 6 to 12 weeks. Our pediatrician Dr. Gordon adds these words: "Get sleep. Somehow."

Take Shifts

This one can be hard when one parent is working. Oftentimes, the one who is staying home with the little one gets no break because the other parent is "working" and "needs their sleep." I get this, as I was the one "working," but ultimately one parent cannot do it all. Teamwork is key. You *both* have to sacrifice now to help each other out, and you both need your sleep—whether your job is to be the stay-at-home parent or the work-away parent.

The shift strategy worked for us, but it did require that Heidi used the ol' breast pump, so I could do the feeding. Many people try to tell you that if your baby takes a bottle, they will never take the nipple. In our experience? Not true. A nipple is a

Dr. Gordon Says . . .

Our expert pediatrician, Dr. Jay Gordon, weighs in on the controversial topic of the family bed, or cosleeping:

Although this is a controversial subject (for some reason) and there are many points of view, I am personally a big advocate of the family bed, or sleeping with the baby. This is the safest place for a healthy, breast-feeding baby. The baby will feel safer and more secure sleeping with the parents, and the mother will get more sleep if she doesn't have to get up and go to another room to breastfeed. People who push back against the family bed are basically telling you not to rest when the baby rests. They make mothering unforgivably harder, and I believe they are wrong.

However, nobody sleeping in bed with an infant (or any child) should ever be taking any drugs or alcohol.

A NOTE ABOUT POSTPARTUM DEPRESSION

Heidi was in an absolute fog and barely remembers anything from those several months right after labor and delivery, but I can tell you without a doubt that she definitely had some postpartum blues. Due to the C-section and pain medication, she was out of it and out of commission physically for a bit. The cacophony of hormones banging around in her body along with the lack of sleep and recovery from delivery literally zombified her for about 6 weeks—and I wasn't doing so awesome in the sleep department myself because I was getting up with the baby, too.

Postpartum depression happens for several reasons. Primarily, after birth, your estrogen and progesterone levels plummet sharply, and that can lead to mood changes, especially depression.[2] Exhaustion also makes the situation much worse, as sleep deprivation has a definite influence on mood. Then there are all those major life changes you've suddenly undergone all at once. Yes, there are plenty of reasons for postpartum depression, but none of them matter as much as how you deal with it when it happens.

The fact is that nearly all the pregnant women I have ever known are terrified of postpartum depression happening to them, and nearly all ended up experiencing it to one degree or another. But in most cases, it wasn't as bad as they had imagined, and they all came through it and are totally fine and healthy, as are their kids.

Postpartum depression manifests itself in a lot of ways, from weepiness at sappy television commercials to outbursts of anger or irritability at anybody who tries to interfere in the mothering process (the Mama Bear mode). You might have mood swings that confuse everyone in your family. You might feel blue, like you are in mourning for the life you have left behind, even as you are excited about the one that lies ahead. However, there is something you should know: If you feel depressed in a way that prohibits you from taking care of yourself or your baby, if you feel irrational thoughts that normally wouldn't make sense to you, if you feel any inclination toward self-harm or violence, or if you just don't feel like you are the same person and you are confused and upset by this, *please call your doctor*. Most postpartum depression is mild and dissipates in a few weeks or sometimes months, but more serious cases can also happen, are not that uncommon, and are *highly treatable*. You can do something about those feelings that are interfering with your life, so please let your doctor help you. Also know that postpartum depression is a biochemical imbalance. It is not a personality flaw and it is not your fault, so please don't be afraid to tell someone and get help. The only wrong thing to do in this situation is to keep it to yourself.

nipple, milk is milk, and you are a human who needs some sleep. Pump so that your significant other can get up with the baby and provide you with some much-needed relief. #NOGUILT!

Specifically, Heidi and I employed the Dream Feed Method, and it worked pretty well for us. She would feed our son and crash out early at around 8:30 p.m. Then I would feed our son around 11:30 p.m, and I'd crash out. He would get up once in the middle of the night, anywhere from around 2:30 to 4:00 a.m, and she would feed him, then go back to bed. I would wake up with him around 7:00, and she would sleep till I left for work. This plan generally allowed each of us to get a minimum of 6 hours of sleep a night, and in some cases even 8. Some sleep, interrupted or otherwise, is better than no sleep.

Support

The next of the three Ss is Support, and this one is *incredibly important*. Women tend to not want to ask for help, even when they need it the most (especially when they need it the most?) But there is absolutely nothing wrong with asking for help, and in fact, it may feel completely impossible to get through the day without it.

Your partner will be an essential support for you, but you may both feel so overwhelmed that you will need some outside help, too. Parents and siblings are great for this purpose, if they are available. Thank God for my mother-in-law. She hadn't even settled back into her home in Florida after meeting her grandkids for the first time when her phone rang—with me on the other end, begging her to come back. She

PUMP IT UP

If you can't make your breasts available for every single baby meal (and these days, this is pretty challenging, especially when you decide to go back to work), you will probably consider using a breast pump. These intimidating contraptions are actually pretty easy to use, once you get the hang of them. Just put the suction cup over your nipple and turn it on. The pump mimics the sucking action of your baby and funnels your breast milk into a bottle, so anyone can feed your baby without having to use formula (or without *always* having to use formula)—allowing you to sleep more (hallelujah!) and the other family members to get in a little baby bonding time. Breast pumps are also very useful when you are away from your baby but your breasts don't know it and start leaking or get uncomfortably full. There are many types, but your lactation consultant can advise you.

Dr. Gordon Says . . .

There is a misconception that in the early months, babies notice only their mothers. The baby is acutely and intensely aware of the other parent! Holding, cuddling, dancing with, and talking to the baby is very important during these early months, so take advantage of this. Just because you didn't give birth to the baby does not mean that you cannot bond with the baby.

came back and stayed with us for a couple of weeks to help us get settled. If you or your birth partner has a parent, family member, or friend to help you during this time, don't be proud. Even if they can do one night a week to help you and yours catch up on sleep, that brief chunk of solid rest can be instrumental during this time. As you get more rested, support can also allow you to get away for a little autonomous time, or time with your partner, both of which are important for your mental health and your relationship.

Also don't be afraid to ask for a break now and then. Once you get done staring at your baby for hours on end (we all do this, just so you don't think you are strange), reach out to friends and family. Having some adult time and conversation can help "normalize" things a bit for you and bring you out of the rabbit hole. Even if the baby is in the carrier while you have coffee with a friend, or you get your sister to come over and hang out with you, or even if you go to a party for a while and hire a (gasp!) babysitter, you will find your sanity slowly returning.

Finally, and this is very, very important: If all of the above measures are not helping, and you find yourself in a very dark place, please seek some professional help. I want to stress this point because even if you don't think you have postpartum depression, if your life isn't working and you can't seem to get out of your rut, there is help available for you. There is no shame in this. Quite the contrary, it's the brave and responsible thing to do. You don't necessarily need to call your doctor. A good therapist or counselor can help you and your family through this time of transition. Dealing with any difficult or depressed feelings is totally normal, and if it isn't going away on its own, don't ignore it. Get yourself any help or support you might need.

About Your Relationship/Sex (or Lack Thereof)

A major part of the support you will need in your new job as a mom is support from the inside—your own partner. And an important part of any romantic relationship is sex. I know, you don't feel like doing that right now, but this is an important subject to consider, even if you aren't cleared by your doctor to "get back into it" (pun intended).

I'm not so sure people really prep you adequately for this one, so let's discuss: Sex after baby will wane for a bit. Doctors say in most cases it's okay to resume sexual activity after 6 weeks, but the waiting period may be potentially longer if you had a C-section. You should be able to push on the scar without pain before resuming intercourse. That said, in most cases, the physical healing from delivery isn't the actual issue at hand—it's everything else. Just because you are told you can resume in 6 weeks doesn't mean you will *want* to resume in 6 weeks. (And as Dr. Gordon has told me, "Hardly anyone gets laid in the first couple of months.")

Your hormone changes can inhibit your sex drive. You are sleep deprived. You may be self-conscious about your body. There is likely a third person in the room (hello tiny peanut). There will be a few temporary changes to your bits and bobs (my immature speak for breasts and vagina) that might make you feel a bit unsure about using them for their former purpose. For example, your boobs will be enormous and they will leak. This might turn on your partner, but it might make you feel extremely self-conscious. Your nether regions will potentially dry up for 6 to 12 weeks, maybe even a bit longer, while you are still breastfeeding, so that can also make you feel *not in the mood*.

Never fear. There are ways to manage this, but it will require a conscious effort on both your parts. Why should you bother? Because intimacy is key for maintaining a relationship, and this is a very important time to maintain your relationship. You need each other now, so keeping an open dialogue and maintaining a loving and nurturing environment between the two of you is extremely important. While things

Dr. Suzanne Says . . .

I always prep the partner, especially if the mom has a history of depression, anxiety, or trauma or had a particularly difficult pregnancy and/or birth, that the mom herself might not recognize postpartum depression, but if the partner sees the signs, s/he can call me. Also, know about Postpartum Support International, postpartum.net, an organization devoted to the treatment of and support for postpartum depression. This is important for folks who may not live near a lot of resources.

can get crazy during this time and sex for some can seem low on the totem pole, I can't stress enough how critical it is to your overall long-term relationship.

As the one who did not give birth in our parenting dynamic duo, I have mentioned that the daddies or parenting partners often feel like outsiders for a while. Making time for one another is so important. Even if you have to schedule sex, while it lacks spontaneity and romance, do it! Scheduled sex will be better than no sex any and every day of the week. Maybe it's not the ideal romantic situation, but it helps. I promise. Think of it like going to the gym. Sometimes you aren't in the mood, but you go anyway. And once you are there, you get into it and afterward you feel great. You know the saying, "Just do it!"

And even if you can't have intercourse, we are all adults here. I think it's obvious there are other things you can do in the bedroom that will bring you both "closer." Do them. When you aren't in the mood, do them anyway.

If you are feeling a bit self-conscious at first, here are some strategies to try that can help bring back the romance:

- **Pump** beforehand if you are feeling self-conscious about "leakage." (Which, honestly, is not a big deal—but if it bothers you, that is a good way to go about managing your concerns.)

- **Lube.** Hello—there is such a thing as lubricant. I think most women are worried their partners will wonder why they aren't getting "turned on" or exhibiting certain physiological indicators of arousal. Simply explain to your partner that this is normal and get some natural lubricants in the bedroom. Coconut oil is a great nontoxic option. Also be sure to hydrate constantly and eat more phytoestrogens (flax, fermented organic soy from tempeh or miso soup, chickpeas, and apples) to boost your lagging estrogen.

- **Dim the lights.** If you are feeling self-conscious, turn off the lights! And it's okay. We've all been there.

Sustenance, or Fourth Trimester Nutrition

Now about your diet. You have been eating, haven't you? And eating well? Don't think that just because the baby is now on the outside, what you eat no longer matters. This is no time to lapse into poor dietary habits. You want quality breast milk, you want to manage your moods, and you want to start getting your body back, don't you?

First let's talk about that last issue. One of the all-time most frequent questions I get is, "How do I lose the baby weight?" The irony of this question is that it implies "baby weight" is different than any other kind of weight. Guess what? It isn't.

Fat is fat. Simple. So the first goal is to simply dispel any notion that there is a secret method in particular that is required to lose baby weight. We lose baby weight by burning fat, and we burn fat the same way we always have as human beings: We create a calorie deficit by eating less and moving more.

Now, where this gets tricky is gauging how *quickly* you should lose any pounds you may have packed on. Our primary goals in this time period are as follows:

1. Nourish your body in a way that facilitates your healing.
2. Keep your energy levels up.
3. Maintain your milk supply (if you're breastfeeding), so you can make sure you pass the optimal amount of nutrients on to your little one.

If we create too great of a calorie deficit by reducing your food intake too much or too soon, we will compromise all of the above.

Remember, the key to getting your "body back" fast after baby is to have had a healthy pregnancy. In all honesty, if you have been with me and have been following this plan through your pregnancy, "bouncing back" will be a snap. But if you haven't, don't stress! We will absolutely get you back in shape—safely and steadily.

However, focusing on weight loss immediately after giving birth is not advantageous. You will be in the process of healing from delivery, exhausted, and possibly breastfeeding. Adding drastic calorie reduction to your plate is a recipe for heightened stress, decrease in breast milk production, and even higher risk of postpartum depression—that is, it's totally counterproductive. Yes, we have all seen the Hollywood actresses and rock stars who drop crazy amounts of weight seemingly overnight—but God only knows what kind of a toll it's taking on them in other areas.

Don't focus on weight loss for *at least* 6 weeks after your baby is born. But don't binge-eat or refuse to get off the couch, either. Just put the notion of weight out of your mind and focus on rest and reverie and some healthy movement with your baby. Enjoy your little one. Keep your attention on your adapting to life as a mommy and on your recovery. This plan will make sure that you don't gain any further weight and that you will gradually lose it in a way that's safe and not stressful.

Maybe you have heard that you need to be taking in 300 to 600 extra calories in a day to breastfeed, since that's how many calories breastfeeding burns. Actually, this is an average and it may not apply to you, but more importantly, as long as you are eating a diet full of nutritious food, you don't need to eat those extra calories. If you burn a few more while you aren't exercising as much, then things will even out.

So how much should you eat? After the 6-week period has passed, we first need to address how much you should be eating by taking into account three different factors.

1. Are you breastfeeding?
2. Do you have weight to lose?
3. Are you exercising?

Calorie Levels

Here are some basics to follow:

- **If you are not breastfeeding and want to lose weight,** I recommend no less than 1,600 calories a day with unlimited green vegetables as "free food." Green veggies require nearly as many calories to digest as they contain, so at any point, you can just eat as many as you want without factoring them into your daily calorie allowance. Low-calorie diets, such as 1,200 a day, I don't recommend. While you must create a calorie deficit to lose weight (roughly 3,500 calories to lose a pound/500 calories a day for 1 pound of weight loss in a week), you shouldn't go for fast and dramatic weight loss at this time in your life. Even if you aren't breastfeeding, you still need enough calories and nutrients to fend off fatigue, mitigate postpartum depression, and aid in recovery from pregnancy and delivery.

- **If you are breastfeeding,** things get a bit more complicated. Are you looking to shed excess pounds that were gained or simply to maintain your weight? When I say excess, I mean you are still *over* 10 to 15 pounds above your pre-pregnancy weight. Remember that your body needed to add roughly 10 pounds of fat for breastfeeding purposes during pregnancy. So, you've already done that extra breastfeeding calorie intake and now you're using it and burning it off. You don't need to gain more. But if you have gained 20 or more pounds of excess fat, then, yes, you are going to want to lose it . . . safely, in a reasonable time frame that doesn't compromise your health and sanity or your baby's milk supply. You will want to eat no less than 1,800 calories, and you will want to lose no more than 2 pounds a week, so gauge your intake by how quickly you are losing weight—and don't be tempted to go faster. I have found, pretty unilaterally, that when breastfeeding women lose more than 2 pounds a week, milk supply can be compromised.

If you are only 10 to 15 pounds or so away from your prebaby weight, this should come off naturally as you continue to breastfeed and exercise over the next 3 months, without reducing your calorie intake much at all. You could eat anywhere from 2,000 to 2,300 calories, going toward the higher end on days you exercise.

At-a-Glance Calorie Chart*

NOT BREASTFEEDING	Want to lose weight	No less than 1,600 calories a day, training or not
	Want to maintain weight	1,800 on nontraining days; 2,000 on training days*
BREASTFEEDING	Want to lose weight	No less than 1,800 training or not
	Want to maintain weight	2,100 on nontraining days; 2,300 on training days*

*As a general rule of thumb for postpartum weight loss, don't lose more than 2 pounds a week—so don't create a calorie deficit of more than 1,000 calories a day. This is applicable if you wish to train intensely and have been cleared by your doctor to do so.

Eating Schedule

Do those nutrition Rules of Thumb still apply? You bet they do. In case your mommy brain has wiped all that out of your head, you can always go back and review Chapter 2, but here's quick recap of the most basic important points.

- **Don't skip meals.** This will help stabilize your blood sugar and energy levels and keep you from bingeing later in the day.

- **Don't snack throughout the day.** Unlike the small meals you may have been taking in throughout the day due to heartburn or even nausea during your pregnancy, you don't need a constant intake of energy now. Snacking throughout the day never allows your body to go into a "postabsorptive" phase, where your body utilizes fat stores for fuel.

- **Focus on four.** The ideal eating schedule for energy and blood sugar stabilization and hormonal harmony is breakfast, lunch, snack, dinner. This means you are eating every 3.5 to 4 hours—the same as you were during pregnancy, unless you were splitting your meals into smaller portions, which you no longer need to do because you have room to digest a full meal again.

Nutrients for You

Again, the nutrition Rules of Thumb apply, both in terms of what to eat and what not to eat. In fact, they apply for the rest of your life, so I hope you will return to Chapter 2 in this book often, even when you aren't pregnant. Eat whole foods, go organic, and so on. Everything I've already said about nutrition remains important. However, in the fourth trimester, you want to focus in particular on nutrients that aid in healing, mitigate postpartum depression, boost milk production, and make that milk as nutrient-dense as possible. Here are some targeted tips.

For a Healthy State of Mind

Follow these guidelines to keep your mood steady and calm and to help ward off or lessen the severity of postpartum depression:

- **Don't skip meals.** Low blood sugar never boosted anyone's mood. I know things can get crazy during this time and it's easy to "forget to eat," but remember: You have a little one to feed, and you also need proper nutrients to heal and sustain yourself.

- **Avoid processed grains and sugars.** These types of foods spike blood sugar and then crash it, which can lead to mood swings and anxiety attacks.

- **Hydrate, hydrate, hydrate.** Water boosts your milk supply, aids in digestion and elimination, and helps to provide you with much needed energy to fend off fatigue.

- **Think nutrient density.** Nutrient deficiencies can have an effect on your mood. We have talked about the importance of vitamins and minerals over the course of your pregnancy for many reasons. The rules still apply.

Nutrients for Mood

Also focus on these nutrients, specifically to ward off postpartum depression and mood swings:

- **Iron:** Get it from red meat, liver, raisins, spinach, broccoli, egg yolks, and iron-fortified breakfast cereals.

- **Folate:** Get it from beans, peanut butter, oatmeal, mushrooms, broccoli, spinach, asparagus, red meat, and liver.

- **Vitamin B$_{12}$:** Get it from fish, milk and milk products, eggs, red meat, poultry, and fortified breakfast cereals.

- **Selenium:** Get it from sunflower seeds, whole grain cereals, and Brazil nuts.

- **DHA/EPA:** Get it from salmon, trout, walnuts, and flaxseeds. Also, cod-liver oil is a supplement many women swear by to help boost mood and milk production.

- **Tyrosine:** Get it from fish, chicken, meat, eggs, legumes, cheese, milk, and yogurt.

Nutrients for Healing

Focus on these nutrients to help fend off infections, heal wounds, and mitigate the effects of any potential blood loss in the event you may have undergone a C-section or episiotomy:

- **Zinc:** Get it from oysters, grass-fed beef or lamb, kale, pumpkin seeds, pork, and chicken.
- **Vitamin A:** Get it from cooked sweet potato, cooked carrots, cooked dark leafy greens like kale, butternut squash, Romaine lettuce, apricots, cantaloupe, mango, and egg yolks.
- **Vitamin C:** Get it from bell peppers, leafy greens, berries, kiwifruit, guava, citrus fruits, tomatoes, and papaya.
- **Vitamin E:** Get it from almonds, pumpkin seeds, kale, hazelnuts, avocado, broccoli, papaya, and olives.
- **Iron:** Get it from red meat, liver, raisins, spinach, broccoli, egg yolks, and iron-fortified breakfast cereals.
- **Probiotics:** Get them from yogurt, kefir, kimchi, and naturally fermented vegetables.

Tips and Nutrients to Maximize Milk Production and Nutrient Density

You can and should still consume any and all the meals and recipes from our Yeah Baby! meal plan. Each and every one has supreme nutrition and appropriate calories to fully support you on a healthy "diet" during this time. A few more nutritional tips to help your kiddo out.

- **Pump and dump—yes or no?** Some people recommend pumping your breastmilk and dumping it out if you have been drinking alcohol, but Dr. Suzanne says there is no science to support this. Instead, if you are drinking alcohol,

---

SHOULD YOU KEEP TAKING YOUR PRENATAL VITAMINS?

If you are eating good, nutrient-dense food every day at every meal, you probably don't need to keep taking your prenatal vitamin, but it can't hurt while you are breastfeeding or just recovering throughout the "fourth trimester." Most doctors recommend it.

just make sure to wait at least 2 to 3 hours before breastfeeding for every 12 ounces, or roughly two drinks, or your baby will get very sleepy. Pumping and dumping doesn't speed the time for it to clear your system either, so no cheating on the clock.

- **Limit caffeine,** as it may interfere with your baby's sleep and dehydrate you. No more than 200 mg a day, which equals roughly one strong cup of coffee.

- **Avoid fish that are high in mercury,** as they may interfere with the development of your baby's nervous system. Tuna, swordfish, mackerel, and tilefish should all be avoided at this time—honestly, you should really limit your consumption of these fish even when you are no longer breastfeeding. Mercury ain't good for *you*, either.

- **Eat plenty of foods rich in calcium and magnesium.** To help baby develop strong bones and teeth, have plenty of cheese, yogurt, kefir, broccoli, kale, almonds, tempeh, blackstrap molasses, and hemp milk.

- **Keep up those omega-3s.** Feed the growing brain and nervous system with salmon, trout, and cod-liver oil.

BREASTFEEDING

Okay, maybe you knew this was coming, and obviously we have to talk about it because it is something that causes so much angst for so many people: breastfeeding. If breastfeeding is a snap for you, awesome. You can pass GO and collect $200. If not, let's dig in.

Numerous women struggle in one way or another with this, and the issues run the gamut. Maybe you aren't producing enough milk. Maybe you are producing too much milk. Maybe there are issues with the "latch." Maybe you have mastitis. Maybe your nipples are cracking and bleeding (fun!). Maybe you just don't like it.

We know by now that things can go wrong with breastfeeding, and they can go wrong for anyone, even the healthiest, most natural-leaning people. Heidi really struggled with the issue of not making enough milk, and it brought up feelings of insecurity and inferiority that I just couldn't relieve her of, no matter how much I tried. That broke my heart. But this happens to a lot of people from all ages and all walks of life. Breasts are "designed" for breastfeeding, theoretically, but the reality doesn't always work out that way.

So should you grin and bear it? And how much is enough? Experts say that the first few weeks really are the hardest, as you get the hang of nursing. It does *not* come naturally to most women, contrary to what you might think.

But it is definitely good for your baby, and it also does good things for your body, so it's definitely worth a good try. (It burns 300 to 600 calories a day![3]) Let's go over some of the most common issues and discuss possible plans of attack.

THE YEAH BABY! FOURTH TRIMESTER SMOOTHIES

Smoothies are awesome for the fourth trimester because they are super fast and easy to digest, and you can really pack in the nutrients. For that reason, I have some special fourth trimester smoothie recipes just for you. These smoothies help you address all of your and your baby's nutrition needs during the fourth trimester as easily and simply as possible. I've given you the names of these very special smoothies here, and you can find them in Appendix A at the end of this book, starting on page 294.

All of these smoothies serve one person: you!

- **Milk Max Smoothie:** A creamy, fruity smoothie that will help boost your milk supply.

- **Super Baby Smoothie:** Optimizes the nutrients in breast milk, so your baby can be a *super baby!*

- **Happy Day Smoothie:** This one boosts your mood and could lessen postpartum depression.

- **Recovery Smoothie:** This smoothie helps to promote healing after delivery.

- **Energizer Smoothie:** This one revitalizes you and gives you a boost of energy, to fend off fatigue.

Ineffective Latch

You'll find plenty of information out there on the Internet, but rather than consulting Dr. Google, I honestly recommend a lactation consultant. There are so many factors to consider! I remember thinking our son was suffocating, when he was actually latching correctly. New moms tend to not put enough of the nipple in the baby's mouth, and a hands-on demonstration (don't be embarrassed) by a lactation consultant is worth a thousand words. Ask to have a lactation consultant visit you as soon as possible after the birth—most hospitals have them available—and keep asking for help while you're in the hospital until you feel comfortable. After you get home, see if you can have your insurance cover the cost of a home visit; if not, attend a breastfeeding seminar for new moms. (Here is a Web site to help you find someone in your area uslca.org/resources/find-an-ibclc.) I highly recommend at least one session to help you and your little one work out the kinks—breastfeeding shouldn't hurt, and if it does, you probably need further instruction. Once you get going, you'll be amazed by how wonderful it feels and how close it helps you feel to your baby.

Mastitis

If you are wondering what this is, you obviously have not experienced it, because you'd know. Mastitis is the swelling of the breasts because of a bacterial infection. Your breasts will get engorged, incredibly painful, and hard to the touch. You may also get a fever and feel like you're getting the flu. The infection can happen when the milk ducts get plugged, or bacteria can get introduced from sore, cracked nipples. This is a serious medical condition and warrants an immediate call to your doctor. It's likely he or she will put you on antibiotics. If the infection is caught early enough, it should clear up fairly quickly.

Mastitis can occur anytime you are breastfeeding, but it's most common in the first month of your pregnancy, before you and your baby get the hang of nursing. Here are a few tips to help you avoid mastitis or manage it (should you get it) in conjunction with treatment from your doctor.

- **Get rest.** Mommies who are fatigued and stressed are more at risk.

- **Make sure your latch is solid.** Good breastfeeding techniques will help prevent sore or cracked nipples.

- **Nurse or pump frequently** to keep the milk flowing and your breasts empty.

- **Drain your breasts thoroughly at each feed.** If your breasts still have milk after your baby is done eating, be sure to use a pump to get the rest of the milk out.

- **Apply wet heat and massage** the affected breast to help get the milk out. Repeat throughout the day.
- **Wear well-fitting nursing bras.** Avoid those that are too small or have an underwire.
- **Above all, keep going!** Even if you have mastitis, continue to breastfeed. It will help empty the milk from your breasts, and it *will not hurt the baby*. (The only exception would be if your infant is in neonatal intensive care. That's because mastitis can increase the amount of sodium in your milk, and it's not recommended for little ones in neonatal intensive care. Otherwise it's perfectly safe.)

Sore or Cracked Nipples

Ouch. In many cases, latch issues cause this because the baby is essentially gumming the end of the nipple instead of mouthing the whole nipple in a way that pushes the milk out. This is when a lactation specialist can be so helpful. Some people try nipple shields for this problem, but a nipple shield can cause latch problems, and most lactation specialists usually recommend against them. However, they have helped some women nurse who might not have nursed otherwise, so the verdict isn't exactly in on these.[4] Before you go that route, however, try applying a bit of breast milk to your nipples after every feed—freshly expressed breast milk can help heal cracked nipples because it offers antibacterial protection. It's an old midwife's trick that's been proven to work![5]

Thrush

Thrush is basically an oral yeast infection that babies often get and pass on to their nursing moms. Then it can get passed back and forth so it is very hard to get rid of.

TONGUE-TIE (ANKYLOGLOSSIA)

Babies use their tongues to nurse correctly, but if they have tongue-tie, they may have problems latching on. Tongue-tie is a condition in which the frenulum (the tissue that connects the bottom of the tongue tip to the floor of the mouth) is tighter and shorter than normal.[6] In some children, tongue-tie does not affect breastfeeding but may cause problems later with speaking or eating. If tongue-tie is seriously interfering with breastfeeding, however, a doctor can easily correct the problem with a simple, mostly painless surgery called a *frenotomy* that snips the tight band of tissue so the tongue is free to move normally. A lactation consultant can check for tongue-tie and advise you on whether the condition requires intervention.

Women who've had C-sections may be more susceptible to this, due to the antibiotics prescribed after the surgery, which tend to let yeast overgrow. To help avoid this, I highly recommend taking probiotics and slipping some baby-appropriate probiotics into your little one's bottle of pumped breast milk. As previously mentioned, BioGaia is a great brand that you can find nearly anywhere. Also back off sugar in your diet, which feeds yeast. You can talk to your doctor about prescription nipple cream, but avoid the ones that can facilitate fungal growth (which is why prescription may be necessary—some over-the-counter brands will be counterproductive). You can also try coconut oil, which is a natural antifungal.

If you already have a bad case of thrush, again, back off on the sugar, eat more foods with natural probiotics like yogurt, drink a lot of water, and air out your boobs when you can[7]—thrush thrives in moist environments. If your baby has oral thrush (a sign is white cheesy-looking lesions in the mouth that look like curdled milk but don't wipe away), your doctor or lactation consultant may recommend treatment, but often it goes away on its own in a couple of weeks.

Overzealous Pump

Your breast pump's level of suction may be up too high and/or the flanges or breast shields may be too small for your nipples. Have your lactation consultant help you to make sure you get this just right.

Low Milk Production

I know this one can bring a lot of anxiety; I have witnessed it firsthand, and it is one of the main reasons why women stop breastfeeding. As I mentioned, Heidi was simply unable to make enough milk to feed our enormous 9-pound son. We had to supplement with formula, and he was happy and able to both breastfeed and be topped off with formula in a bottle. No stress, and no shame! Enough with the perfectionism around 100 percent breastfeeding! I'm telling you this personal tale so that you will not give up on your milk supply, no matter how modest or robust it turns out to be. Either way, it will all work itself out.

That said, there are some things you can do to boost milk supply:

- **Nurse on demand.** Nurse for as long as you can manage. Shoot for 8 to 10 minutes, so the baby gets the nutritious foremilk (the milk at the beginning of the nursing session) and the hydrating hindmilk (the more watery milk at the end of the nursing session). Also nurse as often as possible. I'm not going to lie—this one brought my sweet and exhausted Heidi to tears, so if you can't do it, *that's okay!* But if you can, it will help. As the amazing Dr. William Sears, a well-known pediatrician and author of many classic parenting books has said, the three Bs of breastfeeding are the breast, the baby, and the brain.[8] Essentially, the baby needs to stimulate the breast more often to send signals to the brain to produce more milk. Basic supply and demand: Works in economics and the biology of breastfeeding.

- **Hydrate.** Some say this tip is overrated. I say it can't hurt. You don't need to guzzle gallons, but be sure to prevent yourself from getting dehydrated, which can inhibit milk production.

- **Avoid alcohol.** I know you have been teetotaling for months now. I hate even mentioning this to you. However, if you are having issues making enough milk,[9] research has shown that after drinking one or two glasses of wine, women take longer to release their milk and produce less milk overall.[10] So while you may have heard the old wives' tales about beer enhancing milk production, research suggests the opposite. Be safe, and steer clear.

- **Consider herbs.** Many herbs are touted as having near magical powers when it comes to enhancing breast-milk production. Few have been scientifically tested and proven, but the following may help when taken in moderation while breastfeeding. (That said, *always* talk with your doctor before using any herbal supplement.)

■ Asparagus racemosus	■ Goat's rue
■ Chamomile	■ Milk thistle
■ Fennel	■ Motherwort
■ Fenugreek seeds	■ Red raspberry

- **Stick to your healthy diet.** An overall healthy diet will make a big difference, but the following foods can help boost milk production because they are believed to boost pituitary function and estrogen levels.

- Alfalfa
- Almonds
- Asparagus
- Brewer's yeast in supplement form (not in beer!)
- Carrots
- Chickpeas or hummus
- Coconut and/or olive oil
- Flax
- Garlic
- Oats
- Sesame seeds or tahini sauce
- Spinach
- Wild salmon

And let me reiterate one final breastfeeding fact: Should you need to pump and bottle-feed, supplement with formula, or even feed with formula only, despite all the propaganda, the world won't end. While there are many benefits to breastfeeding, if you are simply unable to do it or choose not to, your child will be fine. My mom was unable to breastfeed me. I love and adore her. We are and have always been utterly bonded. And I am also pretty darn healthy. So try to cut yourself some slack, will ya?

FOURTH TRIMESTER FITNESS

Now for my favorite part! In considering every woman's dream of "bouncing right back" after baby, fitness is the most crucial component. Research shows us that the first 6 months after childbirth are the most crucial to losing the weight and keeping it off, so this is where the magic really happens.

But that doesn't mean blowing it all out at the gym for hours every day. That is not what you need right now. In order to determine what you should be doing, how many times a week, and for how long per session, we need to first establish what your delivery was like.

The American College of Obstetricians and Gynecologists (ACOG) says it's okay to slowly resume exercising as soon as you "feel up to it." That's vague, I know, so let me be a little more specific. As a general rule, it's strongly recommended that no matter what the manner of your baby's birth, 6 weeks off any strenuous training is a must. The body *needs* time to heal.

Understand, exercise stresses the body. The body responds to this stress through a "stress adaptation response," which is how we become more fit. For example: When you lift weights for the first time, you might get blisters. Over time, the body adapts by creating calluses. The same goes for your muscles, tendons, ligaments, cardiovascular system, and so on—all respond to the stress of exercise by becoming stronger, more mobile and flexible, and faster.

Knowing this, please realize that any added stress to your body at this time is *not* advantageous. Your body needs to focus on healing and adapting to parenthood—not recovering from strenuous exercise.

Before you start any training plan, always check with your doctor. Now, let's discuss what is safe with regard to exercise postpregnancy, customized to your particular delivery experience.

Vaginal Birth (No Complications)

In terms of a swift and speedy return to fitness, vaginal birth is definitely the ideal scenario. That said, for many in this position, the expectation is that you will simply return to where you left off prebaby—and this is not the case.

Even if you are super fit and have been super fit throughout your pregnancy, I still don't recommend that you go out and start pounding pavement or grinding away with your Olympic lifts. The reality is that pregnancy does take some toll. I know I told you earlier in this book about how pregnancy can actually improve your athletic performance, and that's all true, but it doesn't happen right away. You still need time to do that healing part—the recovery from the stress of pregnancy will make you stronger, *if* you allow yourself to recover. That means even the fittest pregnant mommies may find their pelvic floor weakened, posture out of alignment, and energy level compromised. In addition, that "loosey-goosey" hormone relaxin that was responsible for softening ligaments and joints during pregnancy can stay in your body for up to 6 months after you've given birth. For all these reasons mentioned and plenty of others, it's important to ease back into your fitness routine.

If you were fit during pregnancy and had a complication-free vaginal delivery, most doctors will allow/recommend light cardio activity (biking, incline walking, swimming, after all bleeding has stopped), stretching, and resistance training with light weights or modified bodyweight exercises during the first 6 weeks. (Again: *Only if you had a complication-free delivery and had a decent level of fitness prior to and during pregnancy.*)

CHILL OUT

During the fourth trimester, it's important to work back to your prepregnancy exercise intensity gradually. For now, avoid any kind of intense training and just maintain steady-state cardio at a moderate intensity. You should be able to carry on a conversation while exercising. If you can't, dial it back.

Andy Says . . .

Again, again, again: If you have had a C-section, be absolutely sure your doctor approves of your workout plan and gives you the thumbs-up when it is okay to start.

Now, once those 6 weeks have passed, you should start to acclimate a bit, and you can begin to push the up button steadily on your regimen.

C-Section Delivery

If you've had a C-section, it's very important to take things even easier. Some doctors will tell you to wait up to 8 weeks before exercising again, depending upon how you are healing.

After the first week post C-section (provided you have your doctor's permission), 10 minutes of walking a day can be very beneficial. Gentle walks help increase circulation, preventing infection and blood clots while bringing in more oxygen and nutrients to the wound to promote healing. (If at any point you notice any bleeding, stop immediately and contact your doctor.)

From the second week forward, you can gradually increase your walking. As the weeks progress, you can build back up to 20 to 30 minutes a day in weeks 4 to 6—again, *as long as your doctor has cleared you to do so.*

Once that tenuous 6-week adjustment and healing period is over, we can begin to kick things up a notch. At this point, you can generally begin to rehab your body. And I use that word literally: You need to rehabilitate. Sadly, this is something that I find is greatly overlooked postpartum.

Specifically, you will need to facilitate proper healing for your core after a C-section. While abdominal muscles are rarely cut (most are separated during a C-section), you can still have scar tissue that can create issues for you down the road, from tenderness and stiffness of skin to abdominal weakness and hip pain. Increased circulation and gentle exercises that safely mobilize and strengthen your core are critical. I have outlined a few for you in this book. I also specifically created a workout program called Hot Mommy Healthy Body, with our expert Andrea Orbeck, to guide you through this time period and get you back into excellent shape. This includes modifications for diastasis recti and for those who have had C-sections (find information about how to purchase this DVD in the Resources section on page 323.)

Also, a good Pilates mat DVD or class, a Level 1 or 2 yoga flow, or a barre class can be very helpful. Be sure to tell your instructor that you have had a C-section so she can help you modify any exercises where necessary.

You should also continue incorporating your cardiovascular conditioning to burn fat and promote circulation. Normally, I like to make resistance training metabolic by doing it in a circuit-training fashion, and I recommend pure cardio (bike, run, swim) only on days off from lifting. But until you can return to that type of strenuous training, I recommend the following schedule:

Week 1: Total recovery. No exercise whatsoever. Even stairs should be avoided.

Week 2: Walk 10 minutes a day.

Week 3: Walk 15 minutes a day.

Week 4: Walk 20 minutes a day.

Weeks 5 and 6: Walk 30 minutes a day.

Weeks 7 to 12: Three gentle-resistance training days + 2 moderate cardio days, which could look something like this:

- 1 day a week Pilates class or Pilates DVD
- 1 day a week level 1 yoga flow class or postpartum yoga DVD
- 1 day a week barre class for postbaby (Pure Barre studios offer a great "Bounce Back" class)
- 2 days a week 30- to 40-minute moderate cardio session of incline walking, biking, or swimming

Diastasis Recti During or After Delivery

Now let's address how you train after baby if you sustained diastasis recti, or abdominal separation. Remember, this means your rectus abdominal muscles (aka, "the 6-pack") separated during pregnancy or during childbirth, and they need to repair themselves.

Generally, if you have sustained this abdominal gap, it will close on its own after about 4 to 8 weeks. However, for those who sustained a more severe separation, it can take up to 3 months (or more) and will require some physical therapy to rehab. (Again, this is only in severe cases—most women don't need to do this.)

As your abdominal muscles are healing, it's a good idea to splint or brace your core while working out. This can help bring the muscles back together and prevent further separation of the abdominal wall under stress. You can find a splint or brace online; here is a good resource for you: diastasisrehab.com.

It's very important not to exacerbate this issue during the fourth trimester because that can prolong healing. With your doctor's permission, you can follow the third

EXERCISE MODIFICATIONS FOR THOSE WITH C-SECTIONS AND/OR DIASTASIS RECTI

Please *avoid* these exercises and movements for at least 3 months if you have had a C-section or diastasis recti:

- Crunches, situps, leg raises, and front planks
- Anything that stretches the abdominal wall (cat cow, up dog, back bends of any kind)
- Running, jumping, stepups
- Torso rotation—twisting lunges or abdominal work like Russian twists, etc.
- Heavily weighted exercises
- Anything with direct downward pressure, such as barbell back squats, overhead presses, etc.

After a roughly 3- to 6-month period, if you consistently and methodically healed your body and conditioned it with bodyweight and or light resistance training and moderate cardio, you should be ready to train more intensely: HIIT intervals, jogging or running, weight lifting, and more. Good rehab exercises include Elevated Heel Slides (page 305) and Mula Bandha (pages 144–145).

trimester pregnancy workout, adhering to all the guidelines previously outlined regarding diastasis recti (see page 201).

Episiotomy or Tearing

As mentioned in the labor and delivery chapter, episiotomy is a surgical cut along the perineum to make more room for the baby to come out, but it should not be done routinely and is actually not very common anymore. However, if you've had one, or if you sustained some tearing to the perineal area during your delivery, please be safe during your postpartum fitness so you can heal and not further aggravate the wound. Generally, you should notice significant healing after 10 days and nearly full recovery after 1 month. Follow the walking regimen established above for C-section recovery for the first 4 weeks. Avoid anything strenuous for the first 4 weeks that can delay healing. Proceed like this:

Week 1: Total recovery. No exercise whatsoever. Even stairs should be avoided.

Week 2: Walk 10 minutes a day.

Week 3: Walk 15 minutes a day.

Week 4: Walk 20 minutes a day.

The 3-Month Mark

No matter what category you fell into above, once you have hit the 3-month post-partum mark, you are generally in the clear to exercise in any *way* you choose—provided you have had no healing complications and have been diligent about your steady return to fitness.

However, many women are not feeling 100 percent until around 6 months. If that's you, that's fine. During this time period, as you think about returning to more aggressive types of fitness (Olympic lifting, HIIT training, Bodyshred, and so on), keep your intensity level at about 70 percent of what it was prepregnancy. If you were running sprints at 10 mph for 1 minute, try them now at 7.5 mph for 1 minute. If you were back-squatting 75 pounds for 12 reps, try it now with around 55 pounds for 10 to 12 reps.

Stay in communication with your doctor, and make sure he or she is in the loop with what you are doing and has given you his blessing.

Most important, listen to your body. If you are struggling with something, dial it back a bit more. Then, as things begin to feel more and more manageable, try amping up your intensity by 5 percent every 2 weeks until you are back at 100 percent—right where you were prepregnancy.

By gradually increasing your reps, weights, and speed every 2 weeks, you will safely and methodically hit your prepregnancy fitness level right on target: at the 6-month mark.

The 6-Month Mark

Now, there's not a ton to say here, and the reason is because, at 6 months, we're no longer talking about "pregnancy fitness." You have currently graduated out of any aspect of pregnancy fitness. At this point, you can return to all the fitness pursuits

Dr. Suzanne Says . . .

Even if you have been working on your pelvic floor strengthening (and if you haven't, you are not alone), you may experience some urinary incontinence during or after labor and delivery. Incontinence is pretty common up to about 6 weeks postpartum, but if you are still having problems after that, you can work with a physical therapist who knows how to do pelvic floor physical therapy. Be forewarned that this involves a gloved hand in your vagina to help you feel exactly what you need to do for your PT exercises, but this can make a big difference in how quickly any pelvic-floor-related issues resolve.

you have always loved to do. You are back to *regular fitness*. Hooray for you!

Meanwhile, if you are looking to achieve any other fitness-related goal, be it aesthetic (toning up problem areas) or athletic (training for a Tough Mudder, running a

Andy Says . . .

Here is what Andy says about strengthening your core to help repair your diastasis recti:

Now is the time when you will really notice if you have experienced an abdominal separation. You will get a small pooch in your stomach when you lie on your side or do an exercise on your hands and knees. This is no time to be doing exercise that puts a lot of strain on the abdominal muscles. Instead, this is a time to heal them. The key is to start working your deep abdominal muscles gently but steadily, to help your body strengthen and start knitting those muscles back together. Do each of these exercises twice, resting for 30 seconds between, once or twice each day.

- *Lie on your side and gently feel for your abdominal muscles. Relax your stomach and feel the area below your navel, between your hip bones. Breathe deeply and hold those lower abdominal muscles so you can feel them contracting. Hold that for 10 seconds (keep breathing) and relax. Repeat. Remember, these muscles have been stretched, so it might take some time to get back in touch with them!*

- *Lie on your back with pillows to make you comfortable. Feel your lower abdominal muscles again, below your navel and between your hip bones. Try to contract and hold those same muscles in this position. Hold for 10 seconds while breathing, then relax and repeat.*

- *Lying on your back with your knees bent, feet on the floor (keep the pillows if it's more comfortable), contract your abdominal muscles, then slowly lower one knee to the side without moving the other leg at all. As soon as your hips start to roll to the side (at first, you won't be able to go very far), slowly bring your knee back to center, and repeat with the other leg. Breathe as you do this, then rest and repeat, for a total of two sets.*

half-marathon), you have entered a whole new category. You have been through pregnancy. You are now officially tough as nails.

This is a time to reevaluate what you want out of your fitness. If it's more on the aesthetic side, like killer buns or 6-pack abs, I have you covered. I have a suite of workouts that will take you anywhere you want to go with regard to your physique. (Check out jillianmichaels.com/collections/dvds to browse through them.) If you just want to get stronger, keep your energy up, or feel great, I highly recommend a membership to Fit Fusion (fitfusion.com). This is an on-demand fitness platform much like Netflix. For about $10 a month, you get access to all my titles and hundreds of other great workouts from many other great trainers (including our own Andrea Orbeck)—anytime, anywhere.

You can also sign up for classes at your favorite boutique gym. You can join a biking group and start training for the AIDS ride. You can buy a good jogging stroller and hit the sidewalk. The options are limitless, and you are in charge. Where you go from here lies beyond the realm of your fourth trimester. It is the realm of your future.

You made it. And look at you! *Yeah, baby.* You are one hot mama.

CONCLUSION

The Rest of Your Lives Together

If you are reading this page, your passage into motherhood is complete. And if you are considering having more kiddos, then we'll just say your adventures in pregnancy have come to an end . . . for now (wink, wink).

Maybe you are reading this or listening to the audiobook while nursing your tiny peanut for the fifth time today. Maybe you are reading this many months postpartum, as you've been too exhausted to read since junior was born. Regardless of when your eyes do grace this page, here we are.

I'm kinda crying right now. Maybe not kinda . . . I totally am. Don't worry—not creepy heaving sobs or anything. But I am tearing up, for sure.

I honestly have felt, with every word written on every page, like I've been there with you. Cheering you on. Holding your hand. Giving you a pep talk. And being a general pain in the ass, which happens to be my specialty—literally and figuratively.

Let me just say how grateful I am that you've allowed me to be a part of your incredible journey. I can't think of a greater honor.

From one mom to another, let me leave you with this.

We all love our kids, but none of us are perfect parents, because none of us are perfect people. I have found that as long as I am honest with myself, take responsibility for my mistakes, and strive to improve myself, it will be good *enough*. Ultimately, that's what kids do—they make us want to be better people. And that is a noble endeavor, provided we can accept our shortcomings lovingly along the way, without any self-loathing.

And as discussed, there will be those who try to shame you . . . for getting the wrong car seat, giving your kid a bottle instead of the boob, for letting your kid have said bottle past the age of 2. Believe me, the list will be endless. Just know in your heart that that casually flung judgment is coming right from that person's own deep-seated insecurities and overwhelming feelings of confusion and cluelessness—in other words, the feelings that parenthood brings out in all of us.

Try not to hate those people, even when they hate on you. Brush it off and empathize. If that doesn't work, just remember the mantra: *They aren't worth the jail time.*

Speaking of overwhelming feelings, you will have many. Ironically, motherhood can leave many of us feeling lonely and lost at times. Just know that you are never alone. We are all out there in the dark with you, trying to figure out this thing called parenthood. We are all going to have moments of joy, and we are all going to disappoint our kids, just like they will disappoint us. But it doesn't make us love one another any less.

Never be ashamed of any feeling you have. Even when you seriously consider stopping the car and letting your kids out—in the middle of nowhere—as I've heard can happen anytime between toddler and teenager. It's normal to miss your autonomy at times, and it's normal to miss the romance you may have had in your relationship when it was just the two of you. Basically, it's normal to miss a lot of things.

Because, the truth is, kids *do* ruin your life. Or, I should say, *life as you knew it*—but out of that ruin, your new life rises with more richness than your prekid self could ever have imagined possible. In time, you will find some semblance of balance. Date nights will resume, thank God. You will eventually get a girls' night out over a few cocktails. The 60-minute yoga class you loved will still be there when Grandma comes to watch the kids on Saturday afternoon. So, no—your life won't be the same. Ever. But it *will* all balance out, into a new place. A better place. In time.

Maybe you have heard people say, "Parenting is hard!" Maybe you've even said it in the past few days or weeks. And it is—it's so hard. Parenting is the hardest thing I have ever worked at in my whole life. But like all things that aren't easy, parenting bears the richest rewards.

I remember before I was a mom, I was watching the series finale of my all-time favorite show, *Six Feet Under*. The mom, Ruth, was talking to her finally grown 20-something daughter, Claire. Their conversation was so poignant and, in my opinion, sums up motherhood beautifully.

> **RUTH:** Oh, Claire, I pray you'll be filled with hope for as long as you possibly can.
>
> **CLAIRE:** Thank you for everything and thank you for giving me life.
>
> **RUTH:** You gave me life.

And so it goes, friend. Wishing you and yours lots of love on the rest of your journey as a beautiful family, through the good times and the bad. Don't forget, you're not alone. We're all right there with you in this zany experience called motherhood.

Hopefully, we will come together again, and I can accompany you on another one of your journeys toward health and happiness.

With love, respect, and admiration.

Yeah Baby! RECIPES

All the Hot Mom, Healthy Baby recipes are designed to help support the growth of your little one, maximize your health over the duration of the pregnancy, and mitigate any unpleasant symptoms of pregnancy such as headaches, acne, bloating, muscle cramps, fatigue, and so on. In addition, they are all calorie-controlled, so you don't have to spend hours on your smartphone app looking up each ingredient one by one.

All of these recipes are fine at any point during your pregnancy. You can swap any of the meals at any time during any trimester.

Remember, these recipes are designed to make your life easier. It is perfectly fine to deviate from them, provided you follow Chapter 2's Nutrition Rules of Thumb over the duration of your pregnancy.

Also note that every recipe in this appendix serves one, unless otherwise noted. However, if you are making smoothies (or whatever) for two, you can always double the recipes.

Enjoy!

Breakfasts

HOT MAMA SMOOTHIE

APPROXIMATELY 300 CALORIES

½ cup organic almond milk

½ cup organic Greek yogurt

½ cup frozen organic blackberries

½ banana

¼ cup organic granola

1 teaspoon chia seeds

Dash of cinnamon

In a blender, combine the almond milk, yogurt, blackberries, banana, granola, chia seeds, and cinnamon. Blend until smooth.

BABY BOOSTER SMOOTHIE

APPROXIMATELY 300 CALORIES

1 banana

1 cup chopped kale

1 cup chopped spinach

⅓ cup chopped pineapple

¼ cup coconut water

1 tablespoon chia seeds

1 tablespoon coconut oil

¼ cup water

In a blender, combine the banana, kale, spinach, pineapple, coconut water, chia seeds, oil, and water. Blend until smooth.

BREAKFAST BOWL

APPROXIMATELY 350 CALORIES

¼ cup bulgur

1 cup coconut milk

Dash of dried goji berries

Pinch of sea salt

1 tablespoon chopped dried apricots

1 tablespoon chopped or slivered almonds

1 teaspoon raw sugar

In a saucepan, combine the bulgur, coconut milk, goji berries, and salt. Bring to a boil over medium-high heat. Reduce the heat to medium and cook for 12 minutes, or until the bulgur is tender, but not mushy. Pour into a bowl and top with the apricots, almonds, and sugar.

B4 POWER PARFAIT

¾ cup organic Greek yogurt

2 tablespoons pomegranate seeds (or handful of berries of your choosing)

2 tablespoons dried coconut slivers

1 teaspoon crushed walnuts

1 teaspoon hemp seeds

1 tablespoon oats

2 tablespoons dried mulberries

Place the yogurt in a bowl. Mix in the pomegranate seeds, coconut, walnuts, hemp seeds, oats, and mulberries. Dig in.

MAPLE PECAN PORRIDGE

¼ cup quinoa

¼ cup coconut milk

½ cup water

¼ teaspoon vanilla extract

1 teaspoon organic grade B maple syrup

½ cup pitted cherries

2 tablespoons chopped pecans

Cook the quinoa with the coconut milk and water according to package directions. Place in a bowl and stir in the vanilla and maple syrup. Top with the cherries and pecans.

Homemade Super Food Mix

I highly recommend making a Super Food Mix and just sprinkling from the container you keep it in. In our house, we mix all the ingredients in the B4 Power Parfait (except the Greek yogurt and pomegranate seeds) in a resealable plastic bag, store it in the fridge, and then sprinkle a bit over yogurt for breakfast. This always makes it quick and easy. You can also multiply the amounts to have enough for lots of smoothies.

APPLE ZUCCHINI FLAP JACKS WITH TURKEY BACON

APPROXIMATELY 350 CALORIES
Makes 3 flap jacks and 2 slices of bacon

½ cup spelt flour

2 teaspoons baking powder

   Pinch of sea salt

   Pinch of ground cinnamon

1 egg white

⅓ cup coconut milk

1 tablespoon apple juice

1 teaspoon olive oil

⅓ cup grated apple (your favorite variety)

½ cup grated zucchini

3 tablespoons ricotta cheese

   Small pat of butter

2 slices Applegate Farms organic turkey bacon

In a medium bowl, mix the flour, baking powder, salt, and cinnamon. Add the egg white, coconut milk, apple juice, and oil and mix until combined. Fold the apple, zucchini, and cheese into the mixture.

In a skillet over medium heat, melt the butter. For each pancake, scoop about 3 tablespoons of batter onto the skillet. Cook for 4 minutes, turning once, or until lightly browned.

Meanwhile, place the bacon on a microwaveable plate and microwave on high power for 4 minutes, turning once.

Serve warm flap jacks with the bacon.

THE CALIFORNIA POACH

APPROXIMATELY 400 CALORIES

1 egg

1 slice multigrain bread (I love Dave's Killer Bread these days. Just a suggestion.)

½ small avocado, sliced

   Ground black pepper

½ grapefruit, sliced

Poach the egg. Toast the bread. Mash the egg and place it on the toast. Lay the avocado slices on the top. Season with pepper to taste. Serve the grapefruit on the side.

FETA FRITTATA

2 eggs

1 teaspoon olive oil

¼ cup chopped cherry tomatoes

1 teaspoon chopped leek

   Pinch of sea salt

Pinch of ground black pepper

3 tablespoons crumbled pasteurized feta cheese

1 cup cubed cantaloupe

In a small bowl, whisk the eggs. Grease a skillet with the oil and heat over medium heat. Cook the tomatoes and leek for 2 minutes, or until softened. Reduce the heat to low and add the eggs, salt, and pepper. Cover and cook for 3 minutes, or until the eggs are firm. Top with the feta and serve with the cantaloupe on the side.

HUEVOS TACOS

¼ avocado, chopped

½ small tomato, chopped

1 teaspoon chopped cilantro

1 egg

2 egg whites

1 teaspoon water

1 teaspoon Earth Balance coconut spread or unsalted butter

½ bell pepper (any color), chopped

¼ cup chopped red onion

   Pinch of salt

2 tablespoons shredded Jack or Cheddar cheese

2 corn tortillas (6" diameter)

In a small bowl, combine the avocado, tomato, and cilantro. Set aside. In another small bowl, whisk the egg and egg whites with the water.

In a skillet over medium heat, melt the coconut spread or butter. Cook the pepper, onion, and salt for 3 minutes, or until softened. Add the eggs and cook, stirring, for 2 minutes. Add the cheese and stir until the cheese is melted and the eggs are fully cooked.

Warm the tortillas according to package directions. Divide the scrambled eggs between the tortillas and top with the reserved avocado mixture. Bon appétit.

BAD A$$ BREAKFAST BURRITO

APPROXIMATELY 425 CALORIES

⅓ yam or sweet potato, cut into pieces

1 teaspoon extra-virgin olive oil

¼ yellow onion, chopped

⅓ cup chopped asparagus spears

1 egg

1 egg white

Pinch of salt

Pinch of ground black pepper

1 whole wheat tortilla (12" diameter)

1 tablespoon grated Gruyère cheese

1 tablespoon shredded pepper Jack cheese

⅓ cup arugula

On a microwaveable plate, microwave the sweet potato on high power for 4 minutes, or until soft.

Meanwhile, in a skillet over high heat, heat the oil. Cook the onion, stirring frequently, for 4 minutes, or until softened. Add the asparagus and cook, stirring frequently, for 2 minutes. Add the egg, egg white, salt, and pepper. Reduce the heat to medium low and cook, stirring, until the eggs are light and fluffy. Place the tortilla on a plate and spread the egg and veggie mixture down the middle. Top with the cheeses, arugula, and cooked yam or sweet potato. Fold over one side and roll into a burrito shape.

LORI AND JAMIE'S FEEL-GOOD MUFFIN

APPROXIMATELY 400 CALORIES PER SERVING
Makes 2 servings

½ cup ground flax mixed with goji berries (you can buy this premixed)

½ banana, mashed

8 tablets of sun chlorella, crushed (available at any health food store, at vitamin shops, or online)

1 egg

1 tablespoon cacao nibs

1 tablespoon almond butter

2 teaspoons ground cinnamon

½ tablespoon pasteurized (not raw) honey (you can add more if you need more sweetness)

1 teaspoon molasses

1 teaspoon coconut oil

1 teaspoon baking powder

1 teaspoon vanilla extract

In a large mug, combine the flax, banana, sun chlorella, egg, cacao nibs, almond butter, cinnamon, honey, molasses, coconut oil, baking powder, and vanilla. Eyeballing it, make sure the mixture is thick like a paste. If it isn't, add more of the flax/goji berry mixture. Microwave for 1 minute, 45 seconds to 2 minutes. Cool for 5 minutes. Remove from the mug and cut in half to make 2 muffins. Top with Earth Balance, butter, more honey, or jam or just eat plain.

Lunches

MEDITERRANEAN CHICKEN SANDWICH

APPROXIMATELY 400 CALORIES

2 slices multigrain bread

1 tablespoon pasteurized goat cheese

1 tablespoon red pepper hummus

1 small grilled chicken breast

Handful of fresh sprouts

1 tablespoon mashed avocado

Toast the bread slices. Spread the goat cheese across 1 slice, then top with the hummus. Add the chicken breast and sprouts. Spread the avocado on the other slice of toast. Place on top of the sandwich and voilà—lunch!

BBQ STEAK SALAD

APPROXIMATELY 400 CALORIES PER SERVING
Makes 2 servings

½ pound grass-fed skirt steak

½ red onion, sliced

1 teaspoon organic barbecue sauce (Amy's is a good brand)

1 teaspoon + 1 tablespoon olive oil

1 teaspoon balsamic vinegar

½ teaspoon Dijon mustard

1 small clove garlic, minced

Pinch of sea salt

Pinch of ground black pepper

3 cups organic baby greens

½ cup halved cherry tomatoes

¼ cup crumbled Parmesan cheese

Heat a large skillet over medium-high heat. In a bowl, coat the steak and onion with the barbecue sauce and 1 teaspoon of the oil. Cook the steak and onion for 6 minutes, turning once, or until a thermometer inserted in the center registers 160°F for medium. Remove the steak and let it rest for a few minutes.

In a small bowl, combine the vinegar, mustard, garlic, salt, pepper, and remaining 1 tablespoon oil. Whisk until thoroughly combined. In a large bowl, combine the greens, tomatoes, and onion. Toss with the dressing. Slice the steak and add it on top of the salad or toss it in. Sprinkle the cheese on top and enjoy.

SLAMMIN' TURKEY SAMMY

APPROXIMATELY 400 CALORIES

2 slices multigrain bread (Dave's Killer Bread or Ezekiel are good)

1 teaspoon Dijon mustard

1 tablespoon fresh fig jam

1 slice aged Cheddar cheese

1 thick slice (2 ounces) turkey breast (not processed deli meat)

Handful of organic baby greens

Toast the bread. Spread the mustard on 1 slice, then spread the fig jam on the other. Place the cheese, turkey, and greens on top of the mustard. Top with the second slice of toast and enjoy.

QUICK AND EASY FISH TACOS

APPROXIMATELY 375 CALORIES

Note: You can make this recipe with wild-caught salmon, rainbow trout, or tilapia.

1 fish fillet (4 ounces)

1 teaspoon olive oil

⅓ cup chopped purple cabbage

1 tablespoon chopped cilantro

¼ cup chopped papaya

¼ cup chopped mango

1 small clove garlic, minced

2 tablespoons fresh lime juice

2 corn tortillas (6" diameter)

Preheat the oven to 350°F. Rub the fish with the oil and place on a baking sheet. Bake for 14 minutes, turning once, or until the fish flakes easily.

Meanwhile, in a medium bowl, combine the cabbage, cilantro, papaya, mango, and garlic. Add the lime juice and toss.

Warm the tortillas according to package directions. Divide the fish between the tortillas. Top with the cabbage mixture and eat up.

CHICKEN CHOP

APPROXIMATELY 400 CALORIES

2 cups fresh spinach

½ apple, chopped

1 tablespoon crushed walnuts

1 tablespoon shredded Cheddar cheese

1 tablespoon balsamic vinegar

1 tablespoon walnut oil

1 small grilled chicken breast, cubed

1 hard-cooked egg, chopped

In a medium bowl, toss together the spinach, apple, walnuts, and cheese. In a small bowl, whisk the vinegar and oil until thoroughly combined. Drizzle over the salad. Toss once more and serve topped with the chicken and egg.

SLAW SALAD

APPROXIMATELY 375 CALORIES

8 ounces or half a can low-sodium chickpeas (from BPA-free can)

¾ cup sliced green cabbage

¾ cup sliced purple cabbage

1 cup shredded carrots

1 rib celery, sliced

2 tablespoons organic low-fat plain yogurt

1 tablespoon water

1½ teaspoons apple cider vinegar

Pinch of salt

Pinch of ground black pepper

½ teaspoon ground turmeric

2 teaspoons toasted sesame seeds

In a medium bowl, combine the chickpeas, cabbages, carrots, and celery. Toss well. In a small bowl, combine the yogurt, water, vinegar, salt, pepper, and turmeric. Whisk until combined. Pour the dressing over the salad and toss again. Sprinkle the sesame seeds on top. For the best flavor, refrigerate for an hour before serving.

SUMMER SHRIMP SALAD

APPROXIMATELY 300 CALORIES

6 shrimp, thawed, washed, peeled, and deveined

2 cups cubed watermelon

½ cup peeled and chopped jicama

1 small jalapeño chile pepper, sliced (optional)

1 teaspoon chopped chives

1 chopped scallion

1 tablespoon chopped cilantro

1 tablespoon lime juice

1 teaspoon lemon juice

1 tablespoon olive oil

Pinch of salt

Pinch of ground black pepper

2 tablespoons crumbled pasteurized feta cheese

Lightly grease a skillet with olive oil and place over high heat. Cook the shrimp for 4 to 5 minutes, stirring occasionally, or until opaque. Transfer to a plate. Cut the shrimp into bite-size pieces.

In a medium bowl, combine the shrimp, watermelon, jicama, chile pepper (if using), chives, scallion, and cilantro. Toss well. In a small bowl, whisk the lime juice, lemon juice, oil, salt, and black pepper until thoroughly combined. Pour the dressing over the shrimp salad. Toss again. Sprinkle the cheese over the top.

CHICKEN ARTICHOKE PIZZA

APPROXIMATELY 300 CALORIES PER SLICE
Makes 6 servings

1 organic whole wheat pizza crust (or dough to make 1 crust)

½ cup pesto sauce

¾ cup chopped grilled chicken breast

1 jar (6 ounces) marinated artichoke hearts, drained

¾ cup sun-dried tomatoes

2 tablespoons chopped red onion

½ cup shredded organic low-fat pasteurized mozzarella cheese

Preheat the oven to 425°F. Lightly coat a baking sheet with olive oil. If using the dough, place it on a floured work surface and roll it out into a circle roughly ¼" thick. Transfer the dough or crust to the baking sheet. Spread the pesto evenly over the top. Arrange the chicken, artichokes, tomatoes, onion, and cheese on top. Bake for 14 minutes, or until the crust is golden brown and the cheese is melted.

CHICKEN BURRITO BOWL

APPROXIMATELY 350 CALORIES

½ cup brown rice

¼ cup cooked black beans

¼ cup cooked corn

1 teaspoon olive oil

½ chicken breast, cut into bite-size pieces

¼ cup chopped red and green bell peppers

1 tablespoon chopped red onion

¼ teaspoon minced garlic

¼ avocado, chopped

1 tablespoon chopped cilantro

½ Roma tomato, chopped

1 tablespoon fresh lime juice

1 tablespoon organic low-fat plain Greek yogurt

Cook the rice according to package directions. Transfer the cooked rice to a bowl and add the black beans and corn. Stir and set aside.

In a skillet over medium-high heat, heat the oil. Place the chicken, peppers, onion, and garlic in the skillet. Reduce the heat to low. Cover the skillet and cook for 10 minutes, or until the chicken is no longer pink and the juices run clear. Place the chicken mixture over the rice mixture. Add the avocado, cilantro, and tomato.

In a small bowl, combine the lime juice and yogurt. Drizzle over the burrito bowl.

CHICKEN PARMESAN ORZO SALAD

APPROXIMATELY 600 CALORIES

⅔ cup orzo

1 tablespoon olive oil

1 half chicken breast, chopped

¼ teaspoon red-pepper flakes (omit if you have heartburn)

1 half clove garlic, minced

4 kalamata olives, pitted and chopped

1 rib celery, chopped

1 tablespoon water

¼ cup chopped parsley

¼ cup grated Parmesan cheese

½ tablespoon pine nuts

Cook the orzo according to package directions. Strain and set aside.

In a large skillet over medium heat, heat the oil. Cook the chicken, pepper flakes (if using), and garlic for 5 minutes. Add the olives, celery, water, and reserved orzo to the skillet. Cook for 3 minutes, or until the water evaporates and the chicken is no longer pink. Transfer to a bowl. Add the parsley, cheese, and pine nuts and toss.

Snacks

THE PBB

APPROXIMATELY 200 CALORIES

1 slice multigrain bread (Dave's Killer Bread or Ezekiel)

1 teaspoon organic peanut butter

⅓ banana

Toast the bread. Smear the peanut butter over the toast. Slice the banana and arrange on top of the peanut butter.

CHOCOLATE CHERRY SMOOTHIE

APPROXIMATELY 225 CALORIES

4 ice cubes

¾ cup almond milk

¾ cup pitted cherries

¼ cup pasteurized ricotta cheese

2 tablespoons apple juice

1 teaspoon unsweetened cocoa powder

In a blender, combine the ice cubes, almond milk, cherries, cheese, apple juice, and cocoa. Blend until smooth and enjoy.

FRUITY GAZPACHO

APPROXIMATELY 160 CALORIES PER SERVING
Makes 3 servings

10 pitted apricots

2 cloves garlic, minced

2 scallions, chopped

½ cucumber, chopped

¾ cup water

1 jalapeño chile pepper, finely chopped

3 tablespoons chopped fresh mint

2 tablespoons olive oil

2 tablespoons apple cider vinegar

1 tablespoon chopped fresh basil

Pinch of ground black pepper

Pinch of sea salt

In a blender, combine the apricots, garlic, scallions, cucumber, water, chile pepper, mint, oil, vinegar, basil, black pepper, and salt. Blend until smooth (or pulse a few times and leave it chunky if you like it better that way). Chill in the refrigerator for at least 2 hours, or overnight.

VEGGIES AND DIP

APPROXIMATELY 200 CALORIES

2 carrots

½ cucumber

½ red bell pepper

1 clove garlic

2 tablespoons fresh lemon juice

2 teaspoons olive oil

½ cup organic low-fat plain Greek yogurt

2 teaspoons white wine vinegar

Wash the carrots, cucumber, and pepper and cut into dipping sticks. In a blender or food processor, combine the garlic, lemon juice, oil, yogurt, and vinegar. Blend or process until smooth. Transfer to a bowl and enjoy with the veggie sticks.

SUPER MOMMY MIX

APPROXIMATELY 250 CALORIES PER SERVING
Makes 2 servings

12 pecan halves

12 walnut halves

2 crushed Brazil nuts

1 tablespoon pumpkin seeds

1 tablespoon sunflower seeds

¼ cup dried golden berries

¼ cup black mulberries

In a bowl, combine the pecans, walnuts, Brazil nuts, pumpkin seeds, sunflower seeds, golden berries, and mulberries.

You can find all these ingredients at thrivemarket.com. However, if making this mix on a busy day is too much of a hassle to handle yourself, there are plenty of super food trail mixes out there that are delicious. Thrive Market has plenty of brands available for you to check out.

COTTAGE CHEESE AND PEACHES

APPROXIMATELY 160 CALORIES

1 small peach, chopped (you can also use an apple or strawberries instead)

½ cup organic low-fat pasteurized cottage cheese

½ teaspoon ground cinnamon

In a bowl, mix together the peach, cottage cheese, and cinnamon. Enjoy!

CHEESE PLATE

APPROXIMATELY 250 CALORIES

10 whole grain crackers (I love Mary's Gone Crackers Super Seed)

2 slices Cheddar cheese

2 slices Gouda cheese

½ apple, sliced

1 sprig of grapes

10 Marcona almonds

On a plate, arrange the crackers, cheeses, apple, grapes, and almonds. Serve.

BANGIN' BRUSCHETTA

APPROXIMATELY 225 CALORIES

2 slices whole grain baguette

2 Roma tomatoes, chopped

2 cloves garlic, minced

1 tablespoon chopped chives

2 teaspoons olive oil

1 tablespoon red wine vinegar

Toast the baguette slices. In a small bowl, combine the tomatoes, garlic, chives, oil, and vinegar. Drain off excess fluid and assemble the bruschetta on the toast slices.

DEVILISH DEVILED EGGS WITH WATERMELON

APPROXIMATELY 200 CALORIES

2 eggs

1 teaspoon Dijon mustard

1 tablespoon organic low-fat plain Greek yogurt

Pinch of paprika

½ cup chopped watermelon

This is an odd combination at the initial sound of it, but you don't eat them together in the same bite. You make the eggs as I will instruct you and have a side of watermelon to provide some additional nutrients and keep your blood sugar up.

Place the eggs in a small saucepan and cover with water. Place over high heat and bring to a simmer. Reduce the heat to low and simmer for 12 minutes. Plunge the eggs into a bowl of ice water and let them cool until you can handle them.

Roll the eggs on the counter to loosen the shells and peel them. Slice each in half. Remove the yolks and place in a small bowl. Add the mustard and yogurt and mash together until creamy. Spoon the yolk mixture into the egg whites. Sprinkle with the paprika. Serve with the watermelon on the side. Devour.

BEAT-THE-BLOAT BAKED POTATO

APPROXIMATELY 150 CALORIES

1 sweet potato

1 small piece ginger, peeled and grated

1 scallion, chopped

½ clove garlic, minced

1 teaspoon coconut oil

⅓ teaspoon sesame seeds

Wash the sweet potato and pierce with a fork about 6 times. Place on a microwaveable plate and microwave on high power for 6 to 7 minutes, or until cooked through. Meanwhile, in a small bowl, combine the ginger, scallion, garlic, oil, and sesame seeds. Slice the cooked sweet potato down the middle. Garnish with the ginger mixture.

RED ANTS ON A LOG

APPROXIMATELY 150 CALORIES

2 celery ribs, trimmed

4 teaspoons almond butter

1 tablespoon dried cranberries

Wash the celery and cut each rib in half. Spread a teaspoon of almond butter on each celery stick. Sprinkle each with the dried cranberries and enjoy.

AWESOME ARTICHOKE

APPROXIMATELY 125 CALORIES

1 artichoke

1 tablespoon organic low-fat plain Greek yogurt

½ teaspoon Dijon mustard

¼ teaspoon olive oil

½ clove garlic, minced

Pinch of ground black pepper

Cut the tips off the artichoke. Rinse the artichoke and steam for 30 minutes, or until the outer leaves fall off.

Meanwhile, in a small bowl, combine the yogurt, mustard, oil, garlic, and pepper. Dip the artichoke leaves and heart into the sauce and enjoy.

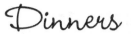

Dinners

ARGENTINE SALMON

APPROXIMATELY 400 CALORIES PER SERVING
Makes 2 servings

- 1 tablespoon organic full-fat plain Greek yogurt
- 1 tablespoon water
- ½ teaspoon Dijon mustard
- Leaves from 2 sprigs fresh oregano
- Pinch of sea salt
- 2 cloves garlic, divided
- 4 tablespoons chopped parsley, divided
- 2 tablespoons apple cider vinegar
- ¼ teaspoon ground black pepper
- 2 teaspoons olive oil, divided
- ½ cup frozen organic corn kernels, thawed
- 1 Roma tomato, chopped
- ½ cup BPA-free canned unsalted chickpeas
- ¼ cup chopped poblano chile peppers
- 2 wild salmon fillets (6 ounces each)
- 1 slice lemon

In a blender, combine the yogurt, water, mustard, oregano, salt, 1 clove garlic, and 2 tablespoons of the parsley. Blend until smooth and set aside.

Mince the remaining clove of garlic. In a medium bowl, combine the garlic, vinegar, black pepper, 1 teaspoon of the oil, the corn, tomato, chickpeas, chile peppers, and the remaining 2 tablespoons parsley. Toss to thoroughly combine. Set aside.

In a medium skillet over medium-low heat, heat the remaining 1 teaspoon oil. Place the salmon skin side up in the pan. Cook for 7 minutes, turning once, or until the fish is opaque.

Divide the veggies between 2 plates and lay a salmon fillet on top of each. Squeeze the lemon slice over the plates. Enjoy with the reserved sauce.

BAKED TROUT

APPROXIMATELY 375 CALORIES

½ butternut squash, halved lengthwise and seeded

1 Roma tomato, chopped

3 tablespoons finely chopped sweet onion

1 tablespoon chopped cilantro

½ jalapeño chile pepper, finely chopped (if you have heartburn, feel free to skip this)

1½ teaspoons lime juice

2 teaspoons coconut oil

1 rainbow trout fillet (5 ounces)

½ teaspoon olive oil

Preheat the oven to 450°F. Line a large baking sheet with foil. Place the squash half on the baking sheet. In a small bowl, combine the tomato, onion, cilantro, pepper (if using), lime juice, and coconut oil. Stir to mix. Fill the squash with the tomato salsa mixture. Save 1 tablespoon of the salsa for garnish. Bake for 45 minutes, or until almost tender.

Remove the baking sheet from the oven. Remove the squash and set aside. Place the trout fillet onto the baking sheet, and brush with the olive oil. Bake for 15 minutes, or until the fish flakes easily. Serve the fish on top of the squash, garnished with the reserved salsa.

MUSSELS MARINARA

APPROXIMATELY 550 CALORIES PER SERVING
Makes 2 servings

1½ teaspoons olive oil

2 cloves garlic, thinly sliced

10 cherry tomatoes, halved

¼ teaspoon red-pepper flakes (feel free to skip this if you have heartburn)

1 teaspoon chopped fresh oregano

1 teaspoon sugar

Pinch of sea salt

¼ pound cleaned mussels

3 ounces spinach linguine (Garden Time is a great brand)

¼ cup chopped fresh flat-leaf parsley

In a pot over medium heat, heat the oil. Cook the garlic for 1 minute. Add the tomatoes, pepper flakes (if using), oregano, sugar, and salt. Reduce the heat to medium low and simmer for 18 minutes, or until the sauce has thickened. Add the mussels, cover, and cook for 5 minutes, or until they open.

Meanwhile, prepare the pasta according to package directions. Drain. Add the pasta and parsley to the sauce and stir to combine.

THAI STEAK

½ teaspoon brown sugar

2 tablespoons ponzu sauce, divided

1 teaspoon wasabi

1 teaspoon coconut oil

¼ pound grass-fed flank steak

⅓ cup organic brown rice

1 piece ginger (1"), peeled and thinly sliced

1 teaspoon sesame seeds

4 scallions, chopped

1 half cucumber, chopped

⅓ cup shredded carrots

1 teaspoon rice vinegar

In a bowl, combine the sugar, 1 tablespoon of the ponzu, the wasabi, and coconut oil. Slice the steak and pierce the slices with a fork. Transfer the steak to the bowl and marinate for 8 minutes.

Meanwhile, cook the rice according to package directions, cooking the ginger along with the rice. Add the sesame seeds to the cooked rice and stir to combine. Set aside.

Lightly grease a skillet with coconut oil and place over medium-high heat. Cook the steak for 4 minutes, turning once, or until a thermometer inserted in the center of a slice registers 160°F for medium. While the steak is cooking, place the scallions in the steak marinade. When the steak is cooked, transfer it to a plate and cook the scallions for 3 minutes, stirring occasionally, or until tender.

In a medium bowl, toss the cucumber and carrots with the vinegar and the remaining 1 tablespoon ponzu. Place the reserved rice on a plate. Top with the cucumber carrot salad. Then top with the steak and scallions.

LEMON LAMB CHOPS

APPROXIMATELY 400 CALORIES PER SERVING
Makes 3 servings

2 tablespoons lemon juice

1 teaspoon olive oil + additional for grilling

½ teaspoon Dijon mustard

½ teaspoon dried oregano

1 small clove garlic, minced

Pinch of sea salt

Pinch of ground black pepper

3 lamb chops

6 cherry tomatoes

6 mushroom caps

½ green bell pepper, cut into squares

½ red bell pepper, cut into squares

¼ red onion, cut into wedges

½ teaspoon dried thyme

Preheat the grill.

In a shallow dish, combine the lemon juice, oil, mustard, oregano, garlic, salt, and black pepper. Poke the lamb chops with a fork and place in the dish. Marinate for at least 8 minutes.

Thread the tomatoes, mushrooms, bell peppers, and onion on 3 skewers. Lightly coat the vegetables with olive oil and sprinkle with salt and black pepper to taste. Grill for 10 minutes, or until the veggies are tender. Transfer to a plate.

Grill the lamb chops for 4 minutes, turning once, or until browned and a thermometer inserted in the center registers 145°F for medium-rare. Sprinkle the thyme on top of the lamb chops. Serve with the veggie kebabs.

VEGGIE PIE

¾ pound sweet potatoes, peeled and cut into chunks

2 teaspoons olive oil

1 large shallot, finely chopped

Pinch of sea salt

Pinch of ground black pepper

¼ teaspoon ground allspice

½ clove garlic, minced

1 tablespoon + 1 teaspoon spelt flour

1 tablespoon Chardonnay, white grape juice, or vegetable broth

¾ cup low-sodium vegetable broth

8 stalks Tuscan kale, stems removed and leaves chopped

6 stalks Swiss chard, stems removed and leaves chopped

½ teaspoon tomato paste

2 ounces mushrooms, chopped

1 cup cooked white beans, drained

1 tablespoon unsalted butter

1 tablespoon organic whole milk

1 large egg

Preheat the oven to 425°F. Place the sweet potatoes in a saucepan and add water to cover the potatoes by 1". Place over high heat and bring to a boil. Reduce the heat to medium low and simmer for 20 minutes, or until tender.

Meanwhile, in a large pot over medium heat, heat the oil. Cook the shallot, salt, pepper, and allspice for 5 minutes, stirring frequently, or until tender. Add the garlic and cook for 1 minute. Add the flour and wine, juice, or 1 tablespoon broth and stir to combine. Add the broth, stir, and bring to a simmer. Add the kale, chard, and tomato paste, cover, and cook for 10 minutes, or until the greens are tender. Stir in the mushrooms and cook, covered, for 6 minutes, or until the mushrooms are almost tender. Add the beans and return the mixture to a simmer. Cook until the consistency of a thick gravy.

Drain the sweet potatoes. Mash with the butter, milk, and egg. Transfer the vegetable mixture to a 6" x 6" pan, patting it into an even layer. Carefully spread the potato mixture on top, covering the vegetable mixture evenly. Bake for 25 minutes, or until the sweet potato crust has turned golden brown in spots and the pie is bubbling.

STEAK CHIMICHURRI

4 ounces grass-fed flank steak

¼ teaspoon ground cumin

¼ teaspoon ground black pepper

½ teaspoon butter

Pinch of sea salt

¼ cup cilantro, chopped

2 tablespoons parsley, chopped

2 teaspoons apple cider vinegar

2½ tablespoons olive oil, divided

1 clove garlic, minced

¼ teaspoon red-pepper flakes (omit if you have heartburn)

½ cup cooked black beans

2 cups arugula

1 tablespoon fresh lemon juice

Rub the steak with the cumin and black pepper. In a skillet over high heat, melt the butter. Cook the steak for 6 minutes, turning once. Reduce the heat to low and cook the steak for 8 minutes, or until a thermometer inserted in the center registers 160°F for medium. Season with salt and set aside on a plate, covered to keep it warm.

Meanwhile, in a blender, combine the cilantro, parsley, vinegar, 2 tablespoons of the oil, the garlic, and pepper flakes (if using). Blend into a paste.

In a small saucepan over low heat, heat the black beans.

Transfer the steak to a plate and top with the chimichurri sauce. Spoon the beans along the side. On a salad plate, arrange the arugula. In a small bowl, whisk the lemon juice with the remaining ½ tablespoon oil. Drizzle over the arugula and serve everything at once.

PEACH PORK CHOPS WITH FENNEL SALAD

APPROXIMATELY 450 CALORIES PER SERVING
Makes 2 servings

¼ cup apple cider vinegar

1½ tablespoons olive oil, divided

2 tablespoons organic grade B maple syrup

1½ teaspoons whole grain mustard

1 large peach

2 boneless center-cut pork chops

1 large fennel bulb, chopped

½ red onion, chopped

¼ cup chopped fresh mint

2 tablespoons lemon juice

In a small bowl, combine the vinegar, 1 tablespoon of the oil, the maple syrup, and mustard. Chop the peach into cubes. In a skillet over medium heat, cook the vinegar mixture and pork chops for 5 minutes. Add the peach, turn the chops, and cook for 5 minutes, or until a thermometer inserted in the center of a chop registers 160°F and the juices run clear.

Meanwhile, in another skillet over medium heat, heat the remaining ½ tablespoon oil. Cook the fennel and onion for 5 minutes, or until tender. Transfer to a bowl and toss with the mint and lemon juice. Plate the pork chops and peach alongside the veggies.

THE ULTIMATE TURKEY BURGER

APPROXIMATELY 500 CALORIES

1 tablespoon chopped fresh basil

1 tablespoon chopped fresh chives

¼ teaspoon mashed anchovy (optional)

¼ teaspoon garlic paste

Pinch of ground black pepper

¼ pound organic ground turkey

½ teaspoon olive oil

1 whole grain hamburger bun

1 teaspoon Dijon mustard

2 large leaves butter lettuce

¼ avocado, sliced

1 slice beefsteak tomato

In a bowl, combine the basil, chives, anchovy (if using), garlic paste, and pepper. Add the turkey and gently mix to combine.

In a skillet over medium-high heat, heat the oil. Cook the burger for 6 minutes, turning once, or until a thermometer inserted in the center registers 165°F and the meat is no longer pink.

Meanwhile, toast the bun. Spread the mustard on the bun bottom. Place the lettuce, avocado, and tomato on top of the mustard. Add the burger and bun top and enjoy!

VEGGIE PASTA

1 cup organic quinoa penne (Ancient Harvest is a good brand. You can find it at thrivemarket.com.)

2 tablespoons olive oil, divided

1 half clove garlic, minced

½ yellow bell pepper, sliced

⅓ cup trimmed and chopped sugar snap peas

⅓ cup spinach leaves

⅓ cup cherry tomatoes

1 tablespoon grated Parmesan cheese

¼ cup pasteurized ricotta cheese

1 tablespoon chopped fresh basil

Pinch of ground black pepper

Prepare the pasta according to package directions.

Meanwhile, in a skillet over medium-high heat, heat 1 tablespoon of the oil. Cook the garlic, bell pepper, and sugar snap peas for 2 minutes, or until tender-crisp. Add the spinach and tomatoes and cook for 2 minutes.

Add the cooked pasta, Parmesan, and the remaining 1 tablespoon oil to the vegetables. Reduce the heat to medium-low and stir for 1 minute, or until combined and heated through. Transfer to a bowl. Top with the ricotta, basil, and black pepper and enjoy!

Special Fourth Trimester Smoothie Recipes

MILK MAX SMOOTHIE

APPROXIMATELY 400 CALORIES

½ cup coconut water

½ cup almond milk

1 tablespoon coconut oil

½ cup chopped kale

½ cup chopped fresh pineapple

½ banana

½ apple (remove core and seeds)

¼ cup rolled oats

2 tablespoons ground flaxseed

1 teaspoon brewer's yeast (you can find this in health food stores)

In a blender, combine the coconut water, almond milk, oil, kale, pineapple, banana, apple, oats, flaxseed, and yeast. Blend until smooth and enjoy immediately.

SUPER BABY SMOOTHIE

APPROXIMATELY 350 CALORIES

1 cup hemp milk

½ cup organic low-fat Greek yogurt

1 teaspoon chia seeds

1 teaspoon blackstrap molasses

1 teaspoon ground cinnamon

1 tablespoon vanilla whey protein powder

1 pear (remove core and seeds)

1 banana

In a blender, combine the hemp milk, yogurt, chia seeds, molasses, cinnamon, protein powder, pear, and banana. Blend until smooth and enjoy immediately.

HAPPY DAY SMOOTHIE

APPROXIMATELY 300 CALORIES

1 cup organic low-fat milk

½ cup organic low-fat vanilla yogurt

1 cup spinach

½ cup raspberries

½ cup blueberries

½ banana

1 teaspoon Barlean's brand orange-flavored fish oil

1 teaspoon hemp seeds

In a blender, combine the milk, yogurt, spinach, raspberries, blueberries, banana, fish oil, and hemp seeds. Blend until smooth. Then enjoy.

RECOVERY SMOOTHIE

APPROXIMATELY 350 CALORIES

½ cup coconut water

½ cup coconut milk

½ cup kefir

⅓ cup chopped mango

1 peeled kiwifruit

¼ cup chopped papaya

⅓ avocado

½ cup chopped kale

1 teaspoon honey

In a blender, combine the coconut water, coconut milk, kefir, mango, kiwi, papaya, avocado, kale, and honey. Blend until smooth and enjoy.

ENERGIZER SMOOTHIE

APPROXIMATELY 150 CALORIES

½ cup coconut water

1 cup cubed watermelon

⅓ cup frozen blackberries

⅓ cup frozen blueberries

1 cup spinach

1 teaspoon chia seeds

1 cup ice

In a blender, combine the coconut water, watermelon, blackberries, blueberries, spinach, chia seeds, and ice. Blend until smooth and enjoy immediately.

Yeah Baby! EXERCISES

Two Important Notes:

1. When an exercise has "Alternating" in the title, the reps listed are total reps for both sides inclusive.

2. When an exercise is pictured with weights, they are optional. If you use them, go light—between 2 and 8 pounds—depending on your strength and comfort level.

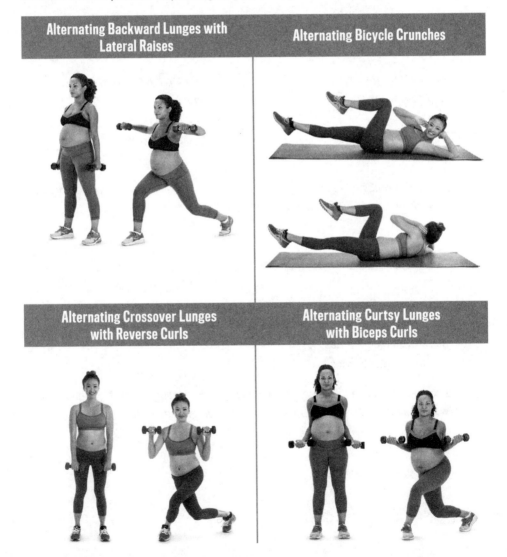

Alternating Backward Lunges with Lateral Raises

Alternating Bicycle Crunches

Alternating Crossover Lunges with Reverse Curls

Alternating Curtsy Lunges with Biceps Curls

Alternating Forward Lunges with Hammer Curls

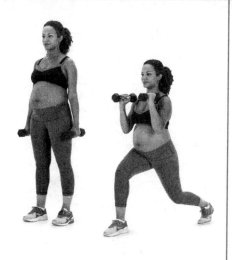

Alternating Hamstring Curls in Ab Hold

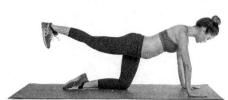

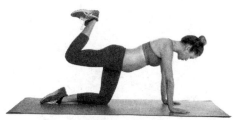

Alternating Heel Drops

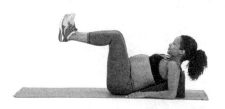

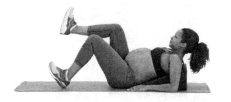

Alternating Knee Switches

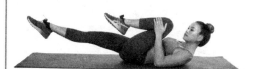

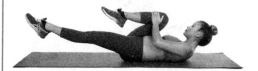

Alternating Low Rows in Table

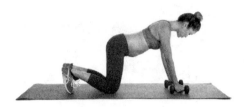

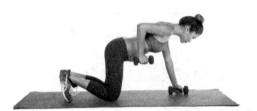

Alternating Renegade Rows

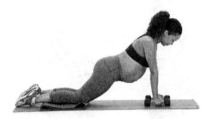

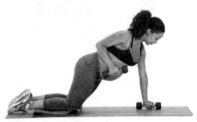

Alternating Reverse Flys in Plank

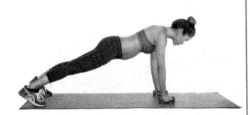

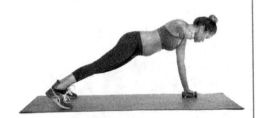

Alternating Reverse Flys in Table

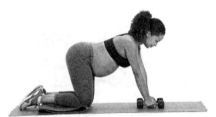

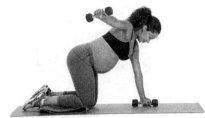

Alternating Side Lunges with Anterior Raises

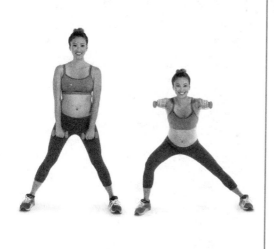

Alternating Side Lunge with Serving Biceps

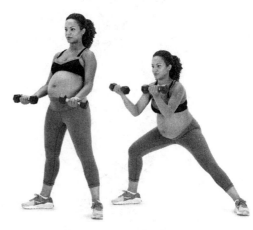

Alternating Standing Toe Tap Crunches

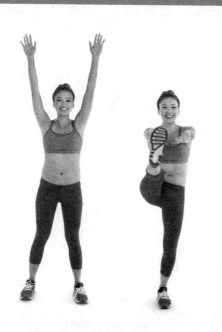

Alternating Stepups

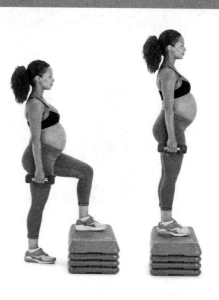

Alternating Sumo Touch Downs

Alternating Surrender Lunges with Shoulder Presses

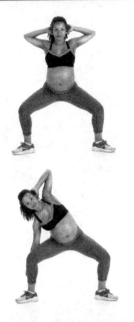

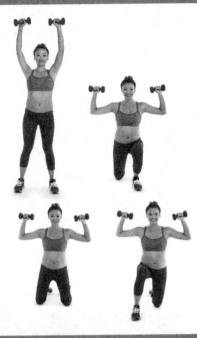

Arm Biceps Stretch

Bear Crawls

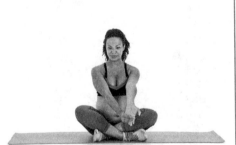

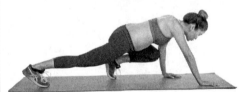

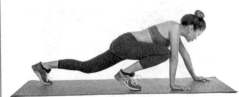

Bent Leg Donkey Kicks

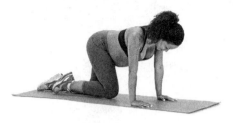

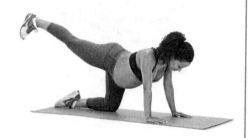

Biceps Curls

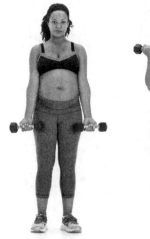
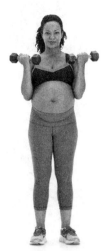

Boat Extensions with Forearms on Ground

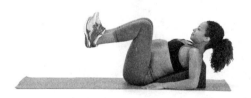

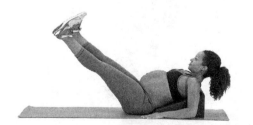

Braced Single Arm Medium Grip Rows

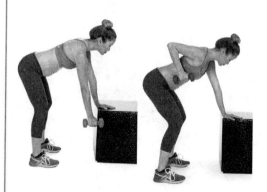

Bridges

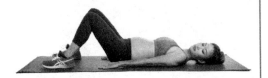

Butterfly Stretch

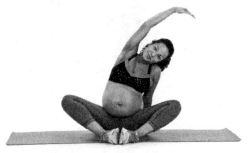

Calf Stretch

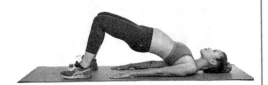

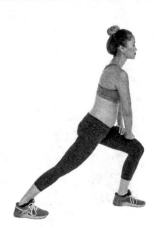

Camel Sitdowns

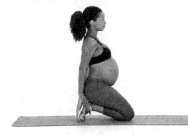

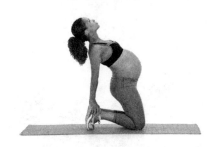

Cat Cow Stretch

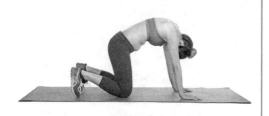

Center Splits Oblique Stretch

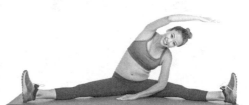

Chair Squats with Anterior Raises

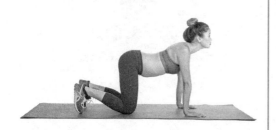

Chest Fly Bridges

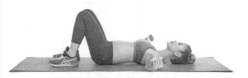

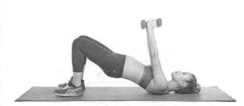

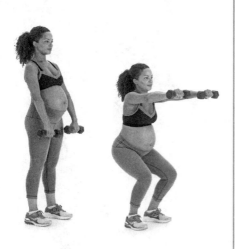

Chest Presses on Physio Ball

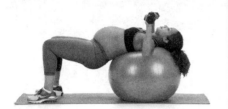

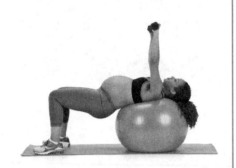

Chest Stretch

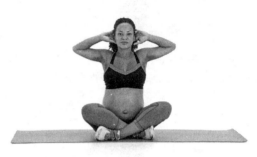

Clams

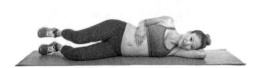

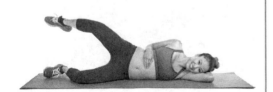

Crescent Pose with Wide Rows

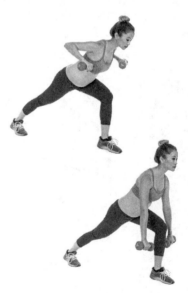

Crunches

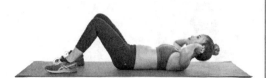

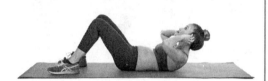

Diamond Pushups on Knees

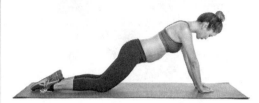

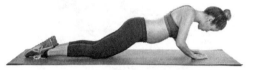

Elevated Heel Slides

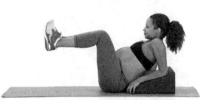

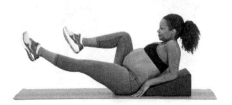

Figure 4 Glute Stretch

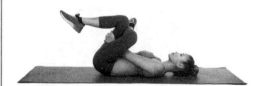

Fire Hydrants

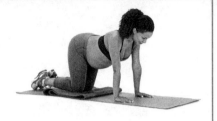

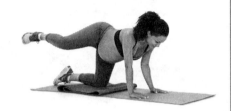

Goddess Squats

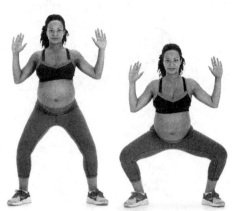

Good Mornings with Arms Crossed on Chest

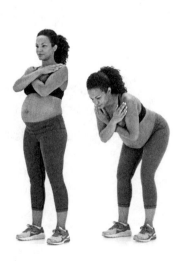

Hammer Curls

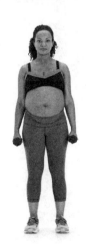
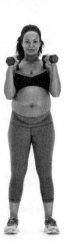

Hamstring Stretch

Head Bangers on Physio Ball

Hip Rotation Stretches, Both Legs Bent

Incline Pushups

Incline Triceps Pushups

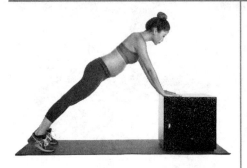

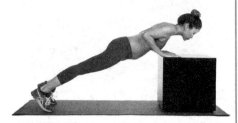

Lat Pullovers on Physio Ball

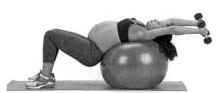

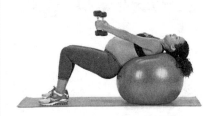

Leaning Oblique Crunches with Alternating Leg Lifts

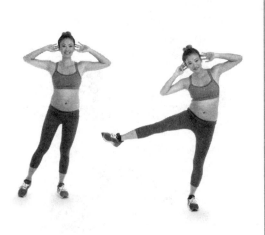

Leg Presses on Physio Ball

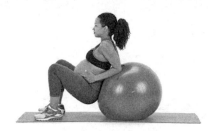

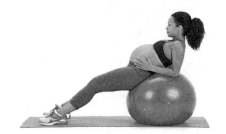

Medium Grip Rows in Crescent Pose

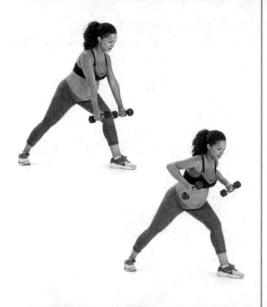

Mermaids

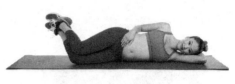

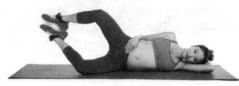

Mermaid Stretch

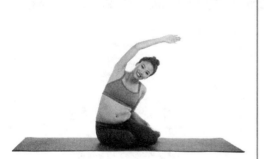

Modified Back Extensions on Knees

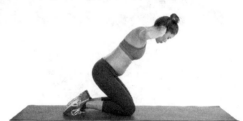

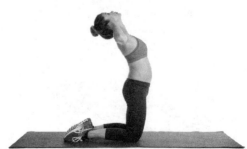

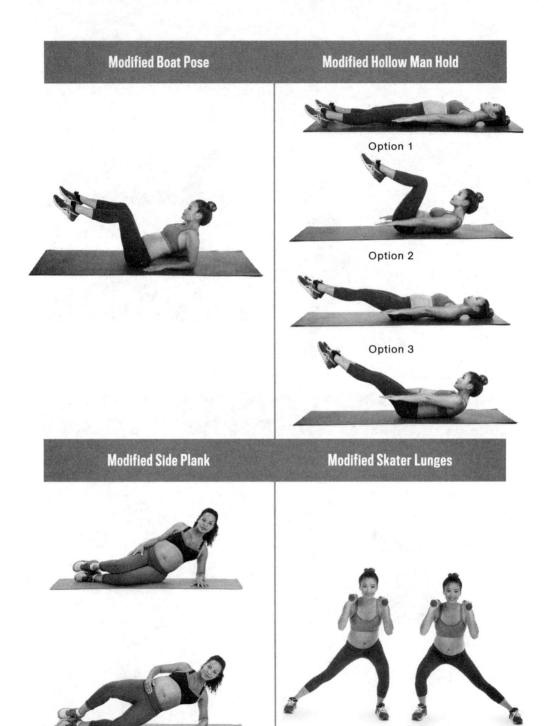

Modified Boat Pose

Modified Hollow Man Hold

Option 1

Option 2

Option 3

Modified Side Plank

Modified Skater Lunges

Mountain Climbers

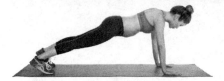

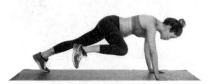

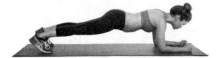

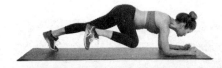

Mula Bandha or Kegels
(see pages 144-145)

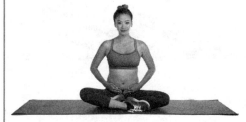

Pelvic Thrusts on Physio Ball

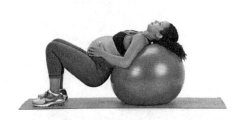

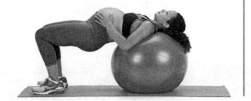

Pigeon Stretch

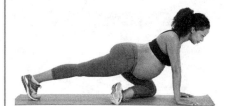

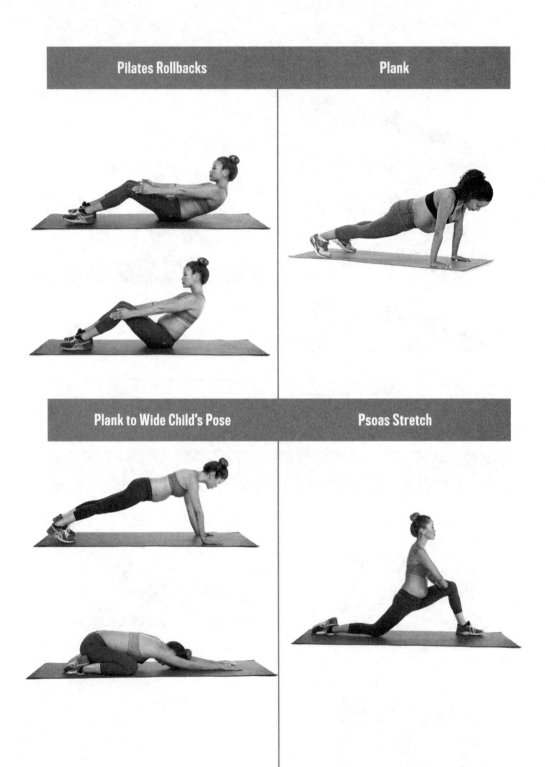

Pilates Rollbacks

Plank

Plank to Wide Child's Pose

Psoas Stretch

Pushups	**Shoulder Stretch**

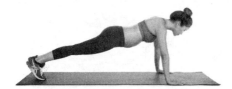

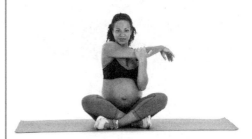

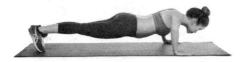

Side Crunches	**Side Lying Inner Thigh Raises**

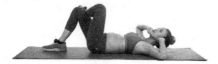

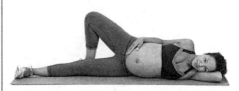

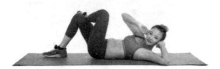

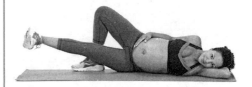

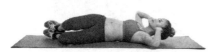

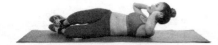

Side Lying Leg Circles

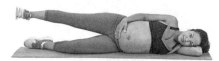

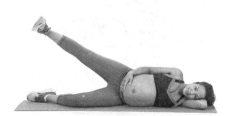

Side Lying Quad Stretch

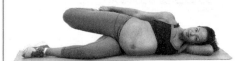

Side Lying Leg Abductions

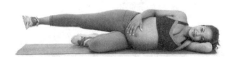

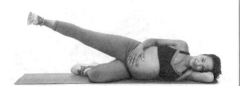

Side Lying Triceps Presses

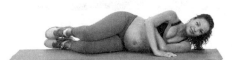

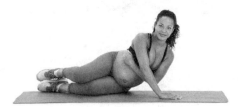

Side Plank

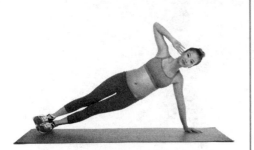

Side Squats with Military Presses

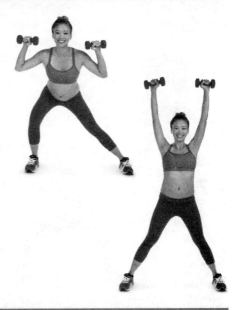

Single Arm Braced Wide Rows in Half Squat

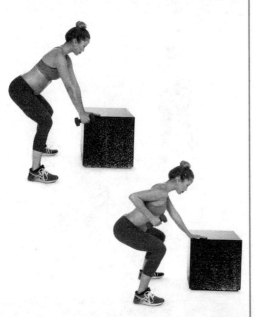

Sitting Trapezius Stretch

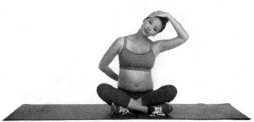

Squats with Biceps Curls

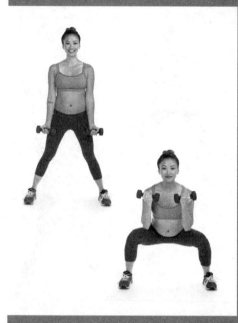

Squats with Goblet Hold

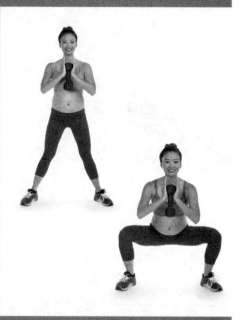

Squats with Serving Biceps

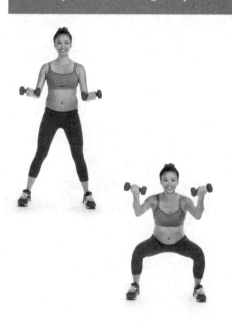

Squats with Wide Rows

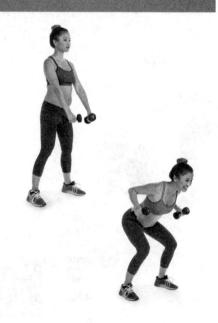

Standing Crunches

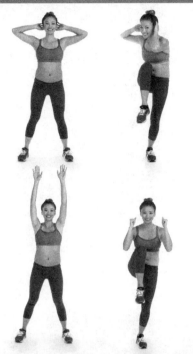

Standing Oblique Crunches

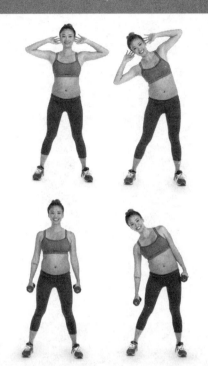

Stationary Lunges with Biceps Drags

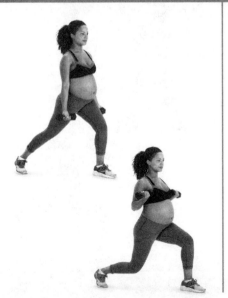

Stationary Lunges with Hammer Curls and Pelvic Tilt

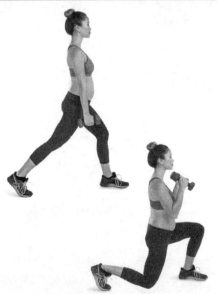

Stiff Leg Deadlifts to Upright Rows

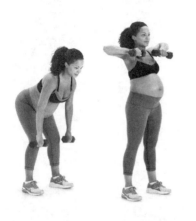

Stiff Leg Deadlifts with Low Rows

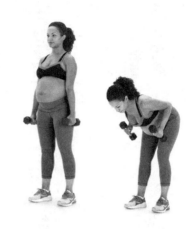

Sumo Squats with Hammer Curls

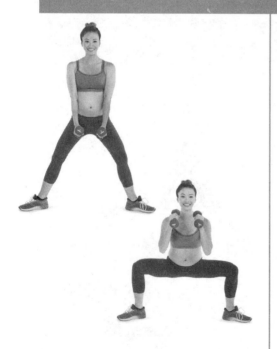

Sumo Squats with Rotator Cuff Flys

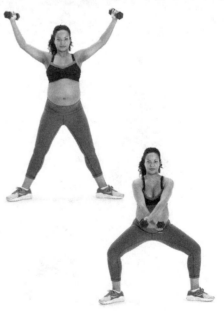

Sumo Squats with Shoulder Presses

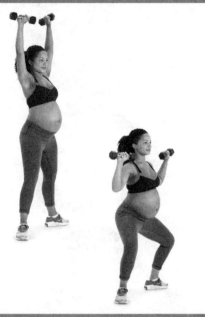

Supported Side Angle

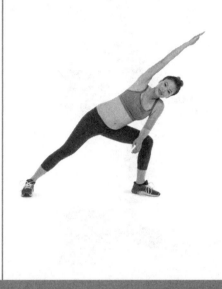

Thoracic Rotation Stretch with One Leg Extended

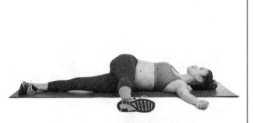

Triangle Presses

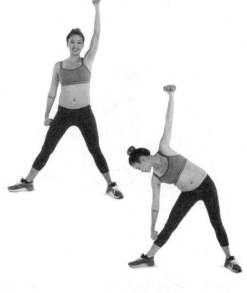

Triceps Dips

Triceps Kickbacks in Crescent Pose

Triceps Stretch

Uneven Table Hold

Walking Plank	Walking Plank (modified on knees)

Wall Squats on Physio Ball	Wide Child's Pose

Woodpecker Pushups

Yeah Baby!
PRODUCTS AND RESOURCES

HOT BOOKS, DVDS, AND OTHER GREAT WORKS BY OUR DREAM TEAM MEMBERS AND OTHER ASSOCIATED EXPERTS

Flavor First, by Cheryl Forberg, RD

The Mindful Mom-to-Be, by Lori Bregman (Heidi's awesome doula)

Hot Mommy Healthy Body DVD, by Jillian Michaels and Andrea Orbeck, shop .jillianmichaels.com/products/jillian-michaels-hot-body-healthy-mommy-dvd

Pregnancy Sculpt DVD, by Andrea Orbeck

A great online workout source: Fit Fusion: fitfusion.com

BELLY SUPPORT

Bellaband: ingridandisabel.com/shop/bellaband

FOOD BRANDS

Ancient Harvest Quinoa Penne: ancientharvest.com/product/supergrain-pasta -penne/

Annie's BBQ Sauce: annies.com/products/condiments-sauces

Applegate Turkey Bacon: applegate.com/products/natural-turkey-bacon

Belcampo Meat Company: belcampo.com

Dave's Killer Bread: daveskillerbread.com/

Earth Balance: earthbalancenatural.com/

Ezekiel bread: foodforlife.com/about_us/ezekiel-49

Mary's Gone Crackers Super Seed Crackers: marysgonecrackers.com

Niman Ranch: nimanranch.com

Organic Prairie: organicprairie.com

Stacy's Pita Chips: stacyssnacks.com/

Sun Chlorella: sunchlorellausa.com

Thundering Hooves: thunderinghooves.net

FOOD SOURCES

American Grass-Fed Association: americangrassfed.org

Certified Humane Raised & Handled: certifiedhumane.org

Environmental Working Group: ewg.org/foodnews/dirty_dozen_list.php

Heritage Foods: heritagefoodusa.com

Organic Trade Association: ota.com

Organic Valley: organicvalley.coop

Thrive Market: thrivemarket.com

USDA National Organic Program: ams.usda.gov/nop

Wild Farm Alliance: wildfarmalliance.org

GREEN HOUSEHOLD AND CLEANING BRANDS AND RESOURCES

Bona: us.bona.com/home.html

Ecover: us.ecover.com

Green cleaning product options: environmentalhomecenter.com

HEPA filters for your furnace or vacuum cleaner: hepa.com

The Honest Company: honest.com

Method: methodhome.com

Mrs. Meyer's: mrsmeyers.com

Safecoat paint: afmsafecoat.com

Shaklee: shaklee.com

Simple Green: simplegreen.com

Skoy Cloth: skoycloth.com/our-products/skoy-cloth

Sources for natural, green furnishings: ecochoices.com, furnature.com, greenguard.org,greenguide.com, greenhome.com

GREEN, NONTOXIC NURSERY PRODUCT COMPANIES

abundantearth.com

babyworks.com

cottontailbaby.com

ecowise.com

humanityinfantandherbal.com

littlemerryfellows.com

shepherdsdream.com

theorganicmattress.com

MIDWIFE AND DOULA RESOURCES

American College of Nurse-Midwives: midwife.org/find-a-midwife

CAPPA (Childbirth and Postpartum Professional Association): cappa.net

Citizens for Midwifery: cfmidwifery.org/find/

DONA (Doulas of North America): dona.org

MORNING SICKNESS AIDS

Sea Band: sea-band.com

Travel Eze: widely available wristbands (they also make tablets, but don't take the tablets while pregnant or breastfeeding) that you can find at places like Wal-Mart or amazon.com

MUSIC FOR BABY

Belly Buds: wavhello.com/products/bellybuds

PAIGE'S BEAUTY PICKS

For Skincare

Burt's Bees 100% Natural Lip Balm, Classic Beeswax: burtsbees.ca/natural -products/lips-lip-care-beeswax-lip-balm/beeswax-lip-balm-tube.html

Derma e Microdermabrasion Scrub: dermae.com/product/245/Microdermabrasion -Scrub.html

Mad Hippie Vitamin C Serum: madhippie.com/shop/vitamin-c-serum/

Osea Eye Gel Serum: oseamalibu.com/eye-gel-serum.html

For Makeup

Burt's Bees Lip Crayons: burtsbees.com/Lip-Crayon/792850028500,default,pd .html

Mineral Fusion Eyeliner: mineralfusion.com/products/liquid-mineral-eyeliner ?variant=4095350851

W3ll People Narcissist Foundation + Concealer Stick: w3llpeople.com/index.php
/narcissist-stick-foundation-5-full.html

For Hair Care

John Masters Dry Hair Nourishment and Defrizzer: johnmasters.ca/dry-hair
-nourishment-defrizzer/

Rahua Voluminous Hair Spray: rahua.com/us/rahua-voluminous-spray.html

Shea Moisture Organic Raw Shea Butter Moisture Retention Shampoo:
sheamoisture.com/Raw-Shea-Butter-Moisture-Retention-Shampoo_p_1302
.html

For Body Care

Andalou Naturals Aloe Mint Cooling Shower Gel: andalou.com/aloe-mint
-cooling-shower-gel

APNO (All Purpose Nipple Ointment) by prescription.

Burt's Bees has many different products for mom and baby that Paige approves of
and that can all be found on their Web site, burtsbees.com:

Burt's Bees Baby Bee Buttermilk Soap

Burt's Bees Baby Bee Nourishing Lotion, Fragrance Free

Burt's Bees Baby Bee Wipes, Fragrance Free

Burt's Bees Baby Bee Diaper Ointment

Burt's Bees Baby Bee Shampoo & Body Wash, Fragrance Free

Burt's Bees Bath & Body Oil with Lemon & Vitamin E

Burt's Bees Doctor Burt's Res-Q Ointment

Burt's Bees Farmer's Friend Hand Salve

Burt's Bees Mama Bee Belly Butter

Burt's Bees Mama Bee Leg & Foot Creme

Burt's Bees Mama Bee Nourishing Body Oil

Burt's Bees Naturally Nourishing Milk & Shea Butter Body Bar

Burt's Bees Peppermint Foot Lotion

Hugo Naturals Vanilla and Sweet Orange Massage and Body Oil: hugonaturals.com

Lansinoh HPA Lanolin Nipple Cream: lansinoh.com

Moom Natural Wax Strips: moom.com

TL Care Organic Cotton Nursing Pads: tlcare.com

For Nail Care

Acquarella Water Color: acquarella.com

Burt's Bees Lemon Butter Cuticle Creme: burtsbees.com (find it under the "Classics" tab)

Deborah Lippmann Intensive Nail Treatment: deborahlippmann.com/it-s-a-miracle

For Baby Care

Burt's Bees Baby has many organic cotton products on their Web site, burtsbeesbaby.com

Butt Naked Baby Soothing Bath Soak: buttnakedbaby.com/#!product/prd1 /918662764/soothing-bath-soak

California Baby Diaper Rash Cream: californiababy.com/calming-diaper-rash -cream-2-9-oz.html

Waxelene The Petroleum Jelly Alternative: waxelene.com

COMPANIES WITH PRODUCTS AND PHILOSOPHIES WE LOVE

Acquarella: acquarella.com

Acure: acureorganics.com

Andalou Naturals: andalou.com

Baby Hugo Naturals: hugonaturals.com/products/baby-hugo

Badger (baby): badgerbalm.com/p-398-baby-balm-organic-baby-skin-care.aspx

Beautycounter: beautycounter.com

Burt's Bees: burtsbees.com

Burt's Bees Baby: burtsbeesbaby.com

Butt Naked: buttnakedbaby.com

California Baby: californiababy.com

Deborah Lippmann: deborahlippmann.com

Deep Steep: deepsteep.com

Derma e: dermae.com

Dr. Bronner's Magic Soaps: drbronner.com

Evan Healy: evanhealy.com

The Honest Company: honest.com

Hugo Naturals: hugonaturals.com

Jane Iredale: janeiredale.com

John Masters Organics: johnmasters.com

Juice Beauty: juicebeauty.com

Little Twig: littletwig.com

Living Nature: livingnature.com

Luminance Skin Care: luminanceskincare.com

Melvita: melvita.com

Mineral Fusion: mineralfusion.com

Moom: moom.com

Morrocco Method: shop.morroccomethod.com

Nature's Baby Organics: naturesbaby.com

Osea: oseamalibu.com

Priti: pritinyc.com

Rahua: rahua.com

Rare El'Ements: rare-elements.com

Shea Moisture: sheamoisture.com

Soapwalla: soapwallakitchen.com

SW Basics: swbasicsofbk.com

Well People: w3llpeople.com

Yarok: yarokhair.com

Zoya: zoya.com

Zuii Organic: zuiiorganic.com

Zuzu Luxe: gabrielcosmeticsinc.com/brand/zuzu-luxe

PROBIOTICS

BioGaia probiotics: biogaia.com

Bio K+: biokplus.com/en_ca

Healthy Trinity: natren.com/healthy-trinity.html

Jarrow Formulas: jarrow.com

RADIATION SHIELDS FOR PREGNANT BELLIES

Belly Armor by Radiashield: bellyarmor.com/radiation/pregnancy-radiation/

DefenderShield: defendershield.com/shop/

RESOURCES FOR YOUR OWN FURTHER RESEARCH

Breastfeeding seminars in your area: uslca.org/resources/find-an-ibclc

Gerald Briggs, pharmacist clinical specialist, who answers many questions on medications and supplements during pregnancy: babycenter.com/expert -gerald-briggs

Information about safe lawn chemicals: safelawns.org

Lead testing: leadlisting.com; National Lead Information Center, 800-424-5323, epa.gov/lead/forms/lead-hotline-national-lead-information-center

Monterey Bay Aquarium's Web site to help you identify the toxicity of various fish species: montereybayaquarium.org/cr/seafoodwatch.aspx

Motherisk research links, for information about safe medications and supplements during pregnancy: motherrisk.com/women/mothernature.jsp

Radon testing: radon.com, radon.info, radonmonitor.com, radon.com/radon /radon_map.html

Resource for finding a splint or brace due to diastasis recti: diastasisrehab.com

Resource for those with postpartum depression: postpartuminternational.org

Resource on safe and unsafe plastics: checnet.org

The U.S. EPA's Web site on water quality reports: epa.gov/drink/local/

SUPPLEMENTS

Barlean's Orange-Flavored Fish Oil: barleans.com/fish-oil-fresh-catch-softgels -orange-flavor-100ct-bfoc100

Best Nest Prenatal Vitamin: bestnestwellness.com/products/best-prenatal-vitamin

Garden of Life *mykind* Multivitamins: gardenoflife.com/content/product/why -choose-mykind-organics/

MegaFood Baby & Me Vitamins: megafood.com/store/en/women-s-health/baby -metm/

New Chapter Organics Perfect Prenatal Vitamins: newchapter.com/content /perfect-prenatal%E2%84%A2-multivitamin

ENDNOTES

Introduction

1 Environmental Working Group, "Body Burden: The Pollution in Newborns, July 14, 2005. ewg.org/research/body-burden-pollution-newborns.

Chapter 1

1 "State Facts about Unintended Pregnancy," Guttmacher Institute, July 2015, guttmacher.org /fact-sheet/state-facts-about-unintended-pregnancy?gclid=CjwKEAjwpfC5BRCT1sKW2qzwq E0SJABkKFKRbVmqGnzD9Jh1NYx5fB7WXTJuuJNCvifD4dWXdSWi2BoCl4jw_wcB.

2 J. Graham, "How to Get Pregnant," Redbook, September 30, 2014, redbookmag.com/body /pregnancy-fertility/advice/a39/get-pregnant-yl/.

3 "Fetal Development Is Dependent on Hormones," Child Health Explanation, childhealth -explanation.com/fetaldevelopment.html.

4 S. Pappas, "The Truth about How Mom's Stress Affects Baby's Brain," Live Science, February 24, 2014, livescience.com/43579-poverty-stress-infant-development.html.

5 "Fetal Development Is Dependent on Hormones," Child Health Explanation.

6 "What Is Hysteroscopy?" Cleveland Clinic, my.clevelandclinic.org/health/treatments _and_procedures/hic-what-is-hysteroscopy.

7 A. Giorgi et al., "Pelvic Laparoscopy," Healthline, December 22, 2015, healthline.com /health/pelvic-laparoscopy.

8 R. W. Harms, MD, "Is It Safe to Have an X-Ray during Pregnancy?" Mayo Clinic, March 19, 2015, mayoclinic.org/healthy-lifestyle/pregnancy-week-by-week/expert-answers/x-ray-during -pregnancy/faq-20058264.

9 M. S. Barros Gomes, "About the Fetal Risks from Diagnostic Use of Radiation during Pregnancy: A Systematic Review and Proposal of Clinical Protocol," *Faculdade de Medicina da Universidade do Porto*, 2015, p. 7, repositorio-aberto.up.pt/handle/10216/78826.

10 A. Scialli, "Is It Safe to Walk through Airport Screening Machines While I'm Pregnant?" Babycenter, March 2016, babycenter.com/404_is-it-safe-to-walk-through-airport -screening-machines-while_2616.bc.

11 R. Antonucci et al., "Use of Non-Steroidal Anti-Inflammatory Drugs in Pregnancy: Impact on the Fetus and Newborn," *Current Drug Metabolism* 13, no. 4 (May 1, 2012): 474–90.

12 M. Trottier, MSc, "Treating Constipation during Pregnancy," *Canadian Family Physician* 58, no. 8 (August 2012): 836–38.

13 "Taking Medicine during Pregnancy," Web MD Health and Pregnancy, webmd.com/baby /guide/taking-medicine-during-pregnancy.

14 "IFPA Pregnancy Guidelines: Guidelines for Aromatherapists Working with Pregnant Clients," 2013, naha.org/assets/uploads/PregnancyGuidelines-Oct11.pdf.

15 "Understanding Vaccines: What They Are. How They Work," U.S. Department of Health and Human Services, January 2008, niaid.nih.gov/topics/vaccines/documents/undvacc.pdf.

16 "Routine Tests during Pregnancy," American College of Obstetricians and Gynecologists, January 2016, acog.org/-/media/For-Patients/faq133.pdf?dmc=1&ts=20150701T1103361014.

17 "Thyroid Disorders and Pregnancy," Children's Hospital of Philadelphia, chop.edu/pages /thyroid-disorders-and-pregnancy#.VfY9Y2RVhBc.

18 "Statistics about Diabetes: Overall Numbers, Diabetes and Prediabetes," American Diabetes Association, April 1, 2016, diabetes.org/diabetes-basics/statistics/?referrer=https://www .google.com/.

19 P. Kristiansson et al., "Reproductive Hormones and Blood Pressure during Pregnancy," *Human Reproduction* 16, no. 1 (2001): 13–17.

20 "High Blood Pressure in Pregnancy," National Heart, Lung, and Blood Institute, nhlbi.nih .gov/health/resources/heart/hbp-pregnancy.

21 "Common Tests during Pregnancy," Stanford Children's Health, stanfordchildrens.org/en /topic/default?id=common-tests-during-pregnancy-85-P01241.

22 E. P. Ben-Joseph, MD, "RH Incompatibility," KidsHealth, October 2014, kidshealth.org /parent/pregnancy_center/your_pregnancy/rh.html.

23 Ibid.

24 M. Bansal et al., "Relationship between Maternal Periodontal Status and Preterm Low Birth Weight," *Reviews in Obstetrics and Gynecology* 6, nos. 3–4 (2013): 135–40.

25 A. Kinney et al., "Smoking, Alcohol and Caffeine in Relation to Ovarian Age during the Reproductive Years," *Human Reproduction* 22, no. 4 (2007): 1175–85.

26 F. Bolumar et al., "Smoking Reduces Fecundity: A European Multicenter Study on Infertility and Subfecundity," *American Journal of Epidemiology* 143, no. 6 (March 15, 1996): 578–87.

27 "Smoking and Infertility: A Committee Opinion," *American Society for Reproductive Medicine* 98, no. 6 (December 2012): 1400–06.

28 M. Mendoza-López et al., "Dietary Intake and Infertility: A Review," *Official Journal of the Federation of American Societies for Experimental Biology* 29, no. 1 (April 2015).

29 R. L. Brent et al., "Evaluation of the Reproductive and Developmental Risks of Caffeine," *Birth Defects Research Part B, Developmental and Reproductive Toxicology* 92, no. 2 (April 2011): 152–87.

30 L. Potter, "Are You Sipping Pesticide Residues in Your Morning Coffee?" Healthy Organic Woman, healthyorganicwoman.com/sipping-pesticides-in-your-morning-coffee/.

31 T. K. Jensen et al., "Does Moderate Alcohol Consumption Affect Fertility? Follow Up Study among Couples Planning First Pregnancy," *British Medical Journal* 317 (May 13, 1998): 505.

32 I. Sample, "Alcohol Hinders Having a Baby through IVF, Couples Warned," Guardian, October 20, 2009, theguardian.com/lifeandstyle/2009/oct/20/alcohol-hinders-baby-ivf.

33 T. K. Jensen et al., "Habitual Alcohol Consumption Associated with Reduced Semen Quality and Changes in Reproductive Hormones; A Cross-Sectional Study among 1221 Young Danish Men," *British Medical Journal Open* 4, no. 9 (October 2, 2014).

34 N. Farahi, MD, and A. Zolotor, MD, "Recommendations for Preconception Counseling and Care," *American Family Physician* 88, no. 8 (October 15, 2013): 499–506.

35 "Weight Gain during Pregnancy," March of Dimes, marchofdimes.org/pregnancy/weight -gain-during-pregnancy.aspx.

36 M. A. Leddy, "The Impact of Maternal Obesity on Maternal and Fetal Health," *Reviews in Obstetrics and Gynecology* 1, no. 4 (Fall 2008): 170–78.

37 Z. Han et al., "Maternal Underweight and the Risk of Preterm Birth and Low Birth Weight: A Systematic Review and Meta-Analyses," *International Journal of Epidemiology* 40, no. 1: 65–101.

38 B. B. Green, MD, MPH, et al., "Risk of Ovulatory Infertility in Relation to Body Weight," *Fertility and Sterility* 50, no. 5 (November 1988): 721–26.

39 "Pregnancy and Nutrition," MedlinePlus, nlm.nih.gov/medlineplus/pregnancyandnutrition.html.

40 A. J. Zolotor, MD, and M. C. Carlough, MD, "Update on Prenatal Care," *American Family Physician* 89, no. 3 (February 1, 2014): 199–208.

41 "Prenatal Care Fact Sheet," Womenshealth.gov, womenshealth.gov/publications/our -publications/fact-sheet/prenatal-care.html.

42 Zolotor and Carlough, "Update on Prenatal Care."

43 E. Group, DC, NP, DACBN, DCBCN, DABFM, "What Is the MTHFR Genetic Defect and How Can It Affect You?" *Global Healing Center*, last updated June 23, 2014, globalhealing center.com/natural-health/what-is-the-mthfr-genetic-defect/.

44 C. D. Lynch et al., "Preconception Stress Increases the Risk of Infertility: Results from a Couple-Based Prospective Cohort Study—the LIFE Study," *Human Reproduction*, January 29, 2014, humrep.oxfordjournals.org/content/early/2014/03/06/humrep.deu032.full.

45 C. L. Harrison et al., "Exercise Therapy in Polycystic Ovary Syndrome: A Systematic Review," *Human Reproduction Update* 17, no. 2 (March 2011): 171–83.

46 Zolotor, and Carlough, "Update on Prenatal Care."

Chapter 2

1 "Of Fat and Fertility," Fit Pregnancy and Baby, fitpregnancy.com/pregnancy/getting-pregnant/fat-and-fertility.

2 "Weight and Fertility," American Society for Reproductive Medicine, 2015, asrm.org/FACTSHEET_Weight_and_Fertility/.

3 C. Bailey, "You Need Body Fat for Conception," Fertility Authority, December 22, 2010, fertilityauthority.com/blogger/cindy-bailey/2010/12/21/you-need-body-fat-conception.

4 D. S. Ludwig and J. Currie, "The Association between Pregnancy Weight Gain and Birthweight: A Within-Family Comparison," *Lancet* 376 (2010): 984–90.

5 E. Oken et al., "Gestational Weight Gain and Child Adiposity at Age 3 Years," *American Journal of Obstetrics and Gynecology* 196, no. 4 (April 2007): 322 e1–8.

6 I. Rogers, "The Influence of Birth Weight and Intrauterine Environment on Adiposity and Fat Distribution in Later Life," *International Journal of Obesity and Related Metabolic Disorders* 27 (2003): 755–77.

7 "Pregnancy and Alcohol: Safety, Effects and Addiction," American Pregnancy Association, July 2015, americanpregnancy.org/pregnancy-health/pregnancy-and-alcohol/.

8 H. S. Feldman et al., "Prenatal Alcohol Exposure Patterns and Alcohol-Related Growth Deficiencies: Prospective Study," *Alcoholism: Clinical and Experimental Research* 36, no. 4 (April 2012): 670–76, online January 17, 2012.

9 C. Leon, "Pesticides in Your Coffee?" Alternet, July 30, 2014, alternet.org/food/coffee-pesticides.

10 K. Sakamoto et al., "Behavior of Pesticides in Coffee Beans during the Roasting Process," *Shokuhin Eiseiqaku Zasshi* 53, no. 5 (2012): 233–36.

11 "Caffeine Intake during Pregnancy," American Pregnancy Association, July 2015, americanpregnancy.org/pregnancy-health/caffeine-during-pregnancy/.

12 Mayo Clinic Staff, "Caffeine Content for Coffee, Tea, Soda, and More," Mayo Clinic Healthy Lifestyle: Nutrition and Healthy Eating, mayoclinic.org/healthy-lifestyle/nutrition-and-healthy-eating/in-depth/caffeine/art-20049372.

13 "Listeria and Pregnancy," American Pregnancy Association, August 2015, americanpregnancy.org/pregnancy-complications/listeria/.

14 "Births and Natality," National Center for Health Statistics, Centers for Disease Control and Prevention, cdc.gov/nchs/fastats/births.htm.

15 J. McGuire et al., "The 2014 FDA Assessment of Commercial Fish: Practical Considerations for Improved Dietary Guidance," *Nutrition Journal* 15, no. 66 (July 13, 2016).

16 K. Kirkpatrick, MS, RD, LD, "Fish Faceoff: Wild Salmon vs. Farmed Salmon," Cleveland Clinic Health Essentials, health.clevelandclinic.org/2014/03/fish-faceoff-wild-salmon-vs-farmed-salmon/.

17 "FDA Cuts Trans Fat in Processed Foods," U.S. Food and Drug Administration, June 16, 2015, fda.gov/ForConsumers/ConsumerUpdates/ucm372915.htm.

18 Y. Smith, "Trans Fat History," News Medical, June 14, 2015, news-medical.net/health/Trans-Fat-History.aspx.

19 M. McEvoy, "Organic 101: What the USDA Organic Label Means," United States Department of Agriculture, March 22, 2012, blogs.usda.gov/2012/03/22/organic-101-what-the-usda-organic-label-means/.

20 E. Ward et al., "Childhood and Adolescent Cancer Statistics," *CA: A Cancer Journal for Clinicians* 64, no. 2 (January 31, 2014): 83–103.

21 "Cancer and Toxic Chemicals," Physicians for Social Responsibility, psr.org/environment-and-health/confronting-toxics/cancer-and-toxic-chemicals.html?referrer=https://www.google.com/.

22 P. Landrigan et al., "Environmental Pollutants and Disease in American Children: Estimates of Morbidity, Mortality, and Costs for Lead Poisoning, Asthma, Cancer, and Developmental Disabilities," *Environmental Health Perspectives* 110, no. 7 (July 2002): 721–28.

23 "Asthma Facts: CDC's National Asthma Control Program Grantees," Centers for Disease Control and Prevention, July 2013, cdc.gov/asthma/pdfs/asthma_facts_program_grantees.pdf.

24 "Chemicals and Our Health: Why Recent Science Is a Call to Action," Safer Chemicals, Healthy Families, 2009, cleanandhealthyme.org/LinkClick.aspx?fileticket=ErDhhofgWmI%3D&tabid=36.

25 J. Hamblin, "The Toxins That Threaten Our Brains," *Atlantic,* March 18, 2014, theatlantic.com/health/archive/2014/03/the-toxins-that-threaten-our-brains/284466/.

26 E. S. Bartlett and L. Trasande, "Economic Impacts of Environmentally Attributable Childhood Health Outcomes in the European Union," *European Journal of Public Health* 24, no. 1 (February 2014): 21–26.

27 R. Krajmalnik-Brown et al., "Gut Bacteria in Children with Autism Spectrum Disorders: Challenges and Promise of Studying How a Complex Community Influences a Complex Disease," *Microbial Ecology in Health and Disease* 26 (March 2015).

28 "Summary Report on Antimicrobials Sold or Distributed for Use in Food-Producing Animals," United States Food and Drug Administration, Department of Health and Human Services, originally published on December 9, 2010, revised and updated September 2014, fda.gov/downloads/ForIndustry/UserFees/AnimalDrugUserFeeActADUFA/UCM231851.pdf.

29 T. P. Van Boeckel et al., "Global Trends in Antimicrobial Use in Food Animals," *Proceedings of the National Academy of Sciences of the United States of America* 112, no. 18 (February 18, 2015): 5649–54.

30 "Biomarkers & Human Biomonitoring," World Health Organization, October 2011, who.int/ceh/capacity/biomarkers.pdf.

31 "The Overuse of Antibiotics in Food Animals Threatens Public Health," Consumers Union, Policy and Action from Consumer Reports, consumersunion.org/pdf/Overuse_of_Antibiotics_On_Farms.pdf.

32 "Bioaccumulation and Eutrophication—Higher Tier," BBC, bbc.co.uk/schools/gcse bitesize/science/triple_ocr_21c/further_biology/ecosystems/revision/6/.

33 A. W. Campbell, "Autoimmunity and the Gut," *Autoimmune Disease,* May 13, 2014, ncbi.nlm.nih.gov/pmc/articles/PMC4036413/.

34 J. F. Shelton et al., "Neurodevelopmental Disorders and Prenatal Residential Proximity to Agricultural Pesticides: The CHARGE Study," *Environmental Health Perspectives* 122, no. 10 (October 2014).

35 K. Feldscher, "Toxic Chemicals Linked to Brain Disorders in Children," *Harvard Gazette,* February 14, 2014, news.harvard.edu/gazette/story/2014/02/toxic-chemicals-linked-to-brain-disorders-in-children/.

36 P. Grandjean et al., "Neurobehavioural Effects of Developmental Toxicity," *Lancet Neurology* 13, no. 3 (March 2014): 330–38.

37 "Dirty Dozen," Environmental Working Group, ewg.org/foodnews/dirty_dozen_list.php.

38 "Clean Fifteen," Environmental Working Group, ewg.org/foodnews/clean_fifteen_list.php .

39 E. Ruppel Shell, "Artificial Sweeteners May Change Our Gut Bacteria in Dangerous Ways," *Scientific American,* April 1, 2015, scientificamerican.com/article/artificial-sweeteners-may-change-our-gut-bacteria-in-dangerous-ways/.

40 J. Suez et al., "Artificial Sweeteners Induce Glucose Intolerance by Altering the Gut Microbiota," *Nature* 514, no. 7521 (October 9, 2014): 181–86.

41 M. B. Azad et al., "Association between Artificially Sweetened Beverage Consumption during Pregnancy and Infant Body Mass Index," *Journal of the American Medical Association Pediatrics*, May 9, 2016.

42 K. R. Tandel, "Sugar Substitutes: Health Controversy over Perceived Benefits," *Journal of Pharmacology and Pharmacotherapeutics* 2, no. 4 (October 2011): 236–43.

43 M. D. Gold, "Reported Aspartame Toxicity Effects," Aspartame Toxicity Information Center, January 12, 2002, fda.gov/ohrms/dockets/dailys/03/jan03/012203/02p-0317_emc -000199.txt.

44 K. Holton, "Actually, MSG Is Not Safe for Everyone," Live Science, September 20, 2014, livescience.com/47931-msg-not-safe-for-everyone.html.

45 K. Michaelis, "MSG Is Dangerous: The Science Is In," Food Renegade, foodrenegade.com /msg-dangerous-science/.

46 S. Preston-Martin et al., "Maternal Consumption of Cured Meats and Vitamins in Relation to Pediatric Brain Tumors," *Cancer Epidemiology, Biomarkers and Prevention* 5, no. 8 (August 1996): 599–605.

47 D. Mozaffarian et al., "Health Effects of Trans-Fatty Acids: Experimental and Observational Evidence," *European Journal of Clinical Nutrition*, 63, suppl. 2 (May 2009): S5–21.

48 L. C. Vinikoor et al., "Consumption of Trans-Fatty Acid and Its Association with Colorectal Adenomas," *American Journal of Epidemiology* 168, no. 3 (August 1, 2008): 389–97.

49 B. A. Golomb et al., "Trans Fat Consumption and Aggression," *Public Library of Science One* 7, no. 3 (March 5, 2012): e32175.

50 F. Trevizol et al., "Cross-Generational Trans Fat Intake Facilitates Mania-Like Behavior: Oxidative and Molecular Markers in Brain Cortex," *Neuroscience* 286 (February 12, 2015): 353–63.

51 L. Yoquinto, "The Truth about Food Additive BHA," Live Science, June 1, 2012, livescience .com/36424-food-additive-bha-butylated-hydroxyanisole.html.

52 F. S. vom Saal, "Evidence That Bisphenol A (BPA) Can Be Accurately Measured without Contamination in Human Derum and Urine, and That BPA Causes Numerous Hazards from Multiple Routes of Exposure," *Environment, Epigenetics and Reproduction* 398, nos. 1–2 (December 2014): 101–13.

53 R. Bhandari et al., "Urinary Bisphenol A and Obesity in U.S. Children," *American Journal of Epidemiology* 177, no. 11 (June 1, 2013): 1263–70.

54 "Study Shows Protective Benefits of DHA Taken during Pregnancy," *Emory University News Release*, August 1, 2011, shared.web.emory.edu/emory/news/releases/2011/08/study-shows -protective-benefits-of-dha-taken-during-pregnancy.html#.V0duEpErKkw.

55 "Pregnancy and Prenatal Vitamins," WebMD Health and Pregnancy, webmd.com/baby/guide /prenatal-vitamins.

56 G. Goedhart et al., "Maternal Vitamin B-12 and Folate Status during Pregnancy and Excessive Infant Crying," *Early Human Development* 87, no. 4 (April 2011): 309–14.

57 "Nutrient Recommendations and Research," VeganHealth.org, veganhealth.org/b12 /vegansources.

Chapter 3

1 "Fetal Stem Cells Can Repair the Mother during Pregnancy," Fight Aging! November 21, 2011, fightaging.org/archives/2011/11/fetal-stem-cells-can-repair-the-mother-during-pregnancy/.

2 S. Wassner Flynn, "Running Mommies: Can Pregnancy Make You Faster?" SheKnows Pregnancy and Baby, pregnancyandbaby.com/moms/articles/945113/running-mommies -can-pregnancy-make-you-faster.

3 "Exercise during Pregnancy," American College of Obstetricians and Gynecologists, May 2016, acog.org/Patients/FAQs/Exercise-During-Pregnancy#pregnancy.

4   D. Symons Downs, "Physical Activity and Pregnancy: Past and Present Evidence and Future Recommendations," *Research Quarterly for Exercise and Sport* 83, no. 4 (December 2012): 485–502.

5   "Exercise during Pregnancy," *American College of Obstetricians and Gynecologists.*

6   "The Benefits of Exercise during Pregnancy," Arizona OBGYN Affiliates, March 12, 2012, aoafamily.com/blog/the-benefits-of-exercise-during-pregnancy/.

7   L. Brin, "How to Exercise When You're Expecting: For the 9 Months of Pregnancy and the 5 Months It Takes to Get Your Best Body Back," *Plume*, March 29, 2011.

8   J. F. Clapp, "Influence of Endurance Exercise and Diet on Human Placental Development and Fetal Growth," *Placenta* 27, nos. 6–7 (June–July 2006): 527–34.

9   A. Park, "Study: Exercise in Pregnancy Benefits Babies," *Time*, April 7, 2010, content.time .com/time/health/article/0,8599,1978193,00.html.

10   P. H. Whincup et al., "Birth Weight and Risk of Type 2 Diabetes: A Systematic Review," *Journal of the American Medical Association* 300, no. 24 (December 24, 2008): 2886–97.

11   J. F. Clapp 3rd, "The Course of Labor after Endurance Exercise during Pregnancy," *American Journal of Obstetrics and Gynecology* 163, no. 6 pt. 1 (December 1990): 1799–805.

12   Ibid.

13   E. May et al., "Aerobic Exercise during Pregnancy Influences Fetal Cardiac Autonomic Control of Heart Rate and Heart Rate Variability," *Early Human Development* 86, no. 4 (March 30, 2010): 213–17.

14   Ibid.

15   "The Benefits of Exercise during Pregnancy," Pure Pharma Pure News, purepharma.com/uk _en/blog/pregnancy-exercise-benefits/.

16   M. Castillo, "Exercise during Pregnancy May Improve Baby's Brain Development," CBS News, November 11, 2013, www.cbsnews.com/news/exercise-during-pregnancy-may-improve-babys -brain-development/.

Chapter 4

1   "Body Burden: The Pollution in Newborns," Environmental Working Group, July 14, 2005, ewg.org/research/body-burden-pollution-newborns.

2   "Indoor Air Quality," US Environmental Protection Agency, epa.gov/indoor-air-quality-iaq.

3   "Carbon Monoxide Detector Requirements, Laws and Regulations," National Conference of State Legislators, April 5, 2016, ncsl.org/research/environment-and-natural-resources /carbon-monoxide-detectors-state-statutes.aspx.

4   W. Jedrychowski et al., "Cognitive Function of 6-Year-Old Children Exposed to Mold-Contaminated Homes in Early Postnatal Period. Prospective Birth Cohort Study in Poland," *Physiology and Behavior* 104, no. 5 (October 24, 2011): 989–95.

5   A. Del Bene Davis, "Home Environmental Health Risks, " *Online Journal of Issues in Nursing* 12 (May 2007): nursingworld.org/MainMenuCategories/ANAMarketplace /ANAPeriodicals/OJIN/TableofContents/Volume122007/No2May07/ HomeEnvironmentalHealthRisks.aspx.

6   "Plants Clean Air and Water for Indoor Environments," NASA Spinoff Technology Transfer Program, spinoff.nasa.gov/Spinoff2007/ps_3.html.

7   T. Fall et al., "Early Exposure to Dogs and Farm Animals and the Risk of Childhood Asthma," *JAMA Pediatrics* 169, no. 11 (November 2, 2015).

8   "Lead and Its Human Effects," King County, kingcounty.gov/healthservices/health/ehs /toxic/LeadGeneral.aspx.

9   A. Del Bene Davis, "Home Environmental Health Risks."

10   "Volatile Organic Compounds' Impact on Indoor Air Quality," US Environmental Protection Agency, epa.gov/indoor-air-quality-iaq/volatile-organic-compounds-impact-indoor-air -quality.

11 "Hundreds of Scientists Issue Warning about Chemical Dangers of Non-Stick Cookware and Water-Repellant Items," Mercola.com, June 3, 2015, articles.mercola.com/sites/articles /archive/2015/06/03/non-stick-cookware-dangers.aspx.

12 "Healthy Home Tips: Tip 6—Skip the Non-Stick to Avoid the Dangers of Teflon," Environmental Working Group, ewg.org/research/healthy-home-tips/tip-6-skip-non -stick-avoid-dangers-teflon.

13 S. S. White et al., "Endocrine Disrupting Properties of Perfluorooctanoic Acid," *Journal of Steroid Biochemistry and Molecular Biology* 127, no. 1–2 (October 2011): 16–26.

14 "Chlorine Free Processing," Conservatree, www.conservatree.org/paper/PaperTypes/CFDisc .shtml.

15 A. Del Bene Davis, "Home Environmental Health Risks."

16 "Why We Don't Sell Miracle-Gro," Organica Garden Supply, organicagardensupply.com /why-we-dont-sell-miracle-gro/.

17 J. Morris, "'Safe' Pesticides Now First in Poisonings," Center for Public Integrity, publicintegrity.org/2008/07/30/8936/safe-pesticides-now-first-poisonings.

18 L. Brown, "Monsanto to Pay $80 Million Civil Penalty for Roundup-Related Accounting Violations," *St. Louis Post-Dispatch,* February 10, 2016, stltoday.com/business/local /monsanto-to-pay-million-civil-penalty-for-roundup-related-accounting/article_21a717ec -5ebf-5376-8278-2a3fe9182208.html.

19 P. Mattera, "Monsanto: Corporate Rap Sheet," Corporate Research Project, corp-research .org/monsanto.

20 "Give Up Fireplaces?" DrWeil.com, drweil.com/drw/u/QAA400892/Give-Up-Fireplaces .html.

21 "How Toxic Are Your Household Cleaning Supplies?" Organic Consumers Association Green Guide, organicconsumers.org/news/how-toxic-are-your-household-cleaning-supplies.

22 "Project TENDR: Targeting Environmental Neuro-Developmental Risks. The TENDR Consensus Statement," *Environmental Health Perspectives* 124, no. 7 (July 2016): : A118–22.

23 "Pregnancy & Radiation," Belly Armor by RadiaShield, bellyarmor.com/radiation/pregnancy -radiation/.

24 "Radiation from Laptop Computers and Televisions during Pregnancy," Radiation Answers, 2007, radiationanswers.org/radiation-and-me/radiation-reproduction/unborn-child/laptop -and-television-radiation-pregnancy.html.

25 C. V. Bllieni et al., "Exposure to Electromagnetic Fields from Laptop Use of 'Laptop' Computers," *Archives of Occupational and Environmental Health* 67, no. 1 (2012): 31–36.

26 "Study Exposes Health Risks from Laptop Radiation, Particularly during Pregnancy," DefenderShield, September 24, 2012, defendershield.com/study-exposes-increased -health-risks-from-laptop-emfs-particularly-during-pregnancy/.

27 "Using a Laptop Computer during Pregnancy," What to Expect, whattoexpect.com /pregnancy/ask-heidi/week-22/laptop.aspx/.

28 F. Flam, "Interrupted: Phthalates Cause Birth Defects in Boys," *Philadelphia Inquirer*, October 27, 2008, as reported on Sott.net, sott.net/article/168448-Male-interrupted -phthalates-cause-birth-defects-in-boys.

29 EWG Verified, ewg.org/ewgverified/.

Chapter 5

1 M. Thomson, MD, et al., "Effects of Ginger for Nausea and Vomiting in Early Pregnancy: A Meta-Analysis," *Journal of the American Board of Family Medicine* 27 (January–February 2014): 115–22.

2 "Morning Sickness," Natural Pregnancy Midwife, natural-pregnancy-midwife.com/morning -sickness.html.

3 "Routine Tests during Pregnancy," The American Congress of Obstetricians and Gynecologists (January 2016), acog.org/patients/FAQs/routine-tests-during-pregnancy.

4 "Immunizations and Pregnancy," *Centers for Disease Control and Prevention* (March 2013), cdc.gov/vaccines/pubs/downloads/f_preg_chart.pdf.

5 "Pregnancy: The Three Trimesters," University of California San Francisco Medical Center, ucsfhealth.org/conditions/pregnancy/trimesters.html.

6 "Pregnancy: Condition Information," National Institute of Child Health and Human Development (December 6, 2013), nichd.nih.gov/health/topics/pregnancy/conditioninfo/Pages/default.aspx#f1.

7 "From Roe to Stenberg: A History of Key Abortion Rulings by the Supreme Court," Pew Research Center, Religion and Public Life (January 17, 2008), pewforum.org/Abortion/From-Roe-to-Stenberg-A-History-of-Key-Abortion-Rulings-by-the-Supreme-Court.aspx.

8 "What Are Some Common Signs of Pregnancy?" National Institute of Child Health and Human Development (July 12, 2013), nichd.nih.gov/health/topics/pregnancy/conditioninfo/Pages/signs.

9 "First Trimester Pregnancy: What to expect," Mayo Clinic (April 22, 2014), mayoclinic.com/health/pregnancy/PR00004.

10 M. Trottier, et al. "Treating Constipation during Pregnancy," *Canadian Family Physician* 58 (August 2012): 836–38.

11 "Morning Sickness," MedlinePlus (November 19, 2014), https://medlineplus.gov/ency/patientinstructions/000604.htm.

12 M. L. Okun et al., "Disturbed Sleep and Inflammatory Cytokines in Depressed and Nondepressed Pregnant Women: An Exploratory Analysis of Pregnancy Outcomes," *Psychosomatic Medicine* 75 (September 2013): 670–81, ncbi.nlm.nih.gov/pubmed/23864582.

13 "What are some common complications of pregnancy?" National Institute of Child Health and Human Development (July 12, 2013), nichd.nih.gov/health/topics/pregnancy/conditioninfo/Pages/complications.aspx#f1.

14 "Pregnancy and Miscarriage," WebMD, webmd.com/baby/guide/pregnancy-miscarriage#1.

15 "Fetal Development," MedlinePlus (September 26, 2015), nlm.nih.gov/medlineplus/ency/article/002398.htm.

16 "Fetal Development: The 1st Trimester," Mayo Clinic (July 10, 2014), mayoclinic.com/health/prenatal-care/PR00112.

17 M. Rashid et al., "Hyperemesis Gravidarum and Fetal Gender: A Retrospective Study," *Journal of Obstetrics and Gynaecology* 32 (July 2012): 475–78.

18 "Pregnancy Calendar Week 6," KidsHealth, kidshealth.org/parent/pregnancy_center/pregnancy_calendar/week6.html.

19 "Pregnancy Calendar Week 7," KidsHealth, kidshealth.org/parent/pregnancy_center/pregnancy_calendar/week7.html.

20 "Pregnancy Week by Week," Mayo Clinic (April 22, 2014), mayoclinic.com/health/pregnancy/PR00004/NSECTIONGROUP=2.

21 "Fetal Development," MedlinePlus (September 26, 2015).

22 "Fetal Development: The 1st Trimester," Mayo Clinic (July 10, 2014).

23 "Stages of Pregnancy," Womenshealth.gov (September 27, 2010), womenshealth.gov/pregnancy/you-are-pregnant/stages-of-pregnancy.html.

24 "Fetal Development," MedlinePlus (September 26, 2015).

25 Ibid.

26 "Pregnancy Week by Week," Mayo Clinic (April 22, 2014), mayoclinic.com/health/prenatal-care/PR00112/NSECTIONGROUP=2.

27 K. A. Costigan et al., "Pregnancy Folklore Revisited: The Case of Heartburn and Hair," *Birth* 33 (December 2006): 311–14.

28 "Pregnant in a Hot Tub," American Pregnancy Association, http://americanpregnancy.org/pregnancy-health/hot-tubs-during-pregnancy/.

29 "Can Pregnant Women Take Baths?" University of Arkansas for Medical Sciences, uams health.com/pregnantwomentakebaths.

30 "Melasma: Overview," American Academy of Dermatology, aad.org/public/diseases/color-problems/melasma.

31 "Fetal Development," MedlinePlus (September 26, 2015).

32 Ibid.

33 "Pregnancy Week by Week," Mayo Clinic (April 22, 2014), mayoclinic.com/health/prenatal-care/PR00112/NSECTIONGROUP=2.

34 "Fetal Development," MedlinePlus (September 26, 2015).

35 "Pregnancy Week by Week," Mayo Clinic (April 22, 2014), mayoclinic.com/health/prenatal-care/PR00112/NSECTIONGROUP=2.

36 "Prenatal Development: How Your Baby Grows during Pregnancy," The American College of Obstetricians and Gynecologists (June 2015), acog.org/patients/faqs/prenatal-development-how-your-baby-grows-during-pregnancy?IsMobileSet=false.

37 "Checklist of Foods to Avoid during Pregnancy," Foodsafety.gov, foodsafety.gov/risk/pregnant/chklist_pregnancy.html.

38 C. Zhang, MD, PhD, et al., "Dietary Fiber Intake, Dietary Glycemic Load, and the Risk of Gestational Diabetes Mellitus," *Diabetes Care* 29 (October 2006): 2223–30.

39 "Chart of High-Fiber Foods," Mayo Clinic (October 8, 2015), mayoclinic.org/healthy-lifestyle/nutrition-and-healthy-eating/in-depth/high-fiber-foods/art-20050948.

40 E. Morales et al., Circulating 25-Hydroxyvitamin D3 in Pregnancy and Infant Neuropsychological Development," *Pediatrics* 130 (October 2012): e913–20; E. Morales et al., "Vitamin D in Pregnancy and Attention Deficit Hyperactivity Disorder-Like Symptoms in Childhood," *Epidemiology* 26 (July 2015): 458–65.

41 "Vitamin D," National Institutes of Health (February 11, 2016), http://ods.od.nih.gov/factsheets/VitaminD-HealthProfessional/; A. Patz, "17 Surprising Ways to Get More Vitamin D," Prevention (December 22, 2014), prevention.com/food/food-remedies/foods-high-vitamin-d.

42 F. M. Rioux et al., "Iron Supplementation during Pregnancy: What Are the Risks and Benefits of Current Practices?" *Applied Physiology, Nutrition, and Metabolism* 32 (April 2007): 282–88.

43 "Swelling during Pregnancy," American Pregnancy Association (July 2015), american pregnancy.org/pregnancy-health/swelling-during-pregnancy/.

44 T. Wolak et al., "Low Potassium Level during the First Half of Pregnancy Is Associated with Lower Risk for the Development of Gestational Diabetes Mellitus and Severe Preeclampsia," *The Journal of Maternal-Fetal & Neonatal Medicine* 23 (September 2010): 994–98.

45 "Dietary Guidelines for Americans" (2005), health.gov/dietaryguidelines/dga2005/document/pdf/Appendix_B.pdf.

46 "Vitamin B_6 (Pyridoxine)," University of Maryland Medical Center (August 5, 2015), umm.edu/health/medical/altmed/supplement/vitamin-b6-pyridoxine.

47 "Vitamin B_6," National Institutes of Health (February 11, 2016), http://ods.od.nih.gov/factsheets/VitaminB6-HealthProfessional/_.

48 "Is It Better to Get Vitamins from Foods or Supplements, and Are Natural Vitamins Better Than Synthetic Vitamins?" ConsumerLab.com, consumerlab.com/answers/ Is+it+better+to+get+vitamins+from+foods+or+supplements,+and+are+natural+vitamins+better+than+synthetic+vitamins%3F/natural_vs_synthetic_vitamin/.

49 Z. S. Lassi et al., "Folic Acid Supplementation during Pregnancy for Maternal Health and Pregnancy Outcomes," *Cochrane Database of Systematic Reviews*, vol. 3 (March 28, 2013); "Anemia of Folate Deficiency," Johns Hopkins Medicine, hopkinsmedicine.org/healthlibrary/conditions/hematology_and_blood_disorders/anemia_of_folate_deficiency_85,P00089/.

50 "Folate: Dietary Supplement Fact Sheet," National Institutes of Health (April 20, 2016), http://ods.od.nih.gov/factsheets/Folate-HealthProfessional/.

51 "Magnesium: Fact Sheet for Health Professionals," National Institutes of Health (February 11, 2016), http://ods.od.nih.gov/factsheets/Magnesium-HealthProfessional.

52 "Quinoa, Cooked Nutrition Facts & Calories," SELF Nutrition Data, nutritiondata.self.com /facts/cereal-grains-and-pasta/10352/2.

53 "Is It True That Flaxseeds Are Not a Good Source of Omega 3s for Some People?" The World's Healthiest Foods, whfoods.com/genpage.php?tname=george&dbid=76.

54 M. B. Zimmermann, "Iodine Deficiency in Pregnancy and the Effects of Maternal Iodine Supplementation on the Offspring: A Review," *American Journal of Clinical Nutrition* 89 (February 2009): 668S–72S; "Iodine," Oregon State University Micronutrient Information Center (August 2015), lpi.oregonstate.edu/mic/minerals/iodine.

55 R. Bowen, "Thyroid Hormones: Pregnancy and Fetal Development," Colorado State University (February 26, 2012), arbl.cvmbs.colostate.edu/hbooks/pathphys/endocrine /thyroid/thyroid_preg.html.

56 "8 DIY Home Remedies for Morning Sickness," Home Remedies for Life (January 6, 2016), homeremediesforlife.com/morning-sickness/.

57 G. Sanabra-Martínez, et al., "Effectiveness of Physical Activity Interventions on Preventing Gestational Diabetes Mellitus and Excessive Maternal Weight Gain: A Meta-Analysis," *British Journal of Obstetrics and Gynaecology* 122, no 9. (August 2015): 1167–74.

58 R. Sovik, "A Beginner's Guide to Mula Bandha (Root Lock)," *Yoga International* (September 26, 2013), yogainternational.com/article/view/a-beginners-guide-to-mula-bandha-root-lock.

Chapter 6

1 "Sleeping by the Trimesters: 3rd Trimester," National Sleep Foundation, sleepfoundation.org /sleep-news/sleeping-the-trimesters-3rd-trimester.

2 "Ultrasound Exams," The American Congress of Obstetricians and Gynecologists (September 2013), acog.org/Patients/FAQs/Ultrasound-Exams.

3 "Routine Tests during Pregnancy," The American Congress of Obstetricians and Gynecologists (January 2016), acog.org/Patients/FAQs/Routine-Tests-During-Pregnancy.

4 Practice Bulletin No. 137: "Gestational Diabetes Mellitus," *Obstetrics & Gynecology* 122 (August 2013): 406–16.

5 "Pregnancy Calendar Week 13," KidsHealth, kidshealth.org/parent/pregnancy_center /pregnancy_calendar/week13.html#cat20733.

6 "Is It Safe to Eat Spicy Foods during Pregnancy?" Baby Center (April 2015), babycenter.com /404_is-it-safe-to-eat-spicy-foods-during-pregnancy_1246919.bc.

7 F. P. McCarthy et al., "Hyperemesis Gravidarum: Current Perspectives," *International Journal of Women's Health* 6 (August 5, 2014): 719–25.

8 "Fetal Development," MedlinePlus (September 26, 2015), nlm.nih.gov/medlineplus/ency /article/002398.htm.

9 "Pregnancy Calendar Week 14," KidsHealth, kidshealth.org/parent/pregnancy_center /pregnancy_calendar/week14.html#cat20733.

10 "Pregnancy Calendar Week 15," KidsHealth, kidshealth.org/parent/pregnancy_center /pregnancy_calendar/week15.html#cat20733.

11 "Pregnancy Calendar Week 16," KidsHealth, kidshealth.org/parent/pregnancy_center /pregnancy_calendar/week16.html#cat20733.

12 "Fetal Development," MedlinePlus (September 26, 2015).

13 "Prenatal Tests," March of Dimes (March 2015), marchofdimes.com/pregnancy/prenatalcare _routinetests.html.

14 "Pregnancy Calendar Week 17," KidsHealth, kidshealth.org/parent/pregnancy_center
/pregnancy_calendar/week17.html#cat20733.

15 "Pregnancy Calendar Week 20," KidsHealth, kidshealth.org/parent/pregnancy_center
/pregnancy_calendar/week20.html#cat20733.

16 "Pregnancy Calendar Week 17," KidsHealth, kidshealth.org/parent/pregnancy_center
/pregnancy_calendar/week17.html#cat20733.

17 "Pregnancy Calendar Week 18," KidsHealth, kidshealth.org/parent/pregnancy_center
/pregnancy_calendar/week18.html#cat20733.

18 K. Korgavkar, et al., "Stretch Marks during Pregnancy: A Review of Topical Prevention,"
British Journal of Dermatology 172 (March 2015): 606–15.

19 "Pregnancy Calendar Week 19," KidsHealth, kidshealth.org/parent/pregnancy_center
/pregnancy_calendar/week19.html#cat20733.

20 "Pregnancy Calendar Week 20," KidsHealth, kidshealth.org/parent/pregnancy_center
/pregnancy_calendar/week20.html#cat20733.

21 "Prenatal Tests," March of Dimes (March 2015).

22 "Glucose Screening and Tolerance Tests during Pregnancy," MedlinePlus (June 11, 2014),
nlm.nih.gov/medlineplus/ency/article/007562.htm.

23 "Gestational Diabetes," American Diabetes Association, diabetes.org/diabetes-basics
/gestational/.

24 "Sex during Pregnancy: What's OK, What's Not," Mayo Clinic (July 31, 2015), mayoclinic
.org/healthy-lifestyle/pregnancy-week-by-week/in-depth/sex-during-pregnancy/art-20045318.

25 "Pregnancy Calendar Week 21," KidsHealth, kidshealth.org/parent/pregnancy_center
/pregnancy_calendar/week21.html#cat20733.

26 "Pregnancy Calendar Week 22," KidsHealth, kidshealth.org/parent/pregnancy_center
/pregnancy_calendar/week22.html#cat20733.

27 "How Many Eggs Are You Born With?" Creative Love Egg Donor and Surrogate Agency,
cledp.com/donate-eggs/how-many-egg-are-you-born-with.html.

28 "Routine Tests during Pregnancy," The American College of Obstetricians and Gynecologists
(January 2016), http://acog.org/-/media/For-Patients/faq133.pdf?dmc=1&ts=20150701T
1103361014.

29 "Prenatal Care and Tests," Womenshealth.gov (September 27, 2010), womenshealth.gov
/pregnancy/you-are-pregnant/prenatal-care-tests.html.

30 Ibid.

31 "Glucose Tolerance Test," American Pregnancy Association (June 2015), americanpregnancy
.org/prenatal-testing/glucose-tolerence-test/.

32 "Common Tests during Pregnancy," Stanford Children's Health, stanfordchildrens.org/en
/topic/default?id=common-tests-during-pregnancy-85-P01241.

33 "Triple Screen Test," American Pregnancy Association (July 2015), americanpregnancy
.org/prenatal-testing/triple-screen-test/.

34 "Sleep during Pregnancy," Mayo Clinic (February 23, 2016), mayoclinic.org/healthy-lifestyle
/pregnancy-week-by-week/in-depth/sleep-during-pregnancy/art-20043827?pg=2.

35 G. N. Koken et al., "Maternal Blood Pressure and Dominant Sleeping Position May Affect
Placental Localization," *The Journal of Maternal-Fetal & Neonatal Medicine* 27 (January 6,
2014): 1564–67.

36 J. Warland et al., "Accuracy of Self-Reported Sleep Position in Late Pregnancy," *Public
Library of Science* (December 23, 2014), journals.plos.org/plosone/article?id=10.1371/journal
.pone.0115760.

37 "Quad Screen Test," American Pregnancy Association (June 2015), americanpregnancy.org
/prenatal-testing/quad-screen/.

38 I. Nehring et al., "Impacts of In Utero and Early Infant Taste Experiences on Later Taste Acceptance: A Systematic Review," *The Journal of Nutrition* (April 15, 2015), jn.nutrition .org/content/early/2015/04/15/jn.114.203976.short.

39 "Maternal Serum Alpha-Fetoprotein Screening (MSAFP)," American Pregnancy Association (July 2015), americanpregnancy.org/prenatal-testing/maternal-serum-alpha-fetoprotein -screening/.

40 "Routine Tests during Pregnancy," The American College of Obstetricians and Gynecologists (January 2015), www.acog.org/-/media/For-Patients/faq133. pdf?dmc=1&ts=20150701T1103361014

41 "Ultrasound: Sonogram," American Pregnancy Association (July 2015) americanpregnancy .org/prenatal-testing/ultrasound/

42 "Pregnancy and Heartburn," University of Rochester Medical Center, urmc.rochester.edu /encyclopedia/content.aspx?ContentTypeID=134&ContentID=10

43 C. Zhang, MD, PhD, et al., "Dietary Fiber Intake, Dietary Glycemic Load, and the Risk of Gestational Diabetes Mellitus," *Diabetes Care* 29 (October 2006): 2223–30.

44 "Vitamins and Other Nutrients during Pregnancy," March of Dimes, marchofdimes.org /pregnancy/omega-3-fatty-acids.aspx

45 L. Wong, "Mommy Brain? 'Smart' Nutrients to Help You Stay Sharp," Holistic Directory, theholisticdirectory.co.uk/articles/story/mommy-brain-smart-nutrients-to-help-you-stay-sharp

46 B. A. Haider et al., "Anaemia, Prenatal Iron Use, and Risk of Adverse Pregnancy Outcomes: Systematic Review and Meta-Analysis," *British Medical Journal* (June 21, 2013); E. C. Eichenwald et al., "Management and Outcomes of Very Low Birth Weight," *The New England Journal of Medicine* 358 (April 17, 2008): 1700–11; R. L. Goldenberg et al., "Low Birth Weight in the United States," *The American Journal of Clinical Nutrition* 85 (February 2007): 5845–905.

47 "Iron: Dietary Supplement Fact Sheet," National Institutes of Health (February 11, 2016), ods.od.nih.gov/factsheets/Iron-HealthProfessional/.

48 S. Daly, "Homocysteine and Folic Acid: Implications for Pregnancy," *Seminars in Vascular Medicine* 5 (May 2005): 190–200, ncbi.nlm.nih.gov/pubmed/16047271; T.O. Scholl et al., "Folic Acid: Influence on the Outcome of Pregnancy," *The American Journal of Clinical Nutrition* 71, no. 5 (May 2000): 1295s–1303s.

49 S. A. Skeaff, "Iodine Deficiency in Pregnancy: The Effect on Neurodevelopment in the Child," *Nutrients* 3 (February 2011): 265–73; "Iodine Fact Sheet for Health Professionals," National Institutes of Health (June 24, 2011), http://ods.od.nih.gov/factsheets/Iodine-HealthProfessional/.

50 "Abdominal Separation (Diastasis Recti)," WebMD, webmd.com/baby/guide/abdominal -separation-diastasis-recti.

Chapter 7

1 "Pregnancy Calendar Week 28," KidsHealth, kidshealth.org/parent/pregnancy_center /pregnancy_calendar/week28.html#cat20733.

2 "Pregnancy Calendar Week 29," KidsHealth, kidshealth.org/parent/pregnancy_center /pregnancy_calendar/week29.html#cat20733.

3 "Pregnancy Calendar Week 30," KidsHealth, kidshealth.org/parent/pregnancy_center /pregnancy_calendar/week30.html#cat20733.

4 "Feeling Your Baby Kick," WebMD, webmd.com/baby/fetal-movement-feeling-baby-kick.

5 Ibid.

6 "Pregnancy Calendar Week 29," KidsHealth.

7 "Pregnancy: The Three Trimesters," University of California San Francisco Medical Center, http://ucsfhealth.org/conditions/pregnancy/trimesters.html.

8 "Pregnancy Calendar Week 28," KidsHealth.

9 "Pregnancy Calendar Week 27," KidsHealth, kidshealth.org/parent/pregnancy_center
/pregnancy_calendar/week27.html#cat20733.

10 M. T. Willis, "Most Pregnant Women Can Fly Safely," abcNEWS, abcnews.go.com/Health
/story?id=117080&page=1.

11 "Travel during Pregnancy," The American College of Obstetricians and Gynecologists
(February 2016), acog.org/Patients/FAQs/Travel-During-Pregnancy#know.

12 "Fetal Development: The Third Trimester," Mayo Clinic, mayoclinic.com/health/fetal
-development/PR00114.

13 "Pregnancy Calendar Week 29," KidsHealth.

14 "Fetal Development: The Third Trimester," Mayo Clinic.

15 "Hemorrhoids Treatment," DrWeil.com, drweil.com/drw/u/ART03032/Hemorrhoids.html.

16 "Pregnancy Calendar Week 31," KidsHealth, kidshealth.org/parent/pregnancy_center
/pregnancy_calendar/week31.html#cat20733.

17 Ibid.

18 "Can You Guess Your Baby's Sex?" WebMD, webmd.com/baby/features/predicting-baby
-gender?page=2.

19 "Is Pregnancy Glow Real?" Mayo Clinic, mayoclinic.org/healthy-lifestyle/pregnancy-week-by
-week/expert-answers/pregnancy-glow/faq-20115104.

20 F. Hytten, "Blood Volume Changes in Normal Pregnancy," *Clinical Haematology* 14
(October 1985): 601–12.

21 "Pregnancy Nail and Hair Growth," What to Expect, whattoexpect.com/pregnancy/hair
-growth/.

22 "Pregnancy: Condition Information," National Institute of Child Health and Human
Development (December 6, 2013), nichd.nih.gov/health/topics/pregnancy/conditioninfo/Pages
/default.aspx.

23 "Pregnancy Week by Week," Mayo Clinic (July 11, 2014), mayoclinic.com/health/fetal
-development/PR00114/NSECTIONGROUP=2.

24 "Fetal Development: The Third Trimester," Mayo Clinic.

25 "Baby's First Dreams: Sleep Cycles of the Fetus," American Institute of Physicians (April 14,
2009), sciencedaily.com/releases/2009/04/090413185734.htm.

26 "Pregnancy Calendar Week 33," KidsHealth, kidshealth.org/parent/pregnancy_center
/pregnancy_calendar/week33.html#cat20733

27 Ibid.

28 "Pregnancy Week by Week," Mayo Clinic (July 11, 2014).

29 "Pregnancy Calendar Week 36," KidsHealth, kidshealth.org/parent/pregnancy_center
/pregnancy_calendar/week36.html#cat20733

30 "Pregnancy Calendar Week 37," KidsHealth, kidshealth.org/parent/pregnancy_center
/pregnancy_calendar/week37.html#cat20733.

31 Ibid.

32 "Pregnancy Calendar Week 39," KidsHealth, kidshealth.org/parent/pregnancy_center
/pregnancy_calendar/week39.html#cat20733.

33 "Pregnancy Week by Week," Mayo Clinic (July 11, 2014).

34 "Prenatal Development: How Your Baby Grows during Pregnancy," The American College of
Obstetricians and Gynecologists (June 2015), acog.org/patients/faqs/prenatal-development
-how-your-baby-grows-during-pregnancy?IsMobileSet=false.

35 "Pregnancy: Condition Information," National Institute of Child Health and Human
Development (December 6, 2013).

36 "Pregnancy Calendar Week 37," KidsHealth.

37 "Pregnancy Week by Week," Mayo Clinic (July 11, 2014).

38 "Pregnancy Calendar Week 38," KidsHealth, kidshealth.org/parent/pregnancy_center /pregnancy_calendar/week38.html#cat20733.

39 "Lifting during Pregnancy," American Pregnancy Association (2014), americanpregnancy .org/is-it-safe/lifting-pregnancy/.

40 "Prenatal Care and Tests," Womenshealth.gov (September 27, 2010), womenshealth.gov /pregnancy/you-are-pregnant/prenatal-care-tests.html.

41 Ibid.

42 Centers for Disease Control and Prevention, "Preventing Early-Onset Group B Strep Disease (GBS)" (May 23, 2016). www.cdc.gov/groupbstrep/about/prevention.html.

43 "Ultrasound: Sonogram," American Pregnancy Association (July 2015), americanpregnancy .org/prenatal-testing/ultrasound/.

44 "Natural Ways to Encourage Labor," OBGYN North, http:// obgynnorth.com/patient _education/childbirth_preparation/natural_ways_to_encourage_labor.

45 S. Corriher, "Marinades Add Flavor but Don't Always Tenderize," *Fine Cooking* 34, finecooking.com/articles/marinades-flavor-tenderize.aspx.

46 J. Yan et al., "Pregnancy Alters Choline Dynamics: Results of a Randomized Trial Using Stable Isotope Methodology in Pregnant and Nonpregnant Women," *The American Journal of Clinical Nutrition* 98 (October 16, 2013): 1459–67.

47 J. A. Greenberg et al., "Omega-3 Fatty Acid Supplementation during Pregnancy," *Reviews in Obstetrics & Gynecology* 1 (Fall 2008): 162–69.

48 J. L. Jacobson et al., "Beneficial Effects of a Polyunsaturated Fatty Acid on Infant Development: Evidence from the Inuit of Arctic Quebec," *Journal of Pediatrics* 152 (March 2008): 356–64.

49 "Vitamin K Deficiency," Oregon State University Micronutrient Information Center (August 2014), lpi.oregonstate.edu/mic/articles/vitamins/vitamin-k#deficiency.

50 "Parsley, Raw, Nutrition Facts & Calories," SELF Nutrition Data, nutritiondata.self.com /facts/vegetables-and-vegetable-products/2513/2.

51 "Vitamin K Fact Sheet for Health Professionals," National Institutes of Health (February 11, 2016), http://ods.od.nih.gov/factsheets/VitaminK-HealthProfessional/.

Chapter 8

1 "Birth Centers: Alternatives to Hospitals," Babycenter Expert Advice, http://www.babycenter .com/0_birth-centers-alternatives-to-hospitals_2007.bc.

2 A. Welch, "No Proven Health Benefits, Unknown Risks of Eating Placenta," CBS News (June 4, 2015), cbsnews.com/news/no-proven-health-benefits-unknown-risks-of-eating-placenta/.

3 "The History of Water Birth," Babycentre, babycentre.co.uk/a542003/the-history-of-water -birth.

4 "Inducing Labor," WebMD Health & Pregnancy, webmd.com/baby/guide/inducing-labor ?page=2.

5 "Pudendal Block," American Pregnancy Association (August 2015), americanpregnancy.org /labor-and-birth/pudendal-block/.

6 G. M. Dileo, "Your C-Section: A Step-by-Step Guide," Babble (2011), babble.com/pregnancy /cesarean-section-guide/.

7 "Caesarean Babies 'Likely to Have Breathing Problems,'" Daily Mail (December 12, 2007), dailymail.co.uk/health/article-501384/Caesarean-babies-likely-breathing -problems.html.

Chapter 9

1   S. M. Matambanadzo, "The Fourth Trimester," *University of Michigan Journal of Law Reform* 48 (2014).

2   "Diseases and Conditions: Postpartum Depression," Mayo Clinic (August 11, 2015), mayoclinic.org/diseases-conditions/postpartum-depression/basics/causes/con-20029130.

3   Z. Barnes, "Q&A: How Many Calories Does Breastfeeding Really Burn?" Women's Health (August 6, 2014), womenshealthmag.com/mom/breastfeeding-burns-calories.

4   N. Mohrbacher, "Nipple Shield: Friend or Foe?" Breastfeeding USA, https://breastfeedingusa .org/content/article/nipple-shield-friend-or-foe.

5   A. Mohammadzadeh et al., "The Effect of Breast Milk and Lanolin on Sore Nipples," *Saudi Medical Journal* 26, (August 2005): 1231–34.

6   "Diseases and Conditions: Tongue-Tie," Mayo Clinic (April 30, 2015), mayoclinic.org /diseases-conditions/tongue-tie/basics/definition/con-20035410.

7   K. Winder, "Nipple Thrush—Treatments for Nipple Thrush," Bellybelly (May 25, 2016), bellybelly.com.au/breastfeeding/nipple-thrush-treatment/.

8   "Increasing Milk Supply," Ask Dr. Sears, askdrsears.com/topics/feeding-eating/breastfeeding /faqs/increasing-milk-supply.

9   C. Huotari, "Alcohol and Motherhood," *La Leche League International* 33 (April–May 1997): 30–31.

10 J. Mennella, PhD, "Alcohol's Effect on Lactation," National Institute on Alcohol Abuse and Alcoholism, pubs.niaaa.nih.gov/publications/arh25-3/230-234.htm.

ACKNOWLEDGMENTS

As I look back on the magnitude of this book, I must acknowledge all of the incredibly brilliant and talented individuals who helped me bring it to life—pun intended. They say when it comes to raising children, "it takes a village," and the same can be said of this project. Many were involved, directly or indirectly, in shaping this book. Therefore, I must shout out the rock-star team that cocreated *Yeah Baby!* Each person has played an important part.

First, I must thank my family for their unwavering support and constant supply of hilarious, heartfelt writing material.

Next, I must recognize the *Yeah Baby!* "dream team" of doctors and experts. There is nothing more sacred than pregnancy and motherhood, and only the best of the best will do when advising mommies on how to best care for themselves and their little ones: pediatrician Dr. Jay Gordon, ob-gyn Dr. Suzanne Gilberg-Lenz, endocrinologist Dr. Katja Van Herle, dietitian Cheryl Forberg, RD, and pregnancy fitness specialist and Olympian Andrea Orbeck. Thanks to your brilliance and expertise, so many women and children will now have all the tools, information, and support they need to make the best choices for themselves and their families.

Thank you to my coauthor, Eve Adamson. You are a bad-ass, hands down. You are the glue that pulled all of this together, shaped the book, and gave it focus. Although I am sure I made you a bit crazy, I am thrilled to say the end result is astounding, so I'm not sorry. ;-) Bravo, friend.

The team at Rodale: Maria Rodale, Marisa Vigilante, Gail Gonzales, and all the other unsung heroes in every facet of publishing—thank you so much for believing in the significance of this project and for all the hard work you've put into the process. I am forever grateful.

Last, thank you to my personal crack team at Empowered Media, especially my tireless assistant Nichole Pellant. I can't wait for the day when you actually have to read this book. Hahaha! To Giancarlo Chersich, business partner extraordinaire: Thank you for never asking me to sell out, always having my back, and making my dreams come true.

PHOTO CREDITS

The following photos are by Matt Rainey: page 296 top left, bottom right; page 297 top left, bottom left; page 298 top right, bottom right; page 299 top right, bottom right; page 300 top left, bottom left; page 301 top left and right, bottom left; page 302 top right, bottom right; page 303 bottom left; page 304 top left, top right; page 305 bottom left; page 306 all photos; page 307 top left, top right; page 308 top right, bottom right; page 309 top left; page 310 bottom left; page 311 bottom left, bottom right; page 312 top right; page 313 top right, bottom right; page 314 all photos; page 317 bottom left; page 318 top left, top right, bottom right; page 319 top left; page 320 bottom left, bottom right; page 321 bottom left; page 322.

The following photos are by Ian Maddox: page 296 top right, bottom left; page 297 top right, bottom right; page 298 top left, bottom left; page 299 top left, bottom left; page 300 top right, bottom right; page 301 bottom right; page 302 top left, bottom left; page 303 top left, top right, bottom right; page 304 bottom left, bottom right; page 305 top left, top right, bottom right; page 307 bottom left, bottom right; page 308 top left, bottom left; page 309 top right, bottom left, bottom right; page 310 top left, top right, bottom right; page 311 top left, top right; page 312 top left, bottom left, bottom right; page 313 top left, bottom left; page 315 all photos; page 316 all photos; page 317 top left, top right, bottom right; page 318 bottom left; page 319 top right, bottom left, bottom right; page 320 top left, top right; page 321 top left, top right, bottom right. Fitness attire for Maddox photos by Fabletics.

INDEX

<u>Underscored</u> page references indicate sidebars and tables. **Boldface** references indicate photographs.

A

Abdominal separation
  exercise and, 176–78, 179, 201–2, 263, 264–65, <u>265</u>
  healing from, 239, 264, <u>267</u>
Acetaminophen, 20
Acne, <u>131</u>
Acupuncture, <u>38</u>, 40, 187–88, <u>224</u>, 226
ADHD, 60, 63
Adoption, 8–9, 38
Advil, 20
Airborne bacteria and viruses, 95
Airport screening, radiation from, <u>19</u>
Air purifiers, 98–99
Air quality, indoor, 95–99
Air travel, in third trimester, <u>188</u>
ALA, food sources of, 136
Alcohol
  breastfeeding and, 254–55, 260
  endocrine effects from, 14
  pregnancy avoidance of, 49–50
  prepregnancy avoidance of, 32–34, 50
Aleve, 20
Allergies
  in children, 60
  dust mite, 100
  mold, 97
  pet, <u>98</u>
Aloe vera gel, for hemorrhoids, 190
Alternating Backward Lunges with Lateral Raises, **296**
Alternating Bicycle Crunches, **296**
Alternating Crossover Lunges with Reverse Curls, **296**

Alternating Curtsy Lunges with Biceps Curls, **296**
Alternating Forward Lunges with Hammer Curls, **297**
Alternating Hamstring Curls in Ab Hold, **297**
Alternating Heel Drops, **297**
Alternating Knee Switches, **297**
Alternating Low Rows in Table, **298**
Alternating Renegade Rows, **298**
Alternating Reverse Flys in Plank, **298**
Alternating Reverse Flys in Table, **298**
Alternating Side Lunges with Anterior Raises, **299**
Alternating Side Lunge with Serving Biceps, **299**
Alternating Standing Toe Tap Crunches, **299**
Alternating Stepups, **299**
Alternating Sumo Touch Downs, **300**
Alternating Surrender Lunges with Shoulder Presses, **300**
Alternative medicine, 40–41
American College of Nurse-Midwives, 218–19
Amniocentesis, 129, <u>129</u>, 130, 164
Amniotomy. *See* Water breaking
Anemia
  megaloblastic, 135
  mold causing, 97
  preterm delivery from, 133
  preventing, 36, 37, <u>72</u>, <u>73</u>
  screening for, 23, 123

Anesthesia, general and local, 228
Ankyloglossia, <u>258</u>
Antibiotics
  for C-sections, 229–30, 259
  in food supply, 60–61, 62
  for Group B strep, 195
  for toxoplasmosis treatment, <u>108</u>
Antiobiotic eye treatment, for newborns, <u>234</u>
APGAR score, 83
APNO, for cracked nipples, <u>259</u>
Apples
  Apple Zucchini Flap Jacks with Turkey Bacon, 274
Apricots
  Fruity Gazpacho, 282
Arm Biceps Stretch, **300**
Artichokes
  Awesome Artichoke, 285
  Chicken Artichoke Pizza, 280
Artificial colors, avoiding, 64
Artificial flavors, avoiding, 66
Artificial sweeteners, avoiding, 64–65, 125
Asbestos, 95
Aspartame, 64–65
Aspirin, 20
Asthma
  in children, 60
  from dust mites, 100
  from mold, 97
Athletic potential, of children of fit mothers, 84
Attention deficit/hyperactivity disorder (ADHD), 60, 63
Autism, 60, 63, 107
Ayurvedic medicine, <u>237</u>

B

Baby care products, chemical-free, 115
Baby's development
  exercise helping, 83–84
  in first trimester, 43
    weeks 1 to 4, 126–27
    weeks 5 to 8, 127–28
    weeks 9 to 12, 130–31
  nutrition influencing, 43, 169
  in second trimester, 43
    weeks 13 to 16, 159
    weeks 17 to 20, 160–61
    weeks 21 to 24, 162
  in third trimester, 43–44
    weeks 25 to 30, 188–89
    weeks 31 to 34, 190–91
    weeks 35 to 40 or delivery, 192, 194
Baby's gender
  "carrying" myth about, 190
  finding out, 155, 159
  ultrasound revealing, 167
Baby's movements, 159, 160, 162, 186, 187, 189, 192
Baby's position, breech, 185–86, 187
Back labor, 226
Back pain
  exercise and, 142
  first trimester, 122
  second trimester, 174
  third trimester, 187–88, 201
Back safety, during exercise, 202–3
Bacon
  Apple Zucchini Flap Jacks with Turkey Bacon, 274
Bacteria, airborne, 95
Bacterial infections, testing for, 18
Bad dreams, 151, 153
Baking soda, for cleaning, 109
Balance, during exercise, 87, 87
Balance problems
  second trimester, 175–76
  third trimester, 201
Bananas
  The PBB, 282

Barrier contraceptives, 30–31, 32
Bear Crawls, **300**
Beauty products
  chemical-free, 114–15
  chemicals in, 113
Bed rest, 186, 188
Belly Alert workout
  modifications, 180, 201
Belly Buds, 187
Bent Leg Donkey Kicks, **301**
Beta-carotene supplements, 136
BHA, avoiding, 66
BHT, avoiding, 66
Biceps Curls, **301**
Bikini incision, for C-sections, 231
Bioflavonoids, 197
BioGaia probiotic, 230, 259
Biophysical profile, 195
Birth control, stopping, 29–31, 32
Birth defects
  from beta-carotene supplements, 136
  choline preventing, 197
  from hot baths, 130
  neural tube defects, 35–36, 37, 86, 165, 166
  screening for, 160, 164, 165, 166–67
Birthing centers, 219–20, 223
Birthing environment, 219–23
Birth plan
  discussing, with doctor, 123
  flexibility with, 214
  guilt about, 216
  items to include in, 193
Bishop's score, 224
Bisphenol A (BPA), 66–67, 105
Bladder infections, 197
Blastocyst, 126
Bleached paper products, 103
Bleach substitute, 109
Bleeding, vaginal, 84, 123, 125, 155
Blood pressure monitoring, 26
Blood sugar stability
  for exercise, 90
  fiber for, 169
  protein for, 197

regular meals for, 252
small meals for, 125, 196
sugar consumption and, 196
Blood sugar testing, 24–25, 27, 155, 161, 163–164, 163
Blood type test, 28–29, 123
BMI, ideal, for conception, 44
Boat Extensions with Forearms on Ground, **301**
Body care products, chemical-free, 114–15
Body mass index (BMI), ideal, for conception, 44
Body temperature, unsafe, 130
Bonding with baby, 247
Borg's Rating of Perceived Exertion (RPE) Scale, 89. *See also* RPE scale, for exercise
Bottled water, 111, 112
BPA (bisphenol A), 66–67, 105
Braced Single Arm Medium Grip Rows, **301**
Brain development, in babies of fit mothers, 84
Bras, 86, 156, 160, 161, 258
Braxton Hicks contractions, 162, 185, 192
Breakfasts
  Apple Zucchini Flap Jacks with Turkey Bacon, 274
  B4 Power Parfait, 273
  Baby Booster Smoothie, 272
  Bad Ass Breakfast Burrito, 276
  Breakfast Bowl, 272
  The California Poach, 274
  Feta Frittata, 275
  Hot Mama Smoothie, 272
  Huevos Tacos, 275
  Lori and Jamie's Feel-Good Muffin, 276
  Maple Pecan Porridge, 273
Breast exam, prepregnancy, 15

definition of, 236
exercise, 261–68
Heidi's experience of, 243
nutrition, 249–55
partner's feelings during, 238
self-doubts in, 241–42
sex in, 247–49
sleep in, 242–44, 246
smoothies, 256, 294–95
support in, 246–47
transitions during, 236
unsolicited advice in, 239–41
Fractionated oils, avoiding, 66
Fragrance, phthalates in, 113
Frenotomy, for tongue-tie, 258
Frittata
Feta Frittata, 275
Fruits. *See also specific fruits*
Fruity Gazpacho, 282
nonorganic vs. organic, 62–64
washing, 57
Furniture
choosing, 102
green, nontoxic, 101
off-gassing from, 96

G

Gas
of babies, 241
from C-section, 233
remedies for, 124, 169
Gazpacho
Fruity Gazpacho, 282
Gender of baby. *See* Baby's gender
General anesthesia, during delivery, 228
Genetic conditions
discussing, with doctor, 124
screening for, 26, 28, 129–30, 129, 164–167
Genetic counseling, 124
Genital herpes, 18
Gestational diabetes
from insulin resistance, 6
overweight newborns and, 83
preventing, 69, 133, 140, 169, 171, 201

risks from, 24–25
screening for, 155, 161, 164
in second trimester, 168
type 2 diabetes after, 27, 83, 134, 161
vitamin D deficiency and, 134
Gilberg-Lenz, Suzanne, xv–xvi
advice on
air travel in third trimester, 188
anesthesia, 228
baby's movements, 189
breech position, 185–86, 187
cord blood banking, 218
cracked, sore nipples, 259
diabetes risk, 161
doulas, 156
episiotomy, 229
glucose tolerance test, 164
herbal and supplement safety, 68
IUI, 9
labor induction, 224, 225, 227
magnesium supplements, 20
noninvasive prenatal testing, 129, 129
pain management for labor, 227
PCOS, 7
placenta eating, 221
postpartum depression, 248
postpartum self-care, 237
prepregnancy health, 10
pumping and dumping breast milk, 254
reasons for forced interventions, 220
shoulder dystocia, 25
sleep position, 165
smoking, 31
stress hormones, 38
urinary incontinence, 266
vaccinations, 21
vaginal birth and baby's microbiome, 230
visitors after delivery, 235
vitamin D₃ test, 23, 36

Ginger, for treating
heartburn, 152
morning sickness, 122, 135
Glowing complexion, 140, 159, 191
Glucola, for glucose tolerance test, 163, 163, 164
Glucose screening test, 161, 163
Glucose tolerance test, 155, 161, 163–64, 163
Gluten-free diet, 77–78
Glute work, 204
Goddess Squats, 306
Gonorrhea, 18, 18
Good Mornings with Arms Crossed on Chest, 306
Gordon, Jay, xvi
advice on
bonding with baby, 247
environmental toxins, 35
family bed, 244
newborn antibiotic eye treatment, 234
newborn vitamin K shots, 234
sex in fourth trimester, 248
sleep, 244
vaccinations, 22
visitors after delivery, 235
Grains
processed, 253
protein in, 70
Graves' disease, 25
Greasy foods, avoiding, 132
Green home products, 98, 101
Green tea, 52
Group B strep, 195
Growth hormones, for dairy cows, 62
Guilt trips, 213, 214, 215, 216
Gum disease, 29
Gynecologist, prepregnancy visit with, 13–19

H

Hair care products, chemical-free, 114
Hair changes, 191
Hammer Curls, 306
Hamstring Stretch, 307
Hashimoto's thyroiditis, 25